Basic Laboratory
Techniques for the
Medical Laboratory
Technician

Basic Laboratory Techniques for the Medical Laboratory Technician

Jean Jorgenson Linné, B.S., M.T. (ASCP)

Karen Munson Ringsrud, B.S., M.T. (ASCP)

Medical Laboratory Assistant Program
Division of Medical Technology
Department of Laboratory Medicine
College of Medical Sciences
University of Minnesota

McGRAW-HILL BOOK COMPANY
The Blakiston Division
New York St. Louis San Francisco London Sydney Toronto Mexico Panama

Basic Laboratory Techniques for the Medical Laboratory Technician

Library of Congress Catalog Card Number 69-19198

ISBN 07-016420-7

7 8 9 0   MAMM   4 3

This book was set in Times Roman by The Maple Press Company, and printed on permanent paper and bound by The Maple Press Company. The designer was William E. Schmidt. The editors were Joseph J. Brehm and Diane Drobnis. Eugene Capriotti and Adam Jacobs supervised the production.

Preface

In the modern medical laboratory a wide variety of analyses ranging from simple to complex are utilized by the physician and are essential to him in the management of his patients. Laboratory personnel, to qualify for such work, require specific training and education. Usually the laboratory is under the direction of a medical doctor, the pathologist, who is a physician specializing in pathology, the study of disease. Under the direction of the pathologist is the medical technologist, who is educated to perform the complex laboratory procedures, to engage in teaching activities, and to handle supervisory and administrative duties. To assist the medical technologist, the medical laboratory technician is specifically trained for routine tasks.

Although the laboratory technician has proper understanding of basic fundamentals and techniques so as to be flexible in the use of his training and skills, he is not qualified to make technical and administrative decisions.

It takes a special type of person to work in a clinical laboratory. He must understand the need for accuracy, be conscientious, and above all, want to be of service to the patient.

The materials for this textbook have been developed from the lectures given students in the medical laboratory assistant program at the University of Minnesota. It is intended to provide the student technician with basic information in the departments of the clinical laboratory where technicians will work; these departments include chemistry, hematology, urinalysis, blood banking, microbiology, electrocardiography, and basal metabolism. In addition to these chapters, a discussion of basic laboratory fundamentals is included.

The authors gratefully acknowledge the contributions of Ruth Hovde, Verna Rausch, Margaret Ohlen Hanson, Elizabeth Lundgren, Ruth Brown Anderson, Marilyn Scovil Cavanaugh, and Mary Lou Kuefner Carlson, people who formerly were associated with the instruction and the administration of the medical laboratory assistant program from which the material for this book evolved.

The authors express their appreciation to Mary Damron, Barbara Merritt, Grace Mary Ederer, Patricia Hanauer Bordewich, Donna Blazevic, Sandra Benson, and Margaret Halsted for their assistance in reviewing the various sections of the book during its preparation, and to Mr. Martin Finch for his assistance in the preparation of the illustrations.

The authors thank Dr. Ellis S. Benson, Professor and head of the Department of Laboratory Medicine, for his encouragement and support of this project.

JEAN JORGENSON LINNÉ
KAREN MUNSON RINGSRUD

Contents

Preface   v

1
Fundamentals of the Clinical Laboratory

Safety in the Laboratory   1
Cleaning Laboratory Glassware   4
Glass Breakage and Replacement   7
Use of the Centrifuge   7
The Microscope   8
Reagent Preparation, Chemicals, and Quantitative Transfer   13
Kinds of Water Used in the Clinical Laboratory   17
Laboratory Calculations   18

2
Chemistry

Introduction   28
The Metric System   29
Glassware   31
Weighing and the Use of Balances   37
Photometry   48
Pipetting   57
Titration   63
Collection, Preservation, and Preparation of Specimens   68
Means of Ensuring Reliable Results   73
Plasma Chloride   80
Blood Glucose   86
Urea Nitrogen   95
To the Student Laboratory Technician   105

3
Hematology

Introduction   107
Approaching the Patient   108

Collection of Samples   110
Specimens for Hematology and the Use of Anticoagulants   115
Formation of Blood Cells and Their Appearance   118
Counting the Formed Elements of the Blood   121
Counting Reticulocytes   139
Cell Morphology—the Preparation, Staining, and Examination
   of Blood Films   142
The Hematocrit Determination   155
The Erythrocyte Sedimentation Rate   157
Coagulation Studies   160
The Hemoglobin Determination   168
Test for Osmotic Fragility of the Red Blood Cell   174
The Red Blood Cell Indices   176
Preparation of Slides for LE Test   178
Examination of Extravascular Fluids   178

4

Urinalysis

Introduction   185
Physical Properties   191
pH   198
Specific Gravity   200
Sugar   208
Protein   216
Ketone Bodies   223
Two By-products of Red Cell Destruction: Bilirubin and Urobilinogen   229
Bilirubin   230
Urobilinogen   232
Hemoglobin in Urine and Feces   236
Urinary Sediment   240

5

Blood Banking

Introduction   262
The ABO Blood Group System   272
The Rh-Hr Blood Group System   279
The Antiglobulin Reaction (Coombs Test)   288

Hemolytic Disease of the Newborn (Erythroblastosis Foetalis)   291
Compatibility Testing or Cross Matching   295
Conclusion   299

6

Microbiology

Introduction   302
Types and Collection of Material for Microbiologic Examination   303
Protection of Laboratory Personnel and Sterilization of Materials   305
Microbiologic Studies   309
Special Equipment and Techniques for Microbiologic Studies   316
Staining Techniques   321
Media Used in Medical Bacteriology   325

7

Basal Metabolic Rate and Electrocardiography Tests

Electrocardiography   337
Basal Metabolic Rate   353

Index   377

1

Fundamentals of the Clinical Laboratory

The aim of the present chapter is to give general information that applies to most laboratory work. The use of certain laboratory equipment (the microscope and the centrifuge, for example) will be discussed as well as the use of laboratory calculations, the importance of laboratory safety, the proper preparation of reagents, and the cleaning of laboratory glassware. Knowledge of these aspects of laboratory work, and of others not specifically discussed in this chapter is necessary as basic information for engaging in the six major areas of laboratory work covered in the six chapters that follow.

SAFETY IN THE LABORATORY

The importance of laboratory safety and the application of the correct first-aid procedures cannot be overemphasized to anyone working in the medical laboratory. Students, as well as laboratory personnel, should be constantly reminded of the need for precautions regarding safety in the laboratory. Most accidents do not just happen—they are usually caused by carelessness. For this reason, laboratory safety should be foremost in the mind of anyone involved in doing laboratory work of any kind.

Most laboratory accidents are preventable by the exercise of good technique and by the use of common sense. Many potential hazards exist in the laboratory, but all these hazards can be controlled by the use of simple precautions and foresight. In every medical institution, the administration supplies the laboratory with many safety devices for equipment and personal use, but it is up to the individual to make use of these safety devices. Safety is a personal thing, and its practice must be a matter of individual desire and accomplishment. Real appreciation for safety requires a "built-in" concern for the other fellow, for an unsafe act may harm the bystander without harming the person who commits the act.

The most serious hazard in laboratory work is the potential of fire and explosion when using flammable solvents, such as ether and acetone. Other sources of injury in the laboratory are poisonous, caustic, or corrosive reagents (such as strong acids and bases), burns and scalds, electric shocks, lacerations from broken glassware or sharp instruments, and infections due to bacterial, viral, or parasitic organisms.

BASIC FIRST-AID PROCEDURES

Because so many of the possible injuries are of such an extreme nature and because in the event of such an injury immediate care is most critical, the application of the proper first-aid procedures must be thoroughly understood by each and every person in the medical laboratory. In many instances, immediate application of correct first aid is extremely essential to the well-being of the victim. A few of the more common emergencies and the appropriate first-aid procedures are listed below. These should be learned well by every student laboratory technician.

1. Alkali or acid burns on the skin or in the mouth. Rinse thoroughly with large amounts of running tap water. If the burns are serious, consult a physician.

2. Alkali or acid burns in the eye. Wash out thoroughly with running water for a minimum of 15 minutes. Help the victim by holding the eyelid open so that the water can make contact with the eye. An eye fountain is recommended for this purpose, but any running water will suffice. The use of an eyecup is discouraged. A physician should be notified immediately, while the eye is being washed.

3. Heat burns. Apply cold running water as soon as possible. If it is a third-degree burn (the skin is burned off), consult a physician immediately, and do not apply any grease or paste.

4. Minor cuts. Wash thoroughly with soap and water. Apply a clean bandage if necessary.

In cases of serious laboratory accidents, such as burns, medical assistance should be summoned while first-aid is being administered. For general accidents, competent medical help should be sought as soon as possible after the first-aid treatment has been completed. In cases of chemical burns, especially where the eyes are involved, speed in treatment is most essential.

GENERAL RULES FOR SAFETY IN THE CLINICAL LABORATORY

1. Know where the fire extinguishers are located, the different types for specific types of fires, and how to use them properly.

2. Pipet organic solvents and concentrated acids and bases by mechanical suction. Do *not* use mouth suction for these reagents.

3. Store and handle all flammable solvents and fuming reagents under a fume hood.

4. Use an explosionproof refrigerator to store ether. Never use ether near an open flame, as it is highly flammable.

5. Do not use *any* flammable substance near an open flame.

6. Wear gloves when handling toxic substances such as bromine or cyanide.

7. Mercury is poisonous. Clean up any spilled mercury immediately. Mercury is also very corrosive to the plumbing apparatus in sinks.

8. If any glass tubing is to be cut, hold the tubing with a towel to prevent cuts of the hands. This precaution also applies to putting a piece of glass tubing through a rubber stopper.

9. Use extreme caution whenever handling laboratory glassware. Broken glassware is probably the greatest source of injury in the laboratory. Immediately discard any cracked or broken glassware, in a separate container, not with other waste.

10. If any strong acids or bases are spilled, wipe them up immediately, using copious amounts of water and great care. Keep sodium bicarbonate on hand to assist in neutralizing acid spillage.

11. Plainly label all laboratory bottles, specimens, and other materials. When a reagent bottle is no longer being used, store it away in its proper place.

12. Put away safely or cover any equipment that is not being used.

13. Replace covers, tops, or corks on all reagent bottles as soon as they are no longer being used. Never use any reagent from a bottle that is not properly labeled. Also label the storage areas.

14. If any water is spilled on the floor, wipe it up immediately. Serious injuries can result from falls caused by slipping on a wet floor.

15. Never taste any chemical. Smell chemicals only when necessary and then only by fanning the vapor of the chemical toward the nose.

16. When handling blades or needles, use extreme caution to avoid possible cuts and infections. Dispose of all blades and needles properly.

17. Always pour acid into water for dilution purposes. Never pour water into acid. Pour strong acids or bases slowly down the side of the receiving vessel to prevent splashing.

18. Use caution when pipetting any specimen coming from a patient. Handle blood, serum, plasma, cerebrospinal fluid, urine, or any other patient specimen with care, as it may be contaminated. Severe infections and illnesses can result if the person handling these specimens does so in a careless manner.

19. Wash your hands frequently while working in the laboratory and especially after handling questionable patient specimens or reagents. *Always* wash your hands before you leave the laboratory.

20. Wear special safety goggles when preparing reagents using strong

Have a log book at front of lab, as sample comes into lab - log time and who delivered it.

chemicals (such as the dichromate acid cleaning solution used to clean laboratory glassware, or aqua regia, another cleaning solution). Some states (Minnesota, for one) have enacted laws which require students, teachers, and visitors who are participating in or observing activities in eye protection areas (defined as an area involving work which is potentially hazardous to the eye) of an educational institution to wear eye-protective devices.

21. Many laboratories have built-in safety showers in the ceiling for use in case of severe fire or burns. Know where this shower is located and how to operate it.

22. Many laboratories have fire blankets, used to smother flames in case of fire. Know where these are to be found.

23. Most hospitals or teaching institutions have some type of fire warning signal and a plan for the procedure to follow in the event of a fire. This plan should be understood thoroughly by any person engaged in working in that institution, whether the person be a student or an employee. Institutions of this type also have some disaster plan with which every worker must be thoroughly familiar.

Every clinical laboratory should have at its disposal a safety reference library. This library should be available to all technical personnel, students, or employees, at all times. References in the safety library should include books or manuals helpful in the prevention of unsafe conditions and for use as a guide to safe procedures to be employed in the event of an accident in the laboratory. The following list includes some of the more pertinent references for a safety library:

1. "Handbook of Organic Industrial Solvents," National Association of Mutual Casualty Companies, 20 N. Wacker Drive, Chicago. This handbook can be obtained free of charge by writing to Frederick H. Deeg at the above address.

2. "Manual of Hazardous Chemical Reactions," Publications Department, National Fire Protection Association, 60 Batterymarch Street, Boston, Mass. 02110. The price of this manual is $1.25.

3. "A Condensed Laboratory Handbook," E. I. du Pont de Nemours & Company, Inc., Wilmington, Del. 19898. This handbook is free of charge.

In summary, the best protection in the clinical laboratory is a healthy awareness of the dangers inherent in the chemicals and materials used in any laboratory and the application of common sense in their use.

CLEANING LABORATORY GLASSWARE

Among the many factors that ensure the reporting of accurate results of the various laboratory determinations is the use of clean, unbroken glassware. There is no point in exerting care in obtaining specimens, handling those specimens, and making the eventual laboratory determination if the glassware used is not extremely clean.

There are various methods of cleaning glassware—depending on its use. In all cases, glassware for the clinical laboratory must be physically clean, in most cases it must be chemically clean, and in some cases it must be bacteriologically clean, or sterile.

Glassware which cannot be cleaned immediately after use should be rinsed with tap water and left to soak in a basin or pail of water to which a small amount of detergent has been added. Glassware that is new is often slightly alkaline and should be soaked for several hours in a dilute hydrochloric or nitric acid solution (about a 1% solution is satisfactory). This glassware should then be washed in the regular manner.

Glassware that is contaminated, as that used in the bacteriology laboratory, must be sterilized before it is washed. This can be done by boiling, autoclaving, or some similar procedure.

General cleaning methods involve the use of a soap, detergent, or cleaning powder. In most laboratories, detergents are used. If the dirty glassware has been soaking in a solution of the detergent water, the cleaning job will be that much easier.

CLEANING GENERAL LABORATORY GLASSWARE

To clean most laboratory glassware, with the exception of pipets (which are cleaned in a special way), the following general method can be used:

1. Put detergent of the specified amount into a dishpan or pail containing medium-hot water. The detergent should dissolve thoroughly.

2. Rinse glassware before placing it in the detergent solution.

3. Using a cleaning brush, thoroughly scrub the glassware, being certain to clean all parts of the glassware. Brushes of various sizes should be available to fit the different-sized test tubes, flasks, funnels, and bottles.

4. Rinse glassware under running tap water; allow the water to run into each piece of glassware, pour it out, and repeat this several times (between seven and ten times is sufficient); rinse the outside of the glassware, too. It is especially important to *remove all the detergent from the glassware before use;* if detergent remains, the alkali in the detergent will interfere with the tests being run in that glassware.

5. After thoroughly rinsing the glassware with tap water, rinse it with deionized or distilled water about three times. Certain glassware for microbiology use requires even more rinsing with deionized water. Use deionized water or distilled water in the final rinsing of all laboratory glassware.

6. Dry the glassware in a hot oven (not to exceed 140°C) or at room temperature. Never dry laboratory glassware with a towel.

7. Check the glassware for cleanliness by observing the water drainage.

Chemically clean glassware will drain uniformly; dirty glassware will drain leaving water droplets adhering to the walls of the glass.

CLEANING PIPETS

Pipets used in the laboratory are cleaned in a special way. Immediately after use, the pipets should be placed in a special pipet container or cylinder containing water; the water level should be such that the pipets are completely covered by it, and the pipets should be carefully placed in the container to avoid breakage. When the pipets are to be cleaned, they are removed from the cylinder and placed in another cylinder containing an acid cleaning solution. This cleaning solution is usually a combination of sulfuric acid and either potassium or sodium dichromate. It is an extremely potent solution, and it must be handled cautiously or serious burns will result (see under Safety in the Laboratory). The pipets are allowed to soak in the cleaning solution for 30 minutes.

The next step involves thorough rinsing of the pipets. This can be accomplished by hand, but more often it is done with the aid of an automatic pipet washer. The pipets are rinsed with tap water, utilizing the automatic pipet washer, for 1 to 2 hours. The pipets are then rinsed in deionized or distilled water two or three times and dried in a hot oven. An alternative cleaning solution used by some is a solution of detergent. However, the acid cleaning solution is recommended.

CLEANING DILUTING PIPETS

Pipets used in the hematology laboratory for diluting purposes are also cleaned in a special way. They should always be rinsed immediately after use, preferably by being placed in a tumbler or beaker of water until cleaned. There are several specific ways of cleaning this type of pipet, but, in general, they are cleaned with solutions of tap water first, then cleaned with distilled water, and finally rinsed with either alcohol or acetone. Acetone assists in drying the inside of the pipet. Usually the cleaning process is done with suction using a special pipet holder which fits onto the suction apparatus. The pipets are also dried with suction. Periodically, the pipets should be cleaned with a detergent solution, rinsed well, and dried.

OTHER CLEANING METHODS

A solution of aqua regia (nitric acid and hydrochloric acid) is often used for special cleaning purposes. It is *very* potent and must be handled with great care.

Another cleaning solution used by some is a dilute nitric acid solution. This can be used to clean glassware but it is not commonly used in most laboratories.

GLASS BREAKAGE AND REPLACEMENT

It is important in the clinical laboratory to check all glassware periodically to ascertain its condition. No broken or chipped glassware should be used. Many laboratory accidents are caused by the use of broken glassware. Serious cuts may result, and infections may set in.

Each time a laboratory procedure is carried out, the glassware used should be checked; equipment like beakers, pipets, test tubes, and flasks should be free from broken edges or cracks. To prevent breakage glassware should be handled carefully, and carrying too much glassware at a time from one place to another in the laboratory is to be avoided.

When glassware is broken, it must be replaced with another like piece. Breakage should be reported to an instructor or department head, so that replacement arrangements can be made. There are several laboratory equipment catalogs available for the purposes of ordering the required items. These catalogs are distributed by the various supply companies handling laboratory equipment and describe the many available items as to quality, capacity, tolerance, and cost. To purchase the needed equipment at the most reasonable price it is advisable to compare specific items as described in several different catalogs.

USE OF THE CENTRIFUGE

Centrifugation is used in the separation of a solid material from a liquid. It is also used in recovering solid materials from suspensions, as in the microscopic examination of urine. Centrifugation is employed in every department of the clinical laboratory, in chemistry, urinalysis, hematology, and blood banking, among others. Proper use of the centrifuge is an important technique for any person engaged in doing laboratory work.

Centrifuges facilitate the separation of particles in suspension by the application of centrifugal force. Several types of centrifuges will usually be found in the same laboratory, each designed for special uses. There are table-model and floor-model centrifuges, some small and others very large; there are even refrigerated centrifuges for special procedures.

Directions for use of a centrifuge are most frequently given in terms of speed, or revolutions per minute (rpm). A rheostat is used to set the desired speed, a given setting on the rheostat dial not necessarily corresponding directly to revolutions per minute. The setting speeds on the rheostat can also change with a variation in weight load and general aging of the centrifuge.

The top speed of most conventional centrifuges is about 3,000 rpm. The microhematocrit centrifuge used in many hematology laboratories for packing red blood cells attains a speed of about 10,000 rpms.

The most important rule to remember in the use of any centrifuge is the following: *always balance the tubes placed in the centrifuge;* that is, in the centrifuge cup opposite the material to be centrifuged, place a container of equivalent size and shape with an equal volume of liquid of the same specific gravity as the load. For most laboratory determinations, water may be placed in the balance tube.

Special centrifuge tubes should be used. These are tubes constructed to withstand the force exerted by the centrifuge. They have thicker glass walls or are made of a stronger, more resistant glass. Some of these tubes are conical, and some have round bottoms.

Whenever a tube breaks in the centrifuge cup, it is most important that both the cup and the rubber cushion in the cup be cleaned well to prevent further breakage by glass particles left behind.

Covers specially made for the centrifuge should be used except in certain specified instances. Using the cover prevents possible danger from flying glass should tubes break in the centrifuge.

Centrifuges should be checked, cleaned, and lubricated regularly to ensure proper operation.

THE MICROSCOPE

Of the equipment in the clinical laboratory, the microscope receives the most use. Microscopic work is a basic part of many areas of the laboratory—hematology, microbiology, urinalysis, and blood banking—to name a few. Because the microscope is such an important piece of equip-

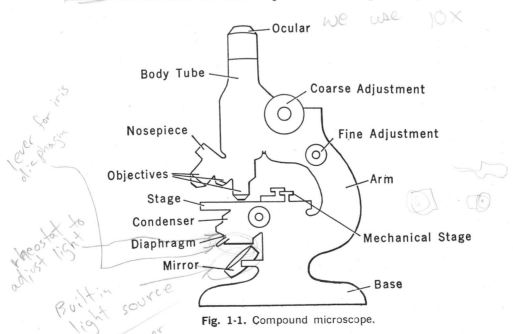

Fig. 1-1. Compound microscope.

ment and a precision instrument, it must be kept in excellent condition optically and mechanically.

The structure basic to all types of compound microscopes (the type used in most clinical laboratories) consists of four main categories: (1) the framework, (2) the illumination system, (3) the magnification system, and (4) the adjustment system (Fig. 1-1).

PARTS OF THE MICROSCOPE

The framework of the microscope consists of several units. The *base* is a firm, horseshoe-shaped foot on which the microscope rests. The *arm* is the structure which supports the magnifying and adjusting systems. The arm also is the handle by which the microscope can be carried without injury to the delicate parts. The *stage* is the horizontal platform, or shelf, on which the object being observed is placed. In some types of microscopes, a "mechanical stage" is added, making the manipulation of the object to be observed much easier. *All microscopes we use have mechanical stage. (moves the slide + necessary for complete and thorough scanning)*

Good microscopic work cannot be accomplished without proper illumination. The illumination system is therefore an important part of the compound microscope. The mirror is part of the illumination system. The mirror reflects the beam of light directed at it from the microscope light upward. The mirror has two sides; one is flat and the other concave. The concave side should be used for clinical microscopy work. In order to be certain that the mirror is at the correct angle, the ocular is removed and the light centered while the technician is looking through the body tube. *so fills your whole area* *Flat side of mirror used for directing sunlight if that is your only light source.*

Another part of the illumination system is the condenser. This is used to focus the light from the mirror on the material under examination. The condenser is a conical lens system with the point planed off. It can be raised and lowered beneath the stage by means of an adjustment knob. By using the condenser properly, the image field is evenly lighted. *no dark or hot spots*

The third and last unit of the illumination system to be discussed in this section is the *iris diaphragm*. This diaphragm consists of a series of horizontally arranged interlocking plates with a central aperture. It can be opened or closed as necessary to adjust the intensity of the light by means of a lever. The size of the aperture, and consequently the amount of light permitted to pass, is regulated by the person using the microscope. The arrangement is similar to the diaphragm on most cameras. *mirror reflecting light thru condenser*

The magnification system contains several important parts. This system too plays an extremely important role in the use of the microscope. The *ocular,* or *eyepiece,* is a lens which magnifies the image formed by the objective. The usual magnification of the ocular is five times ($5\times$) or ten times ($10\times$). Other oculars, however, can be obtained with other magnifications. Most modern microscopes have two oculars and are called *binocular* microscopes. Some student microscopes have only one ocular, and these are called *monocular* microscopes. The magnification produced by the ocular, when multiplied by the magnification produced by the objective, gives the total magnification of the subject being viewed.

The *objectives* are the major part of the magnification system. There are usually three objectives on each microscope. They are designated according to focal length: 16 mm, 4 mm, and 1.8 mm. The objectives are mounted on the nosepiece, which is a pivot, enabling a quick change of objectives. The 16-mm objective is the shortest one and is sometimes called the *low-power* objective. The 4-mm objective is often called the *high-power* objective. The 1.8-mm objective is the longest one and is called the *oil-immersion* objective. The distance from the bottom of the objective and the material being studied on the microscope stage is called the *working distance*. The working distance is very short for the 4-mm and 1.8-mm objectives, and for this reason correct focusing habits are necessary to prevent injuring the objectives against the slide on the stage. Often the term *parfocal* is used in speaking about a microscope. This term means that if one objective is in focus and a switch is made to the use of another objective, the focus will not be lost. The usual magnification of the 16-mm objective is 10×. For the 4-mm objective the usual magnification is 43× and for the 1.8-mm objective 97×. To obtain the total magnification for a microscope, the magnification of the objective is multiplied by the magnification of the ocular. Each type of microscope can have slightly different magnifications, depending on the ocular and the objective used. The actual magnification of an objective is inscribed directly on the outside of the objective itself.

The *body,* or *mechanical, tube* is the part of the microscope through which the light passes to the ocular. This is the tube which actually conducts the image.

The adjustment system enables the body tube to move up or down for focusing the objectives. This system usually consists of two adjustments, one coarse and the other fine. The coarse adjustment gives rapid movement over a wide range and is used to obtain an approximate focus. The fine adjustment gives a very slow movement over a limited range and is used to obtain exact focus after prior coarse adjustment.

To understand thoroughly the intricate workings of the lens system of the microscope would require a much more detailed study than is deemed feasible for a student laboratory technician. Rather it is more important at this time to learn the mechanics in general and to understand how to use and care for the microscope properly.

CARE OF THE MICROSCOPE

The microscope is a precision instrument and must be handled with great care. When it is necessary to transport the microscope, it should always be carried with both hands; it should be carried by the arm and supported under the base with the other hand. When not in use, the microscope should be covered and put away in a microscope case, or *with a dust cover — should be moved as little as possible* in a desk or cupboard. It should be left with the low-power objective *+ have* in place, the body tube barrel adjusted to the lowest position possible, *its own designated* and the condenser down. *place in the lab,*

The surface of most microscopes is finished with a black or gray enamel and metal plating which is resistant to most laboratory chemicals. These surfaces may be kept clean by washing with a neutral soap and water. To clean the metal and enamel surfaces of the microscope, a gauze should be moistened with the cleaning agent. Rubbing the surface with a circular motion will clean the enamel and metal. These should be dried immediately with a clean, dry piece of gauze. The mirror can also be cleaned in this manner. Gauze should *never* be used to clean any of the optical parts of the microscope. *Don't use GAUZE ON LENSES or OPTICAL PARTS*

The glass surfaces of the ocular, the objectives, and the condenser are hand-ground optical lenses. These lenses must be kept meticulously clean. Optical glass is softer than ordinary glass and should never be cleaned with paper tissue or gauze. These materials will scratch the lens. To clean the lenses of the microscope, use lens paper. If a lens is especially dirty, a small amount of xylol may be put on the lens paper. Xylol should be used sparingly, because it can damage the lens mounting if it is allowed to get beyond the front seal. The oil-immersion lens will require the use of a small amount of xylol on the lens paper in order to clean it properly. When xylol is used, the lens should be dried with a clean piece of lens paper. The lenses should never be touched with the fingers.

recommended

Dust can be removed from the lens of the ocular with a camel's hair brush. The oculars should not be removed for more than a few minutes, as dust can collect in the tube and settle on the rear lens of an objective. At regular intervals the ocular can be taken apart and cleaned on the inside with a camel's hair brush. The ocular can be checked for additional dirt by looking through it, using the microscope lamp for light. Dirt on any part of the ocular will rotate with the ocular when it is turned.

The stage of the microscope should be cleaned after each use by moistening a piece of gauze with a little xylol. After being cleaned thoroughly, the stage should be wiped dry. *with soap + water — Dry well*

The coarse and fine adjustments occasionally need attention. When there is unusual resistance to any manipulation of these knobs, force must not be used to overcome the resistance. Instead, the cause of the problem must be found first. A small drop of oil may be necessary. It is best to call in a repairman specializing in microscopes when a serious problem occurs. *A good binocular microscope with a built in light source costs about $1,500.00*

USE OF THE MICROSCOPE

Most microscopes utilize a lamp of some sort to assist in the illumination system. Some lamps are built into the microscope, and others are separate.

So that one doesn't ruin objectives
by running them into the slides. one must
know these lighting controls so they can see properly

2 BASIC TECHNIQUES FOR THE MEDICAL LABORATORY TECHNICIAN

The biggest concern in learning how to use a microscope for the first time is the lighting and fine adjustment maneuvers. One must be certain that the mirror, condenser, and diaphragm are in correct adjustment. Light adjustment is made before any focusing is done. The light adjustment is accomplished by raising and lowering the condenser and opening and closing the diaphragm. At the start of this initial lighting adjustment, the condenser should be all the way up and the diaphragm all the way open, with the low-power objective in place. While looking through the ocular, the diaphragm can be closed until the field is just beginning to be closed off. Next, the condenser should be lowered until the light is even.

The object to be examined is placed on the stage and secured. Usually the object to be observed is placed on a glass microscope slide. Care must be taken to avoid injury to the objectives while placing specimens on the stage. The barrel, or tube, of the microscope should be raised by means of the coarse-adjustment knob to prevent damage to the objectives.

Focusing is the next technique to be mastered. With the object on the stage and while watching from the side, the low-power objective is brought down as far as it will go, so that it almost meets the top of the specimen to be studied. The coarse adjustment is used for this procedure. The objective must not be in direct contact with the specimen. This must be watched from the side, as stated previously, to avoid damage to the objectives. Once the objective is just at the top of the specimen to be examined, the object is slowly focused upward using the coarse-adjustment knob, looking through the ocular while this is being done. When the object is nearly in focus, it is brought into clear focus by use of the fine-adjustment knob. When changing to another objective, the barrel distance must not be changed. As stated previously, most microscopes are parfocal. The only adjustment necessary should be that using the fine-adjustment knob. The fine adjustment is used continuously during the microscopic study.

If a greater magnification is needed, more light is necessary. Additional light is provided by the use of immersion oil placed on the viewing slide when the oil-immersion lens (1.8-mm objective) is used. The oil directs the light rays to a finer point. When the oil-immersion lens is to be used, the desired area on the slide is first found by using the $10\times$ (16-mm) objective. Once this area is located, the body tube is raised by using the coarse-adjustment knob, a drop of immersion oil is placed on the slide, and the oil-immersion lens is lowered into the oil while the technician looks at it from the side. The ocular should not be looked through during this adjustment procedure. When the initial adjustment has been made, the fine adjustment is made while looking through the ocular. The oil remaining on the lens of the objective after the study has been completed must be cleaned off using lens paper.

TYPES OF MICROSCOPES

There are other types of microscopes used for special microscopy procedures. The compound microscope is the one used in routine clinical observations and the one with which a laboratory technician should become most familiar. A dark-field microscope is one in which the light illuminating the object to be magnified is reflected rather than transmitted light. As a result, the object under study appears light against a dark background.[1] Any compound microscope may be converted to a dark-field microscope by use of a special dark-field condenser in place of the usual condenser. The dark-field microscope is used to observe the spirochetes in the exudates from leptospiral or syphilitic infections.

Another type of microscope which is used in the laboratory is the phase microscope. The optical system of the phase microscope is such that materials with different densities appear to differ from each other in the intensity and the shade of the light transmitted through them.[2] The need for staining is therefore eliminated. The phase microscope has found a use in the hematology laboratory in the counting of platelets using a direct method.

REAGENT PREPARATION, CHEMICALS, AND QUANTITATIVE TRANSFER

For the various clinical laboratory determinations many types of glassware, equipment, specimens, and reagents are used. It is important to understand fully just how valuable the reagents are in the clinical laboratory, as the accuracy of the determinations depends to a great extent on the accuracy of the reagents used. A reagent is defined as any substance employed to produce a chemical reaction. In preparing reagents, instructions should be followed exactly. Often certain reagents will be purchased in a fully prepared state; in this case it is important that the reagents be obtained only from reputable chemical companies. To repeat a most important precept, *instructions must be followed;* this is a strict rule in the laboratory. One should never rely on memory in preparing a reagent but, rather, follow a specific set of instructions or directions devised for the preparation of each reagent needed.

As stated in the definition of a reagent, a reagent is a substance used to produce a chemical reaction. Instructions for preparing a reagent resemble a cake recipe in that they tell what quantities of ingredients to mix together. Instructions tell the names of the chemicals needed, the number of grams or milligrams needed, and the total volume to which the particular reagent should be diluted. The most commonly used solvent used for dilution purposes is deionized or distilled water.

Chemical supply companies furnish "ready-made" reagents which fill the needs of some laboratories. These reagents usually cost more money, and therefore in large laboratories and in teaching institutions ready-made reagents are not often used. For students it is important that the preparation of reagents be practiced, as this is one of the fundamentals of the clinical laboratory.

REAGENT PREPARATION

Preparation of reagents involves the use of a balance (analytical, triple-beam, or centigram, for example) and other special volumetric measuring devices (such as volumetric flasks and graduated cylinders). The various types of available volumetric glassware are discussed in Chapter 2.

Since chemicals are used in the preparation of reagents and the accuracy of the laboratory determinations depends on the quality of the reagents employed, it is essential that only chemicals from reliable companies be used.

GRADES OF CHEMICALS

A chemical is a substance occurring naturally or obtained through a chemical process; it is used to produce a chemical effect or reaction. Chemicals are produced in various purities or grades. It is essential that the user of chemicals in reagent preparation understand the many grades of chemicals available and which grade or type should be used for which reagent. A system is used to indicate the purity of a chemical, and anyone engaged in doing laboratory work should know what this system is. The most common designations of degrees of purity are listed below:[3]

1. Pure. Entirely unadulterated.

2. Reagent grade, or analytical reagent grade (A.R.). These chemicals are of a high degree of purity and are used often in the preparation of reagents in the clinical laboratory.

3. American Chemical Society (A.C.S.). The American Chemical Society has developed many reagent grade, or A.R., chemicals, and those which meet their standards are designated by the letters "A.C.S."

4. Chemically pure (C.P.). These chemicals are usually sufficiently pure to use in most analyses done in the clinical laboratory.

5. Pharmacopeia of the United States (U.S.P.). Those reagents which meet the specifications set up by the Pharmacopeia of the United States (a book of standards and potency for drugs and chemicals prepared by the United States Pharmacopoeial Convention, Inc., an officially recognized organization) are labeled "U.S.P." They are generally less pure than the C.P. grade.

6. Technical, practical, or commercial grade. These chemicals are used only for industrial purposes and are generally not used in the preparation of reagents for the clinical laboratory.

Chemicals used in the laboratory take various forms. It is necessary that persons using these chemicals know the chemical forms and which form should be used in the preparation of the specific reagent desired. Some of the common forms are lumps, sticks, pellets, granules, fine granules, crystalline powder, crystals, fine crystals, powder, and liquid. There are some special forms such as chips, scales, and flakes, but these are not frequently used in reagent preparation. *Don't often see these last in AR grade.*

It is important that chemicals kept in the laboratory be stored properly. Chemicals that require refrigeration should be immediately refrigerated. Solids should be kept in a dry place. Chemicals that produce fumes (such as ammonia and hydrochloric acid) should be stored in a special place where these fumes will not contaminate other chemicals. Fuming chemicals should be opened only under a hood, so that the vapors will not escape into the room. Chemicals that are flammable should be kept not only away from flames but also in a cool place. Chemicals that absorb water should be weighed only after dessication or drying in a hot oven; otherwise their weight will not be accurate. *STORING REAGENTS*

QUANTITATIVE TRANSFER

In preparing any solution in the clinical laboratory, it is necessary to utilize the practice known as *quantitative transfer*. It is essential that the *entire* amount of the weighed or measured substance be used in preparing the solution. In using quantitative transfer, the entire amount of the measured substance is transferred from one vessel to another for dilution purposes. The usual practice in preparing most laboratory reagents is to weigh the chemical in a beaker (or other suitable vessel) and quantitatively transfer this chemical to a volumetric flask for dilution with deionized water. The volumetric flask chosen must be of the correct size; that is, it must hold the amount of solution that is desired for the total volume of the reagent being prepared.

Procedure for Quantitative Transfer and Dilution

1. Place a clean, dry funnel in the mouth of the volumetric flask.
2. Carefully transfer the chemical in the measuring vessel into the funnel.
3. Wash the chemical into the flask with small amounts of deionized water or the required solvent for the reagent.
4. Rinse the measuring vessel (beaker) three to five times with small portions of deionized water or the required solvent until *all* of the chemical has been transferred from the vessel into the volumetric flask (add each rinsing to the flask).

5. Rinse the funnel with deionized water or the required solvent, and remove the funnel from the volumetric flask.

6. Dissolve the chemical in the flask by shaking it. Some chemicals are more difficult to dissolve than others. On occasion, more special attention must be given to the problem of dissolving the chemical.

There are several methods by which dissolving of solid materials can be hastened. Heating usually increases the solubility of a chemical, and heat also causes the fluid to move (the currents set up help in dissolving). Even mild heat, however, will decompose some chemicals, and therefore it must be used with caution. Agitation by using a stirring rod or swirling by means of a mechanical shaker increases solubility by removing from contact with the chemical the saturated solution which hinders further solution of the substance. Rapid addition of the solvent is another means of hastening the solution of solid materials. Some chemicals tend to cake and form aggregates as soon as the solvent is added. By adding the solvent quickly and keeping the solids in motion, this aggregation may be prevented.

7. Add deionized water or the required solvent to about ½ in. below the calibration line on the flask, allow a few seconds for drainage of fluid above calibration line, and then carefully add deionized water or the required solvent to the calibration line (the *bottom* of the meniscus must be exactly on the calibration mark).

8. Stopper the flask with a ground-glass stopper, and mix well by inverting at least twenty times.

9. Rinse a properly labeled reagent bottle with a small amount of the mixed reagent in the volumetric flask. Transfer the prepared reagent to the labeled reagent bottle for storage.

Containers for storage of reagents, usually a reagent bottle, should be labeled before the material is added. Never should a reagent be placed in an unlabeled bottle or container. If an unlabeled container is found, the reagent in it must be discarded. Proper labeling of reagent bottles is of the greatest importance. All labels should include the name and concentration of the reagent, the date the reagent was prepared, and the initials of the person making the reagent (Fig. 1-2).

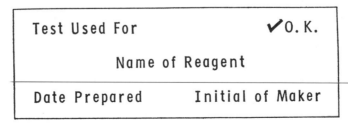

Fig. 1-2. Sample label.

After the prepared reagent is in the reagent bottle, it must be checked by some means before it is put into actual use in any procedure. This can be done in one of several ways, depending on the reagent itself. After the reagent has been checked, this is noted on the label, and the solution can then be put into active use in the laboratory.

The most common amount of solution prepared at one time is 1 liter. If 1 liter of reagent is needed, the measured chemical must be transferred quantitatively to a 1-liter volumetric flask and diluted to the calibration mark with deionized water or the required solvent. The method of quantitative transfer requires a great deal of care and accuracy.

Using solutions of the correct concentration is of the greatest importance in attaining good results in the laboratory. Quantitative transfer, along with accurate initial measurement of the chemical, helps to ensure that the solution will be of the correct concentration.

KINDS OF WATER USED IN THE CLINICAL LABORATORY

For use in the clinical laboratory, all water should be free from substances which could interfere with the tests being performed. Interference due to particles in the water must therefore be eliminated. It is important that any person involved in doing clinical laboratory procedures understand the reasons for the special emphasis placed on the kinds of water used.

Many minerals are found in natural water. Among those commonly found in water are iron, magnesium, and calcium. Water from which these minerals and others have been removed by distillation is known as *distilled water*. In the process of distillation, water is boiled, and the resulting steam is cooled; condensed steam is distilled water. Distilled water is often used in the laboratory.

Another kind of water used is known as *deionized water*. In the process of deionization, water is passed through a resin column containing positively (+) and negatively (−) charged particles. These particles combine with ions present in the water to remove them. Therefore, only those substances which can ionize will be removed in the process of deionization. Organic substances and other substances which do not ionize are not removed. Both deionized and distilled water are used widely in the clinical laboratory.

A third type of water available is called *double-distilled water*. This is water which has gone through the distillation process twice, so that more constituents are removed. In the second distillation process, the main constituent removed is ammonia. This type of water must be used in doing tests for nitrogen compounds (for example, the test for urea nitrogen, a common chemistry determination) or any other procedures where ammonia could contaminate the test and thereby alter the results. Sometimes double-distilled water is known as *ammonia-free water*.

Rarely is tap water used in the clinical laboratory, the exception being for the initial washing of glassware. Whenever water is needed in any procedure or reagents are to be made and diluted with water, care should be taken to use the type of water best suited to the test or reagent. Plain tap water is not used in any procedures or in the making of reagents.

LABORATORY CALCULATIONS

A sound background in basic mathematics (including algebra), an understanding of the units in which quantities are expressed, and a knowledge of the methods of analysis are all necessary in performing laboratory calculations. There are no simple formulas enabling a person to solve all such problems, but certain basic fundamentals are a part of many of the problems encountered in a clinical laboratory.

PROPORTIONS

These are a device often used for determining a quantity from a given ratio. Setting up proportions for solving a problem is common in laboratory calculations.

Example:

A formula calls for 5 g of sodium chloride $(NaCl)/1,000$ ml of solution. If only 500 ml of the solution is needed, how much NaCl is needed?

$$\frac{5 \text{ g}}{1,000 \text{ ml}} = \frac{x \text{ g}}{500 \text{ ml}}$$
$$x = 2.5 \text{ g of NaCl}$$

RELATING EQUAL CONCENTRATIONS

To relate equal concentrations, a most useful formula is concentration $(C_1) \times$ volume (V_1) = concentration $(C_2) \times$ volume (V_2). If any three of the values are known, the fourth may be determined. Several applications of this formula are used in the clinical laboratory, one of these being in titrations, where equal concentrations of reactants are present at the end point (see under Titration in Chapter 2), and in the preparation of weaker solutions from stronger solutions.

Example:

To calculate the milliliters of 10% sodium hydroxide solution (NaOH) required to prepare 1,000 ml of 2% sodium hydroxide:

$$C_1 \times V_1 = C_2 \times V_2$$
$$10\% \times x \text{ ml} = 2\% \times 1,000 \text{ ml}$$
$$x \text{ ml} = \frac{2(1,000)}{10} = 200 \text{ ml}$$

DILUTION FACTORS

In most laboratory determinations, a small sample is taken for analysis, and the final result is expressed as concentration per some convenient standard volume.

To derive a factor by which the determination answer (for the small sample) may be multiplied to give an answer in the desired units, one must first determine the amount of specimen actually analyzed in the procedure and then multiply this by a factor that will express the concentration in terms of the desired standard volume.

Example:

In a certain procedure, 0.5 ml of blood is diluted to a total of 10 ml with various reagents. 1 ml of this dilution (expressed as a 1:20 dilution; e.g., 0.5 ml in a total of 10 ml is the same ratio as 1 ml in 20 ml) is used in the next step in the analysis. The final answer is to be expressed in concentration per 100 ml of blood. The dilution factor by which the determination answer is multiplied to give the concentration per 100 ml of sample (blood) is

$$\frac{10 \text{ ml (volume of total dilution)}}{1 \text{ ml (volume of dilution used)}} \times \frac{100 \text{ ml (volume of blood required for expression of result)}}{0.5 \text{ ml (volume of blood used)}}$$

or

$$10 \times 200 = 20,000 = \text{dilution factor}$$

SIGNIFICANT FIGURES

Using more digits than necessary ·to calculate and report the results of a laboratory determination has several disadvantages. It is important that the number used contain only the digits necessary for the precision of the determination. Using more digits than necessary is misleading in that it ascribes more accuracy to the determination than is actually the case. There is also the danger of overlooking a decimal point and making an error in judging the magnitude of the answer. Digits in a number which are needed to express the precision of the measurement from which the number is derived are known as *significant figures*. Judgment must be exercised in determining how many figures should be used. Some rules to assist in making such decisions are:

1. Use the known accuracy of the method to determine the number of digits that are significant in the answer, and, as a general rule, retain one more figure than this.

Example:

A urea nitrogen result was reported as 11.2 mg%. This would seem to indicate that the laboratory is capable of determining the urea nitrogen concentration this closely. In reality, the accuracy of most urea nitrogen methods is $\pm 10\%$ (the result, 11.2 mg% could vary from 10 to 12 mg%). In addition, if the decimal point were omitted or overlooked, the result could be taken as 112 mg%.

2. Take the accuracy of the least accurate measurement, or the measurement with the least number of significant figures, as the accuracy of the final result.

Example:

In the addition of

$$
\begin{array}{r}
206.1 \\
7.56 \\
0.8764 \\
\hline
\end{array}
$$

rewrite as

$$
\begin{array}{r}
206.1 \\
7.6 \\
0.9 \\
\hline
\end{array}
$$

In this example, the least accurate figure is accurate to one decimal place; this is therefore the determining factor.

Another practice for the use of significant figures is in rounding off decimal values to the proper place. As a general rule, when the figure next to the last one to be retained is less than 5, the last figure should be left unchanged. When the figure next to the last one to be retained is 5 or greater than 5, the last figure is increased by 1.

Examples:

2.31463 g is rounded off to 2.3146 g.
5.34659 g is rounded off to 5.3466 g.

EXPRESSIONS OF SOLUTION CONCENTRATION

Concentration of solutions of reagents may be expressed in one of three general ways: by *proper name,* by *physical units,* or by *chemical units.*

There are very few instances where a solution is described by *proper name,* as far as its concentration is concerned. In Chapter 4, Urinalysis, the use of Benedict's solution is discussed. This solution is prepared with specific amounts of ingredients according to a series of instructions or directions. When Benedict's solution is needed, one knows exactly what is meant and which chemicals in specific amounts are used in its preparation. Another example of a reagent described by proper name is Wright's stain used in the hematology laboratory.

Physical units are commonly used to express concentration. The units used are either of *weight* or of *volume.* One way of expressing concentration is by *weight per unit volume* (or W/V). When weight per unit volume is used, the amount of solute (the substance which goes into solution) per volume of solution is expressed. Weight per unit volume is used most often when a solid chemical is diluted in a liquid. The usual way to express weight per unit volume is as grams per liter (g/liter) or milligrams per milliliter (mg/ml). If a concentration for a certain solution is given as 10 g/liter, it means that there are 10 g of solute for every liter of solution. If a solution with a concentration of 10 mg/ml is desired and 100 ml of this solution is to be prepared, the use of a proportion formula can be applied.

Example:

$$\frac{10 \text{ mg}}{1 \text{ ml}} = \frac{x \text{ mg}}{100 \text{ ml}}$$
$$x = 1,000 \text{ mg, or 1 g}$$

One gram of the desired solute is weighed and diluted to 100 ml. (See under Reagent Preparation.)

In working with *standard solutions* (see Chapter 2), it will be seen that their concentrations, almost without exception, are expressed as milligrams per milliliter.

Another way of expressing concentration using physical units is by *volume per unit volume* (V/V). When using volume per unit volume to express concentration, a liquid chemical is diluted with another liquid; the concentration is expressed as the number of milliliters of liquid chemical per unit volume of solution. The usual way of expressing volume per unit volume is as milliliters per milliliter (ml/ml) or milliliters per liter (ml/liter). The number of milliliters of liquid chemical in 1 milliliter or 1 liter of solution utilizes the volume per unit volume expression of concentration. If 10 ml of alcohol is diluted to 100 ml with water, the concentration is expressed as 10 ml/100 ml, or 0.1 ml/ml, or 100 ml/liter. If a solution with a concentration of 0.5 ml/ml is desired and 1 liter is to be prepared, a proportion can again be used to solve the problem.

Example:

$$\frac{0.5 \text{ ml}}{1 \text{ ml}} = \frac{x \text{ ml}}{1,000 \text{ ml}}$$
$$x = 500 \text{ ml}$$

Five hundred milliliters of the liquid chemical is measured accurately and diluted to one thousand milliliters (1 liter).

To express concentration in milliliters per liter, one needs to know how many milliliters of liquid chemical there are in 1 liter of the solution.

Any chemical (liquid or solid) can be made into a solution by diluting it with a solvent. The usual solvent is deionized or distilled water (see under Kinds of Water Used in the Clinical Laboratory). If the desired chemical is a liquid, the amount needed is measured in milliliters or liters (on occasion, liquids are weighed, but the usual method is to measure them); if the desired chemical is a solid, the amount needed is weighed in grams or milligrams.

A third way of expressing concentration using physical units is by _weight per unit weight_ (W/W). This expression is not commonly used. There are not many reagents prepared using only solid chemicals and no liquid solvent. When the desired chemical is a solid and it is mixed with, or diluted with, another solid, the expression of concentration is weight per unit weight. The usual ways to express weight per unit weight is as milligrams per milligram (mg/mg) or as grams per gram (g/g). The number of milligrams or grams of one solid in the total number of milligrams or grams of the dry mixture is the weight per unit weight.

An example of a chemical reagent using this expression of concentration is Rothera's reagent (see under Ketone Bodies in Chapter 4), which is used in the detection of acetone in the urine. Rothera's reagent is prepared by mixing two dry chemicals together in specific amounts.

Another commonly used expression of concentration utilizing physical units is the _percent solution_ (%). A definition of percent is _parts per hundred parts_ (the part can be any given unit). Unless otherwise stated, a percent solution usually means grams or milliliters of solute per 100 ml (g/100 ml or ml/100 ml) of solution. Percent solutions can be prepared using either liquid or solid chemicals. Percent solutions can be expressed either as weight per unit volume percent (W/V%) or volume per unit volume percent (V/V%), depending on the state of the solute (chemical) used, e.g., whether it is a solid or a liquid. When there is a solid chemical dissolved in a liquid, percent means _grams of solid in 100 ml of solution_. If 10 g of NaCl is diluted to 100 ml with deionized water, the concentration is expressed as 10%. If 2.5 g is diluted to 100 ml, the concentration is 2.5%. The following is an example of concentration expresssed in percent:

Example:

Ten grams of NaOH is diluted to 200 ml with water. What is the concentration in percent? A proportion can be set up to solve this problem.

$$\frac{10 \text{ g}}{200 \text{ ml}} = \frac{x \text{ g}}{100 \text{ ml}}$$
$$x = 5\% \text{ solution}$$

Remember that the percent expression is based on how much solute is present in _100 ml_ of the solution.

When specifically stated, some concentrations of solutions are expressed as the milligrams of solute in 100 ml of solution (mg%). When this is used, "mg%" is always stated. If 25 mg of chemical is diluted to 100 ml, the concentration in milligrams percent would be expressed as 25 mg%.

If a liquid chemical is used to prepare a percent solution, the expression of concentration is as volume per unit volume percent, or milliliters of solute per 100 ml of solution. If 10 ml of hydrochloric acid is diluted to 100 ml with water, the concentration is 10%. If 10 ml of the same acid is diluted to 1 liter (1,000 ml), the concentration is 1%.

The third main category of expressing concentration is using *chemical units*. In the following discussion of the use of chemical units, the terms *molarity (M)* and *normality (N)* will be explained.

The molarity of a solution is defined as the number of gram molecular weights of a compound per liter of solution. Another way of defining molarity is the number of moles per liter of solution. A *mole* is the molecular weight of a compound in grams (one mole equals one gram molecular weight, or 1 GMW). The number of moles of a compound equals the number of grams divided by the gram molecular weight of that compound. One gram molecular weight equals the sum of all atomic weights in a molecule of the compound expressed in grams.

To determine the gram molecular weight of a compound, the correct formula must be known. This formula known, the sum of all the atomic weights in the compound can be found by consulting a periodic table of elements or a chart with the atomic weights of the elements.

Examples:

1. Sodium chloride has 1 sodium ion and 1 chloride ion; the formula is written NaCl. The gram molecular weight is derived by finding the sum of the atomic weights:

$$Na = 23$$
$$Cl = 35.5$$
$$GMW = 58.5 \text{ g}$$

If the gram molecular weight of NaCl is 58.5 g, a 1 M solution of NaCl would contain 58.5 g of NaCl/liter of solution, because molarity equals moles per liter, and 1 mole of NaCl equals 58.5 g.

2. For $BaSO_4$, the gram molecular weight equals 233 (the formula indicates that there is 1 barium, 1 sulfate, and 4 oxygen ions).

$$1 \text{ Ba} = 137 \times 1 = 137$$
$$1 \text{ S} = 32 \times 1 = 32$$
$$4 \text{ O} = 16 \times 4 = \underline{64}$$
$$233$$

Knowing the gram molecular weight to be 233, a 1 M solution of $BaSO_4$ would contain 233 g of $BaSO_4$/liter of solution.

Not always will the quantities of solutions needed be in units of whole liters, and often concentrations using fractions or multiples of a 1 M concentration will be desired. Parts of a molar solution are expressed as decimals. If a 1 M solution of NaCl contains 58.5 g of NaCl/liter of solution, a 0.5 M solution would contain ½ of 58.5 g, or 29 g/liter, and a 3 M solution would contain 3×58.5 g, or 175.5 g/liter.

Example:

What is the molarity of a solution containing 10 g of NaCl/liter? Molarity equals the number of moles per liter, and moles equal the grams divided by the gram molecular weight.

Step 1: Find the gram molecular weight for NaCl: It is 58.5 g (Na = 23 and Cl = 35.5).

Step 2: Find the moles per liter.

$$10 \text{ g}/(58.5 \text{ g/mole}) = 0.171 \text{ moles of NaCl}$$

Step 3: Knowing that the number of moles per liter of solution equals the molarity, the molarity of the example solution is therefore 0.171 M.

Equations might prove useful to some in working with molarity solutions. Some of these equations are listed below:

1. $\text{Molarity} = \dfrac{\text{no. of moles of solute}}{\text{liters of solution}}$

2. $\text{Molarity} = \dfrac{\text{no. of grams of solute}}{\text{gram molecular weight}} \times \dfrac{1}{\text{liters of solution}}$

3. Moles of solute = molarity $\times$ liters of solution

4. Grams of solute = molarity $\times$ gram molecular weight $\times$ liters of solution

NOTE: These equations are all on the basis of a liter of solution; if something other than 1 liter is used, refer back to the 1-liter basis (500 ml = 0.5 liter, or 2,000 ml = 2 liters, for example).

Unfortunately, molarity does not provide a basis for direct comparison of strength for all solutions. An example of this is that 1 liter of 1 M NaOH will exactly neutralize 1 liter of 1 M HCl, but it will neutralize only ½ liter of 1 M H_2SO_4. It is therefore more convenient to choose a unit of concentration that *will* provide a basis for direct comparison of strengths of solutions. Such a unit is referred to as an *equivalent* (or equivalent weight), and this term is used in describing the next unit of concentration to be discussed—normality.

The *equivalent* (equiv) is the weight in grams that will liberate, combine with, or replace one gram atom (g atom) of hydrogen ion (H+). By using equivalents, the numbers of units of all substances involved in a reaction are made numerically equal.

Examples:

Reaction 1:

$$1 \text{ equiv NaOH} + 1 \text{ equiv HCl} \rightarrow 1 \text{ equiv } H_2O + 1 \text{ equiv NaCl}$$

Reaction 2:

1 equiv NaOH + 1 equiv $H_2SO_4 \rightarrow$ 1 equiv H_2O + 1 equiv Na_2SO_4

The balanced equation for this reaction is

$$2NaOH + 1H_2SO_4 \rightarrow 2H_2O + 1Na_2SO_4$$

This same reaction expressed using moles is

1 mole NaOH + ½ mole of $H_2SO_4 \rightarrow$ 1 mole H_2O + ½ mole Na_2SO_4

One equivalent of any acid will neutralize one equivalent of any base.

In discussing molarity the term moles per liter (moles/liter) is used; in units of normality, the terms equivalents per liter (equiv/liter), milliequivalents per milliliter (meq/ml), or milliequivalents per liter (meq/liter) are used. The normality of a solution is defined as the number of equivalents (or equivalent weights) per liter of solution, or the number of milliequivalents per milliliter of solution. The *equivalent weight* is the weight in grams that will liberate, combine with, or replace one gram atom of hydrogen. The equivalent weight may be found by dividing the gram molecular weight by the total combining power, or valence, of the positive ion (ions) of the substance.

Examples of Equivalent Weights:

HCl has 1 atom of H+ and 1 atom of Cl⁻; therefore, equivalent weight equals molecular weight.

H_2S has 2 atoms of H+ and only 1 atom of S⁼, *or* 1 atom of H+ with ½ atom of S⁼; therefore, equivalent weight equals one-half the molecular weight, or

$$\text{Molecular weight/Total positive valence} = {}^{34}\!/_2 = 17$$

NaCl has 1 atom of Cl⁻ and 1 atom of Na+ (Na+ replaces H+); therefore, equivalent weight equals molecular weight.

A liter of a 1 *N* solution of H_2SO_4 contains the same number of equivalents as 1 liter of 1 *N* HCl, or 1 *N* NaOH, or 1 *N* Ba(OH$_2$). Again, equations might prove useful in working with normality solutions; some of these are:

1. Normality = equiv solute/liters solution
2. Normality = $\dfrac{\text{g solute}}{\text{GMW/combining power (valence)}} \times \dfrac{1}{\text{liters solution}}$
3. Normality = $\dfrac{\text{moles}}{\text{combining power}} \times \dfrac{1}{\text{liters solution}}$
4. Normality = $\dfrac{\text{g solute}}{\text{equiv weight}} \times \dfrac{1}{\text{liters solution}}$
5. Normality = equival/liter
6. Normality = meq/ml

On occasion, it is necessary to convert an expression of concentration in molarity to one in normality and vice versa. Two simple formulas are available for this purpose:

1. Molarity = normality/total positive combining power (valence)
2. Normality = molarity × total positive combining power

To prepare 1 liter of a 2 N NaCl solution, first calculate the gram molecular weight using the known formula for the compound: Na = 23, Cl = 35.5, the gram molecular weight thus being 58.5 g. In working with normality problems, the equivalent weight is used; therefore, the next step is to calculate this: The gram equivalent weight equals the gram molecular weight divided by the valence, or 58.5 g divided by 1; the gram equivalent weight is therefore 58.5 g. For 1 liter of a 1 N solution of this compound, 58.5 g would be weighed; for 1 liter of a 2 N solution, 58.5 g × 2, or 117 g, of NaCl/liter is needed.

An example of another such problem follows:

Example:

Prepare 200 ml of a 0.5 N $CaCl_2$ solution.
Step 1: Calculate the gram molecular weight.

$$Ca = 40 \times 1 = 40$$
$$Cl = 35.5 \times 2 = \underline{71}$$
$$111 \text{ g GMW}$$

Step 2: Calculate the gram equivalent weight.

$$\text{Equivalent weight} = \text{GMW/valence} = 111\tfrac{1}{2} = 55.5 \text{ g}$$

Step 3: Solve for normality.
A 1 N solution would contain 55.5 g/liter.
A 0.5 N solution would contain only half as much chemical per liter of solution, or 27.8 g.
a proportion could be set up to solve this:

$$\frac{55.5 \text{ g/liter}}{1 \text{ } N \text{ solution}} = \frac{x \text{ g/liter}}{0.5 \text{ } N \text{ solution}}$$
$$x = 27.8 \text{ g}$$

However, only 200 ml of this solution is needed. Therefore another proportion could be set up for this:

$$\frac{27.8 \text{ g}}{1,000 \text{ ml}} = \frac{x \text{ g}}{200 \text{ ml}}$$
$$x = 5.6 \text{ g}$$

Step 4: Actual preparation of solution: 5.6 g of $CaCl_2$ is weighed and diluted to 200 ml volumetrically (see under Reagent Preparation).

REFERENCES

1. R. P. MacFate, "Introduction to the Clinical Laboratory," p. 344, The Year Book Medical Publishers, Inc., Chicago, 1961.
2. Lot B. Page and Perry J. Culver, "A Syllabus of Laboratory Examinations in Clinical Diagnosis," rev. ed., p. 69, Harvard University Press, Cambridge, Mass., 1960.
3. MacFate, *op. cit.*, p. 75.

BIBLIOGRAPHY

Allen, Joe E.: An Exploratory Study of the Attitudes of Laboratory Workers toward Accident Prevention: Safety in the Chemical Laboratory, *J. Chem. Educ.*, October, 1966.

Annino, Joseph S.: "Clinical Chemistry: Principles and Procedures," 3d ed., Little, Brown and Company, Boston, 1964.

Brooks, Stewart M.: "Integrated Basic Sciences," The C. V. Mosby Company, St. Louis, 1962.

Davidsohn, Israel, and Benjamin B. Wells: "Clinical Diagnosis by Laboratory Methods (Todd-Sanford)," 13th ed., W. B. Saunders Company, Philadelphia, 1962.

Ederer, Grace Mary, and Barbara Tucker: Accident Survey and Safety Programs in Two Hospital Clinical Laboratories, *Am. J. Med. Technol.*, 26:219, 1960.

Routh, Joseph I.: "Fundamentals of Inorganic, Organic, and Biological Chemistry," 4th ed., W. B. Saunders Company, Philadelphia, 1960.

Testing of Glass Volumetric Apparatus, *Natl. Bur. Std. Circ.* 602, 1959.

Tucker, Barbara: Safety Programs in the Hospital, *Safety Newsletter,* National Safety Council, Chicago, August, 1965.

2

Chemistry

The field of laboratory medicine is expanding rapidly, and with it the specialty of clinical chemistry. Perhaps chemistry is the area where changes are occurring more rapidly than in any other. For this reason there is an increased demand for well-trained, qualified laboratory personnel to perform the routine clinical chemistry determinations.

The techniques of most chemical procedures performed in the laboratory are not in themselves difficult, but their proper execution requires genuine interest, reliability, and a good basic knowledge of the principles involved. It is essential, therefore, that the basic principles as well as techniques used in clinical chemistry be mastered by the student.

From studying this chapter, the student should gain enough knowledge and basic skill instruction to be able to perform accurately and conscientiously the routine chemical determinations done in a clinical laboratory. This instruction involves basic theory of chemical determinations, use and care of laboratory equipment and apparatus, application of quantitative measurement, proper preparation of reagents, recognition of problems when they arise, proper collection and handling of laboratory specimens, reporting of results obtained, and, perhaps more important than anything else, the appreciation of the necessity for care and accuracy when performing any procedure in the laboratory.

If the basic knowledge is adequate, other, more complicated chemistry determinations can more easily be learned. Also in this chapter, certain specific methods are discussed for the determination of urea nitrogen, glucose, and chloride. These procedures are carried out routinely in most clinical laboratories, and in each the general principles of most other laboratory determinations in chemistry are applied.

To maintain any degree of proficiency, practice and experience are necessary. Repeated practice with the laboratory tools discussed in this chapter will result in a much better understanding of clinical chemistry and, eventually, a keen appreciation of honest and accurate performances in the chemistry laboratory.

Clinical application will be discussed throughout the chapter. In this way it is hoped that the student will not lose sight of the most important aspect of the chemistry determinations performed—the reason for making the determination in the first place—the patient.

THE METRIC SYSTEM

The ability to measure accurately is the keystone of the scientific method in general. Therefore, a student in any scientific course must have a working knowledge of the systems and units of measurement.

There are two generally used systems of measurement, the metric system and the English system. In chemistry and other related scientific fields the metric system is used as the basis of all measurement. The metric system differs from the one used in measurements outside the laboratory (the English system). Instead of units such as feet, inches, pounds, pints, and quarts, the metric system uses units of grams, liters, centimeters, and meters, among others.

The metric system is readily mastered and much more convenient to use than the English system, because it is based on a decimal system in which the divisions and multiples are in a *ratio of tens*.

It is necessary to set up certain standards for use in the metric system. The International Bureau of Weights and Measures is responsible for setting up the necessary standards. It is also necessary that the student of chemistry understand how the English and metric systems correlate with each other. Since in everyday life the English system is used in most measurements, it is important that the methods of converting English system units to those in the metric system be understood for scientific use. The metric system units used most commonly in the laboratory will be discussed in this chapter.

There are three main categories used in measurement: weight (or mass), length, and volume. The standard unit in the metric system for measurement of *length* or distance is the *meter* (m). The "standard meter" is the distance between two lines on a platinum-iridium bar kept at the International Bureau of Weights and Measures near Paris, France. Copies of this "standard" are to be found at the National Bureau of Standards in Washington, D.C. One meter equals 39.37 inches, slightly longer than a yard in the English system. There are 2.54 centimeters (cm) in one inch (in.).

The meter is divided into tenths, called *decimeters* (dm); into hundredths, called *centimeters;* and into thousandths, called *millimeters* (mm). One thousand meters equals a *kilometer* (km).

According to the metric system theory of decimals or tenths, the following examples are shown for measurement of length:

$$25 \text{ mm} = 0.025 \text{ m}$$
$$10 \text{ cm} = 100 \text{ mm}$$
$$1 \text{ m} = 100 \text{ cm}$$
$$0.1 \text{ m} = 100 \text{ mm}$$

The standard unit in the metric system for the measurement of weight is the *kilogram* (kg). This is the basis for all other weight measurements in the metric system. The "standard kilogram" is determined by the weight of a block of platinum-iridium kept at the International Bureau of Weights and Measures. One kilogram weighs approximately 2.2 pounds (lb). Conversely, one pound equals approximately half a kilogram.

The kilogram is divided into thousandths, called *grams* (g), the gram being the measurement unit used much more often than the kilogram in the clinical laboratory. The gram is divided into thousandths, called *milligrams* (mg). Milligrams and grams are units used in all weighing that is necessary for a clinical chemistry laboratory. Some examples of metric system weight measurement equivalents are:

$$10 \text{ mg} = 0.01 \text{ g}$$
$$0.055 \text{ g} = 55 \text{ mg}$$
$$25 \text{ g} = 25,000 \text{ mg}$$
$$1.5 \text{ kg} = 1,500 \text{ g}$$

The standard unit for the measurement of *volume* in the metric system is the *liter* (often abbreviated "l" but spelled out in this book). The "standard liter" is the volume occupied by a kilogram of pure water at 4 degrees centigrade (4°C, the temperature at which a volume of water weighs the most) and at normal atmospheric pressure. A liter is slightly more than one quart (qt) in the English system. The liter is divided into thousandths, called *milliliters* (ml). Some examples of volume equivalents in the metric system are:

$$500 \text{ ml} = 0.5 \text{ liter}$$
$$0.25 \text{ liter} = 250 \text{ ml}$$
$$2 \text{ liters} = 2,000 \text{ ml}$$

The term *cubic centimeter* (cc) is often used to describe a milliliter, and for all practical purposes they mean the same thing in routine laboratory measurements; that is, one cubic centimeter equals one milliliter. The abbreviation "cc" is a common means of expressing measurement of volume in the laboratory.

In measuring *temperature* there are two scales commonly used, *Fahrenheit* (F) and *centigrade* (C). The temperature used in scientific study is centigrade. It is a rare case when readings on one scale must be converted to the other, as almost without exception readings taken and used in the clinical laboratory will be on the centigrade scale. Examples of comparative readings on the two scales are given below:

	°F	°C
Freezing point of water..........	32	0
Boiling point of water.............	212	100

It is possible, however, to convert from one scale to the other, and a student in the chemistry laboratory should be able to do this if the need arises. The basic conversion formulas are:

1. $1°C = \frac{9}{5}°F$
   $1°F = \frac{5}{9}°C$
2. To convert Fahrenheit to centigrade:
   Method A: Add 40, multiply by $\frac{5}{9}$, and subtract 40 from the result.
   Method B: $C = \frac{5}{9}(F - 32)$
3. To convert centigrade to Fahrenheit:
   Method A: Add 40, multiply by $\frac{9}{5}$, and subtract 40 from the result.
   Method B: $F = \frac{9}{5}C + 32$

GLASSWARE

Since it is most commonly in the chemistry department that the greatest variety and amount of glassware is used for laboratory determinations, the general discussion of laboratory glassware will be found in this chapter. It is important, however, to realize that glassware is used in all areas of the clinical laboratory, and where special glassware is employed, the information concerning its use will be found in the chapter dealing specifically with that area of the laboratory.

There are many different types of glass which can be used to make laboratory glassware. Some of these are soda lime, borosilicate glass (known by the commercial names of Kimax or Pyrex), 96 percent silica, and fused silica and quartz. Pyrex or Kimax are widely used in laboratory glassware because of their high qualities of resistance. If the various pieces of glassware in a laboratory are examined, it will be seen that one or the other of these brands of glass is used to make many different kinds of glassware. It is essential always to choose glassware of a reliable composition and one which will be resistant to laboratory chemicals and conditions. Borosilicate glass is a high-thermal-resistance glass with a low alkali content. In this type of glass, mechanical strength and thermal and chemical resistance are well balanced. This type of glass should be used whenever heating or sterilization by heat is employed. Since heating, both by physical means and by chemical reactions, makes up such an important part of the chemistry laboratory, it can easily be seen why glassware made from borosilicate is so often used.

There are two main categories into which most laboratory glassware can be separated: (1) *containers and receivers* and (2) *volumetric* apparatus. Examples of containers and receivers are beakers, test tubes, erlenmeyer flasks, and reagent bottles. Examples of volumetric glassware are volumetric flasks, pipets, graduated cylinders, and burets.

CALIBRATION OF VOLUMETRIC GLASSWARE

Calibration is the means by which glassware or other apparatus used in quantitative measurement is checked to determine its exact volume. To calibrate is to divide the glassware or mark it with graduations (or other indexes of quantity) for purposes of measurement. Calibration marks will be seen on every piece of volumetric glassware used in the laboratory. Specifications for calibration of glassware are set up by National Bureau of Standards.[1]

Each piece of volumetric glassware must be individually checked and must comply with these specifications before it can be accurately used in the clinical laboratory. Pipets, burets, volumetric flasks, and other volumetric glassware are supposed to hold, deliver, or contain a specific amount of liquid. This specified amount, or volume, is known as the *units of capacity* and is indicated by the manufacturer directly on each piece of glassware.

Volumetric glassware is usually calibrated by weight, using distilled water. The units of capacity determined will therefore be the volume of water contained in, or delivered by, the glassware at a particular temperature. The manufacturer knows what the weights of various amounts of distilled water are at specific temperatures. They use this information in the calibration of volumetric glassware. If a manufacturer wants a volumetric flask to contain 100 ml, a sensitive balance is used, such as an analytical balance. The weights corresponding to what 100 ml of distilled water weighs at a specific temperature are placed on one side of the balance. Gradually, distilled water is added to the flask to be calibrated (placed on the other side of the balance), until equilibrium is achieved. The manufacturer then makes a permanent mark on the neck of the flask at the bottom of the water meniscus level. This flask is then calibrated to contain 100 ml. Other sizes and types of volumetric glassware are similarly calibrated.

The volume of a particular piece of glassware varies with the temperature. It is for this reason that it is necessary to specify the temperature at which the glassware was calibrated. Glass will swell or shrink with changes in temperature, and the volume of the glassware will therefore vary with changes in temperature. Most volumetric glassware for routine clinical use is calibrated at 20°C. This means that all the calibration process and checking took place at a controlled temperature of 20°C. On all volumetric glassware the inscription "20°C" will be seen. Although 20°C is almost universally adopted as the standard temperature for calibration of volumetric glassware, each piece of glassware will have the temperature of calibration inscribed on it. As the diameter of a ring gets shorter as the ring gets colder, at a low temperature the volume of a volumetric flask is less than it is at a higher temperature. A 50-ml volumetric flask which has been calibrated at 20°C would at 10°C contain less than 50 ml.

Since the laboratory depends to such a great extent on the quality of its glassware in producing reliable results, it is necessary to be certain that the glassware is of the *very best quality*. Glass used for volumetric glassware must meet certain standards of quality. It must be transparent and free from striations and other surface irregularities. There should be no defects present which would distort the appearance of the liquid surface or portion of the calibration line seen through the glass.

The *design and workmanship* for volumetric glassware is also specified by the National Bureau of Standards. The shape of the glassware must permit complete emptying and thorough cleaning, and it must stand solidly on a level surface.

The *designation of use* for the glassware is indicated on each piece of volumetric glassware. There are two main classifications of usage, and these are based on how the glassware is to measure a given volume of liquid. In the clinical laboratory, the two classifications for usage of volumetric glassware are (1) to deliver and (2) to contain. These are indicated directly on the glassware by their initials, "T.D." (to deliver) or "T.C." (to contain). The to-contain volumetric glassware is designed and calibrated to contain a given volume of liquid. The units of capacity indicated on the glassware is the volume which to-contain glassware must contain. The to-deliver volumetric glassware is calibrated to deliver the specified, or indicated, volume of liquid into a receiving vessel. For example, a 5-ml to-deliver volumetric pipet, when used properly, will deliver exactly 5 ml into a test tube or other receiving vessel. More will be explained concerning this designation of usage under Pipetting.

CONTAINERS AND RECEIVERS

This category of laboratory glassware includes many of the most frequently used and most common pieces of glassware known to the student. Containers and receivers must be made of good-quality glass. They are not calibrated to hold a particular or exact volume but, rather, are available for various volumes, depending on the use desired. Beakers, erlenmeyer flasks, test tubes, and reagent bottles are made in many different sizes (Fig. 2-1). This glassware, like the volumetric glassware described

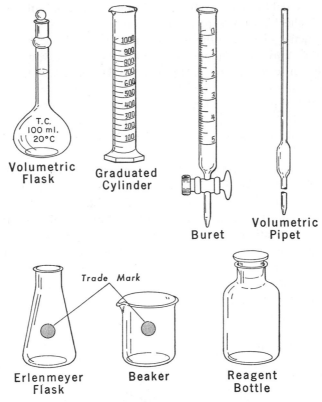

Fig. 2-1. Laboratory glassware.

previously, has certain information indicated directly on the vessel. The volume size and the brand name, or trademark, are two pieces of information found on items such as beakers and test tubes. Containers and receivers are not as expensive to purchase as volumetric glassware, because the process of exact volume calibration is not necessary.

Beakers are available in many sizes and in several forms. The most common form used in the clinical laboratory is known as the *Griffin low form*. Beakers should be made of glass which is resistant to the many chemicals used in them and also resistant to heat.

Erlenmeyer flasks are used commonly in the laboratory for preparing reagents, for titration procedures, and for preparing blood filtrates. They too come in various sizes and must be made from a resistant form of glass.

Test tubes come in many sizes, depending on the use for which they are intended. Test tubes without lips are the most satisfactory, because there is less chance of chipping and eventual breakage. Since chemical reactions occur in test tubes used in the chemistry laboratory, test tubes intended for use in this laboratory should be made of borosilicate glass. This type of glass is resistant to thermal shock.

All reagents should be stored in a reagent bottle of some type. These can be made of glass or some other material. Some of the more commonly purchased ones now are made of polyethylene. They are made in various sizes. The one used should meet the needs for the particular situation.

VOLUMETRIC GLASSWARE

As discussed previously, volumetric glassware must go through a vigorous process of volume calibration. This calibration process is quite lengthy and time-consuming for the manufacturer; therefore, the cost of volumetric glassware is relatively high as compared with the cost of noncalibrated glassware (beakers, test tubes, etc.).

Volumetric flasks are flasks with a round bulb at the bottom which tapers to a long neck on which the calibration mark is found. The specifications set up by the National Bureau of Standards apply to all volumetric glassware and therefore to volumetric flasks (Fig. 2-1). Volumetric flasks are calibrated to contain a specific amount or volume of liquid, and therefore a "T.C." is inscribed somewhere on the neck of the flask. There are many different sizes of volumetric flasks, depending on the volume of liquid to be used. The following are some of the sizes in which volumetric flasks can be purchased: 10 ml, 25 ml, 50 ml, 100 ml, 500 ml, 1 liter, and 2 liters.

Each flask, depending on the stated units of capacity, has been calibrated individually to contain the specified volume. For each size of volumetric flask there are certain allowable limits within which the volume of the flask must lie. This is called the *tolerance* for the flask. All volumetric glassware has a specific tolerance, that is, the capacity tolerance, which is dependent on the size of the glassware. For example, a 100-ml volumetric flask has a tolerance of ±0.08 ml.[1] Conditions during the calibration of a 100-ml volumetric flask are controlled so as to guarantee these limits. A tolerance of ±0.08 ml indicates that the allowable limits for the volume of a 100-ml volumetric flask are from 99.92 ml to 100.08 ml. A tolerance of ±0.05 ml for a 50-ml volumetric flask indicates allowable limits ranging from 49.95 to 50.05 ml for the volume of the flask. Volumetric flasks are used in the preparation of specific volumes of reagents, or laboratory solutions.

A *graduated measuring cylinder* is a long cylindrical piece of glassware with calibrated markings on it. Graduated measuring cylinders are used to measure volumes of liquids. These graduated cylinders can be made from plastic or polyethylene as well as from glass (Fig. 2-1). Graduated cylinders come in various sizes according to the volumes they measure: 10 ml 25 ml, 50 ml, 100 ml, 500 ml and 1,000 ml. A 100-ml graduated cylinder can measure 100 ml or a fraction thereof, depending on the calibration, or graduation, marks on it. Most graduated cylinders are calibrated to deliver. This will be indicated directly on the glassware by the inscription "T.D."

Graduated cylinders can be used to measure a specified volume of liquid, such as water, in the preparation of laboratory reagents. A graduated cylinder has calibration markings on it which indicate the capacity of the cylinder at different points. If 450 ml of water is to be measured, the most satisfactory cylinder size to use would be one of 500 ml capacity. Graduated cylinders are not calibrated with the accuracy of volumetric flasks. Therefore, the capacity tolerance for graduated cylinders allows a greater variation in volume for a specific cylinder. The capacity tolerance is greater for the larger graduated cylinders. A 100-ml graduated cylinder (T.D.) has a tolerance of ±0.40 ml, meaning that the allowable limits extend from 99.60 to 100.40 ml.

Another type of volumetric glassware used extensively in the laboratory is the *pipet*. There are many types of pipets available. It is important, however, to use only those pipets manufactured by reputable companies. Care and discretion should be used in selecting pipets for use in the chemistry laboratory, since their accuracy is one of the determinants of the accuracy of the procedures carried out. A pipet is a glass cylindrical tube used in measuring fluids. It is calibrated to deliver, or transfer, a specified volume from one vessel to another (Fig. 2-1).

Each pipet has at least one calibration or graduation mark on it, as does all volumetric glassware. In general, a pipet may be filled by using mouth suction or some other suction apparatus. When strong acids, bases, or solvents are measured, mouth suction is *never* used. These solutions are far too potent to risk using the mouth. Caustic liquids and some solvents are very dangerous; some destroy tissue immediately on contact. Some solvents have harmful vapors. Even when pipetting noncaustic liquids it is necessary to avoid contact of the liquid with the mouth. To help prevent getting the pipetted fluid into the mouth while filling the pipet, the top graduation mark is placed at a reasonable distance from the mouth hole. The National Bureau of Standards requires that the suction tube (that part of the pipet between the top graduation mark and the mouth hole) be at least 16 cm long. This minimum distance is to help prevent getting liquids into the mouth when pipetting them.

The opening (orifice) at the delivery tip of the pipet is of a certain size so as to give a specified length of time for drainage when the pipet is held vertically. Whenever a pipet is drained, it must be held in a vertical position to ensure proper drainage. A pipet will not drain as fast when held at a 45-degree angle as when held vertically. More will be discussed pertaining to the actual pipetting procedure under Pipetting.

Pipets, being volumetric glassware, are classified in the two main categories, to contain and to deliver, according to how the pipet is to be

TD pipet would be like frosted band serological type pipet in which the last drop is extractable and should be extracted.

used. To identify a to-contain pipet, for instance, the manufacturer has again inscribed the initials T.C. on the pipet itself. As for most other volumetric glassware, the temperature of calibration for pipets is usually 20°C.

Since the use of pipets and the technique of pipetting is so important to the overall performance of procedures in the chemistry laboratory, more pertinent information on the types of pipets available and their uses will be covered under Pipetting.

A fourth category of volumetric glassware is the *buret*. A buret is a long cylindrical piece of glassware with graduation divisions, or marks, on it and a stopcock closing at one end (Fig. 2-1). The stopcock closing on the delivery tip of the buret serves to control the flow of liquid. A buret is used to deliver measured quantities of fluids or solutions. Like all other volumetric glassware, burets are carefully calibrated according to the specifications set up by the National Bureau of Standards.

Burets also have a specific capacity tolerance depending on the size of the buret. The allowable limits of volume variation are dependent on the size of the buret. Burets come in different sizes, the smaller ones being the most accurate (as they have the smaller tolerance variation). Some common capacities for burets are 5 ml, 10 ml, and 25 ml. The capacity tolerances for burets are similar to those for graduated pipets (see under Pipetting for discussion of this type of pipet), as burets resemble this kind of pipet very closely. For a 5-ml buret, the tolerance is ±0.02 ml. This means that the allowable limits for the volume of this particular buret range from 4.98 to 5.02 ml. The chief difference between the buret and the graduated pipets is that the buret has a special closing on the delivery tip, called a *stopcock*. The stopcock controls the flow of liquid from the buret. Burets are used in titration, a means of quantitative measurement (see Titration for more information on the use of the buret).

WEIGHING AND THE USE OF BALANCES

There are many and varied pieces of laboratory apparatus used in performing chemical determinations, and the knowledge of the proper use and handling of this equipment is an important part of any course of study dealing with laboratory work. Probably some of the most important instruments are the various types of balances used in the laboratory. Almost every procedure performed in the chemistry laboratory depends to some extent on the use of a balance. The one balance considered to be the "backbone" of the clinical chemistry laboratory is the analytical balance. This balance, along with other types, namely, the triple-beam, the Cent-O-Gram, and the torsion types of balances, will be discussed in this section. A single laboratory is likely to have each of these types, and for this reason a student in a laboratory training course should understand how the various balances operate. Every laboratory should have some type of analytical balance and at least one other less sensitive type of balance. These are the minimum for essential weighing instruments.

Balances are used to weigh the necessary chemicals used in the preparation of the many chemical solutions needed in the laboratory. Some solutions require more accurately weighed chemicals, and some do not. The accuracy needed depends on what the solution is to be used for.

ANALYTICAL BALANCE

There are many different types of analytical balances made by different companies and made with various degrees of automatic operation. For the purposes of this discussion, the analytical balances will be divided into two types, the manually operated analytical (Fig. 2-2) and the automatic analytical (Fig. 2-3). Each company manufacturing analytical balances has its own special name for each of the various automatic analytical balances produced. Every analytical balance is used to weigh very small amounts of substances with a high degree of accuracy, but just how this is accomplished differs slightly with the various types of balances available. Some require little or no manual operation, and some are more time-consuming and require much manipulation on the part of the operator of the balance. Some of the fine analytical balances manufactured for use in the clinical laboratory, are the Ainsworth, the Voland, The Gram-atic, the Christian-Becker, the Mettler, and the Sartorius. Others are also available. It is important to investigate carefully several different analytical balances before deciding on one for use in a particular laboratory.

As stated previously, almost every procedure performed in the labora-

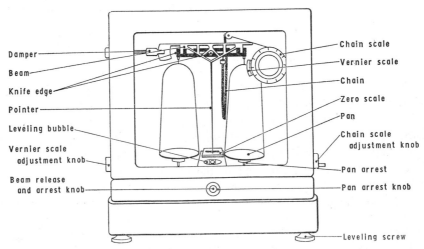

Fig. 2-2. Manual analytical balance.

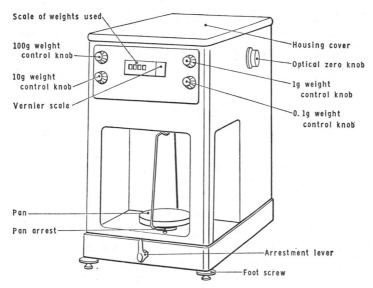

Fig. 2-3. Automatic analytical balance.

tory depends on the use of balances, the most important one being the analytical balance. Before any procedure is started, reagents must be prepared and standard solutions made. Standard solutions are always very accurately prepared, and the use of the analytical balance is employed in weighing the necessary chemicals for the standard. The analytical balance might be called the starting point of each method used in the chemistry laboratory. On the accuracy of the analytical balance depends the accuracy of all the chemical determinations. An instrument which is so sensitive and so essential must be constructed with high-quality workmanship and treated very carefully by those persons using it.

The analytical balance should be cleaned and adjusted at least once a year to ensure its continued accuracy and sensitivity. The accuracy of the analytical balance is what makes this instrument so essential in the clinical laboratory. The accuracy to which most analytical balances used in the clinical laboratory should weigh chemicals is commonly 0.1 mg, or 0.0001 g. Whenever this accuracy is needed, the analytical balance must be used. Differences between automatic and manual analytical balances lie mainly in the manner in which the weights are added in the weighing procedure. In the manual balance the weights are actually placed on one of the balance pans by hand. In the automatic analytical balance the weights are added by the manipulation of a series of dials.

It is essential that the parts of the analytical balance be thoroughly understood, so that the weighing process can be carried out to the degree of accuracy necessary. Once the correct use of an analytical balance has been mastered, one should be able to use any of the available types, as they all have the same basic parts. Each manufacturer supplies a complete operating direction manual, as well as information on the general use and care of the balance, with each balance purchased. These directions should be followed closely.

Basic Parts

1. Glass enclosure. The analytical balance is enclosed in glass to prevent currents of air and collection of dust from disturbing the process of weighing.

2. Balancing screws. Before doing any weighing on the balance, it must be properly leveled. This is ascertained by observing the leveling bubbles, or spirit level, located near the bottom of the balance. If necessary, adjust the balancing screws located on the bottom of the balance case (usually found on each leg of the balance).

3. Beam. This is the structure from which the pans are suspended.

4. Knife edges. These support the beam at the fulcrum during weighing and give sensitivity to the balance. Knife edges are vital parts and are constructed of hard metals to give a minimum amount of friction.

5. Pans for weighing. In the manually operated analytical balance, there are two pans: on the right-hand pan the weights are placed; on the left-hand pan the object to be weighed is placed. In the automatic analytical balance, there is only one pan. On this pan the object to be weighed is placed. The pans are suspended from the ends of the beam.

6. Weights. In the manual balance, the weights are found in a separate weight box. These weights are never handled with the fingers but are removed from the box and placed on the balance pan by using ivory-tipped forceps. Mishandling of weights, either by using fingers or by dropping, can result in an alteration of the actual and true mass of the weight. These weights come in units ranging from a 50-g to a 100-mg weight. The values of the weights are stamped directly on top of the weights. In the automatic analytical balance, the weights are inside the instrument and are not seen by the operator unless there is need to remove the casing for repair or adjustment purposes. The weights are added by manipulation of specific dials calibrated for the weighing process. In the automatic analytical balance, the built-in weights are on the same end of the beam as the sample pan and are counterbalanced by a fixed weight at the opposite end; they are removed from above the pan when an object is weighed. There is always a constant load on the beam, and the projected scale has the same weight regardless of the load. The total weight of an object is registered automatically by a digital counter or in conjunction with an optical scale.

7. Pan arrest. This is a means of arresting the pan so that sudden movement or addition of weights or chemical will not injure the delicate knife edges. The pan arrests (usually found under the pans) can absorb

any shock due to weight inequalities, so that the knife edges are not subjected to this shock. The pan must be released to swing freely during actual weighing. In the automatic analytical balance the arresting mechanism for both the pan and the beam is operated by a single lever. Partial release or full release can be obtained depending on how the lever is moved.

8. Damping device. This is necessary to arrest the swing of the beam in the shortest practical time, thus cutting down the time consumed for the weighing process.

9. Vernier scale. This is the small scale used for obtaining precise readings to the nearest 0.1 mg. It is used in conjunction with the large reading scale to obtain the necessary readings.

10. Reading scale. In the manual analytical balance, this scale is actually the reading scale for the chain which is used for weighing 100 mg or less. It is used in conjunction with the vernier scale to obtain readings to the nearest 0.1 mg. In the automatic analytical balance, this is usually a lighted optical scale, giving a high magnification and sharp definition for easier reading. The total weight of the object in question is registered automatically on this viewing scale.

General Rules for Use of the Analytical Balance

Weighing errors will develop if the balance is not properly positioned. It is, therefore, very important that the balance be located and mounted in an optimal position. The balance must be level. This is usually accomplished by adjusting the movable screws on the legs of the balance. The firmness of support is also important. The bench or table on which the balance rests must be rigid and free from vibrations. Preferably a room should be chosen for setting up the balance which provides a constant temperature and humidity. Ideally, the analytical balance should be in an air-conditioned room. The temperature factor is most important. The balance should not be placed near hot objects such as radiators, flames, stills, or electric ovens. In like manner, the balance should not be placed near cold objects, especially not near an open window. Sunlight or illumination from high-powered lamps should be avoided in choosing a good location for the analytical balance.

The analytical balance is a delicate precision instrument which will not function properly if abused. When learning to use an analytical balance, students should make themselves responsible for the knowledge of, and adherence to, the rules for the use of the particular balance with which they are provided. The following general rules apply:

1. Set up the balance where it will be free from vibration.

2. Load and unload the balance only when the pans are arrested; if the pans are not arrested, the delicate knife edges can be damaged.

3. Close the balance case before observing the reading; any air currents present would affect the weighing process.

4. Never weigh any chemical directly on the pan; a container of some type must be used for the chemical.

5. Never place a hot object on the balance pan. If an object is warm, its weight will be too light because of convection currents set up by the rise of the heated air.

6. Whenever the shape of the object to be weighed permits, handle it with tongs or forceps. Round objects such as weighing bottles may be handled with the fingers, but take care to prevent weight changes caused by moisture from the hand. Do not hold any object longer than necessary.

7. On completion of weighing, remove all objects, and clean up any chemical spilled on pans or within the balance area. Close the balance case.

Speed in weighing is obtained only through practice.

Procedure for Weighing Using a Manual Analytical Balance

1. Sitting directly in front of the center of the balance, dust off the pans and the inside of the balance with a soft brush.

2. Check to see that the balance is level by observing the leveling bubbles. Make any necessary adjustment by means of the leveling screws on the legs of the balance.

3. To adjust the balance to a beginning reading of zero, lower the beam and release the pan arrests, making certain that the chain reading scale and the vernier scale are both set at zero. Note where the pointer comes to rest, and slowly move the chain until the pointer rests exactly on zero. Arrest the pans and raise and lock the beam. Recheck by repeating these same steps once again. The pointer should still rest exactly at zero. By use of the vernier scale adjustment knob, adjust the zero of the vernier scale to match the zero of the chain reading scale.

4. With the beam raised and locked and the pans arrested, place the weighing vessel on the left-hand pan, using tongs if possible.

5. From the box of weights provided with the balance, transfer the first weight to the right-hand pan, using the special forceps. Choose a rather large weight as the first weight. A 20-g weight would be satisfactory for most purposes as the first weight used. Lower the beam and release the pan arrests. Note where the pointer swings, in relation to the zero point. If the pointer swings to the left, the weight is heavier than the vessel. If the pointer swings to the right, the weight is lighter than the vessel. Arrest the pans, and raise and lock the beam.

6. Depending on the direction of the pointer's swing in the previous step, either add another weight from the box of weights, or remove the 20-g weight and replace it with a lighter one (10 g). Repeat this process

by adding and removing weights (being certain to raise and lock the beam and arrest the pans before each change of weights) until the addition of the smallest weight in the box (100 mg) causes the pointer to swing to the left. Close the balance window.

7. At this point add weight from the chain. The chain has a total weight of 100 mg and is used when no further weights from the box can be used. With the beam locked and the pans arrested, add 50 mg from the chain by moving the chain-scale adjustment knob. Lower the beam and release the pans. Observe the pointer. Again, if the pointer swings to the left, the chain weight is too light, and more weight must be added. Raise the beam and arrest the pans. Depending on the swing of the pointer either add weight by moving the chain by 20-mg steps until the addition of 20 mg causes the pointer to swing to the left, or remove weight by 20-mg steps until the pointer swings to the right. When the weight using the chain has been narrowed down to within 10 mg of true balance, leave the beam lowered and the pans released, and gradually add or remove weight until balance is obtained. The weighing vessel has now been weighed, and the actual weighing of the desired chemical can commence. Record the weights used to obtain balance of the weighing vessel. To obtain the reading to the nearest 0.1 mg the vernier scale (Fig. 2-4) must be used in conjunction with the chain scale. Raise the beam and arrest the pans.

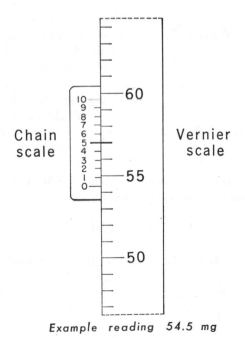

Example reading 54.5 mg

Fig. 2-4. Reading obtained using vernier scale.

8. To the weight of the weighing vessel add the amount of chemical to be weighed. For example, if the weighing vessel weighs 35.5646 g and the amount of chemical to be weighed is 10.5555 g, the total weight is 46.1201 g. This total weight should be on the right-hand pan. To accomplish this, add the necessary weights from the box of weights and the chain scale to make up the difference.

9. Add the chemical in small amounts, using a clean spatula until balance is achieved. Before each addition of chemical raise the beam and arrest the pans. When balance is obtained, the given amount of chemical has been weighed in the weighing vessel. Then transfer it quantitatively to a flask for dilution (see under Quantitative Transfer in Chapter 1).

10. Return all weights to the box, return the chain to zero, and clean up any spilled chemical from the balance area. Leave the beam in a raised and locked position, and arrest the pans.

Procedure for Weighing Using an Automatic Analytical Balance

1. Before doing any weighing, make certain that the balance is properly leveled. Observe the spirit level (leveling bubble), and adjust the leveling screws of the legs of the balance if necessary.

2. To check the zero point adjustment, fully release the balance and turn the adjustment knob clockwise as far as it will go. The optical scale zero should indicate three divisions below zero on the vernier scale. Using the same adjustment knob, adjust the optical scale zero line so that it aligns exactly with the zero line on the vernier scale. Arrest the balance.

3. With the balance arrested, place the weighing vessel on the pan, using tongs if possible, so that no humidity or heat is brought into the weighing chamber by the hands. Close the balance window.

4. Weigh the vessel in the following manner: partially release the balance and turn the 100-g weight control knob clockwise. When the scale moves up, turn the knob back one step. Repeat this operation with the 10-g knob, 1-g knob, and 0.1-g knob, in that order. Arrest the balance. After a short pause, release the balance, and allow the scale to come to rest. Read the result and arrest the balance. With the balance arrested, unload the pan, and bring all knobs back to zero.

5. Add the weight of the sample chemical amount desired to the weight of the vessel just weighed to get the total to be weighed. Set the knobs (100 g, 10 g, 1 g, and 0.1 g) to read the correct total weight needed. When the 0.1-g knob has been set at its proper reading, the balance should be placed in partial release. Slowly add the chemical to the vessel until the optical scale begins to move downward. When the optical scale starts downward, fully release the beam, and continue to add chemical until the optical scale registers the exact position desired. To obtain the reading to the nearest 0.1 mg (the sensitivity of most analytical balances),

the vernier scale must be used in much the same manner as it was used in the manual analytical balance readings.

6. With the balance arrested, unload the pan, and bring all the knobs back to zero. Clean up any spilled chemical in the balance area.

TORSION BALANCE

These modern balances are used mainly for weighing chemicals in the laboratory. They are sensitive, responsive instruments with an exceptionally long service life during which there is no significant deterioration in performance. In normal use, they require very little maintenance. The unique attributes of the torsion balance movement, which is assembled as a single flexible structure by means of highly tensed torsion bands of watch-spring alloy, eliminate the use of knife edges, bearings, and other loose parts which become dull, misaligned, and soiled. Having no knife edges to dull or other loose parts to be adjusted accounts for the popularity of the torsion balance. Little or no adjustment is required, and this is important in a laboratory, where the time element is so important.

The torsion balance features high sensitivity under a heavy load, permits fast weighing, and is relatively inexpensive. Care must be taken to avoid overloading these balances. Some models have a dial-controlled torque spring to eliminate the use of smaller loose weights. Other models are offered with dial-controlled built-in weights which may reduce still further the number of loose weights required. Many weighing determinations can be completed in about one-fifth the time formerly required. There is a sliding tare weight provided to counterbalance the weighing vessel used. The beam is operated by a lever on the balance case. Some torsion balances are enclosed completely in glass or metal cases. Several of these balances have a damping feature, which brings the balance to equilibrium quickly. One such damping device is an oil dashpot which is factory-filled with silicon oil. These damping devices provide for an even faster weighing process than is obtained by the torsion balances lacking them.

There is usually a means by which the torsion balance can be arrested. This need only be done when the balance is to be moved to a new location or otherwise transported.

The sensitivity of the torsion balance varies with the model chosen. For most clinical laboratories, however, balances with a sensitivity of readings to the nearest 0.01 g are satisfactory. The manufacturer supplies a complete manual with directions on the setting up, proper use, and care of the particular torsion balance ordered. These directions should be followed closely.

Procedure

1. Check to be sure that the balance is level, and adjust the leveling screws, if necessary.

2. Check the zero adjustment. The optical reading scale should read zero with the pan empty and clean; adjust the optical zero with the small control knob, if necessary.

3. Place the weighing vessel on the pan. Turn the weight control knob until the optical reading scale reads zero.

4. Add the chemical to the vessel until the desired weight registers on the optical scale. A vernier scale is present on most models in order that the weight may be read to the accuracy needed. Torsion balances used in clinical laboratories have accuracies of either 0.1 g or 0.01 g.

5. Remove the vessel with the weighed chemical from the pan. Turn the control knob to zero, and wipe up any spilled chemical immediately.

TRIPLE-BEAM BALANCE

Another common piece of laboratory apparatus for weighing purposes is the triple-beam, or "trip," balance (Fig. 2-5). This is a less sensitive balance with accuracy to the nearest 0.1 g. Whenever reagents are to be prepared using 0.1-g accuracy or less, the triple-beam balance can be used most satisfactorily. As the words "triple-beam" and "trip" suggest, there are three beams present on the balance. Each beam is of a different weighing scale. A 0- to 100-g scale, 0- to 500-g scale, and 0- to 10-g scale are the usual scales provided on the triple-beam balance. These scales are provided with movable weights. The two larger scales have weights which lock into accurately milled notches at each calibration to ensure absolute accuracy at each position.

Some models of the triple-beam balance (called the *Harvard triple-beam balance*) have two pans, and some have a single pan. The principle of the weighing process is the same whether there are two pans or only one.

Some type of less sensitive balance such as the triple-beam or torsion type balance is an essential piece of equipment for every clinical laboratory,

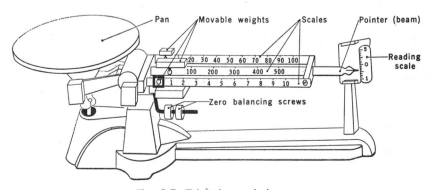

Fig. 2-5. Triple-beam balance.

as there are many reagents prepared which do not need the accuracy of the analytical balance. When reagents to be made do not need an accuracy of more than 0.1 g, the triple-beam balance can be used. It is a simple and rapid balance to operate and one which gives accurate weighings when used properly. Even with a balance of less sensitivity, it is essential that it be used carefully and according to the directions established for the particular model.

The triple-beam balance should be placed on a reasonably flat and level surface. The beam should be near a zero balance with all the movable weights at their zero points. A final zero balance is attained by adjusting the balancing screws. It is advisable to check the zero balance periodically, especially if the balance has been moved. If an object is to be weighed, the balance must be set at zero before any weighing is begun. If a vessel is weighed in preparation for addition of chemical, it is not necessary to set the balance at the exact zero reading.

Procedure

1. Place the weighing vessel on the balance pan without previously bringing the balance to zero.

2. With the weighing vessel on the pan, bring the balance to zero by adjusting the movable weights on the three scales. Record the sum of the weights required for balance.

3. To the recorded weight add the amount of chemical to be weighed. For example, if the reagent to be prepared requires 10.5 g of sodium chloride and the weighing vessel weighs 35.5 g, the total weight is 46.0 g. Move the movable weights on the scales to give this total weight.

4. Gradually add the chemical until the pointer of the balance rests exactly at the zero mark on the vertical reading scale. Remove the weighing vessel, and return the movable weights to their zero positions. Transfer the chemical quantitatively to the flask for dilution.

5. Wipe up any spilled chemical immediately from the balance area.

A special type of triple-beam balance is known as the *Cent-O-Gram balance*. This balance has three beams also, but they are tiered on three levels, so that the readings can be obtained from a single eye level. The three beams on the Cent-O-Gram balance are each of a different weighing scale. The center beam is graduated to 100 g with calibrated notches at 10-g intervals. The front beam is graduated to 1 g in 0.01-g notches. The rear beam is graduated to 10 g in 1-g notches. As the name would imply, the sensitivity of this balance is to the nearest 0.01 g. The Cent-O-Gram balance has a level for arresting the balance when placing objects on the pan.

On any type of triple-beam balance, the balance position of an object on the pan can be determined by observing the swing of the pointer. A swing of an equal number of divisions on either side of the zero mark on the dial indicates that the scale is balanced. It is not necessary to wait for the oscillation to stop to determine the correct weight. This observation enables the weighing process to be a simple and rapid one.

PHOTOMETRY

In chemistry, as in the other clinical laboratory areas, there is a need for using quantitative techniques. By using a quantitative method, the exact amount of an undetermined substance can be determined accurately, and this is the basis for most chemistry determinations. There are various methods for measuring substances by a quantitative technique, and one of the techniques used most frequently in the chemistry laboratory involves the use of photometry. Photometry is a quantitative technique in that it can measure the exact amount of the substances desired in a particular procedure. Photometry, or, to use a synonym, colorimetry, employs color and color variation to ascertain the concentration of substances.

Photometry is perhaps the most frequently used quantitative device in the laboratory, and for this reason it is imperative that any student engaged in learning clinical laboratory techniques know and understand thoroughly the principles of photometry. There is probably no measurement technique used as much but understood as little as photometry. The procedures involving the use of photometry are numerous in the laboratory. Although many of the photometry procedures are less precise, they offer a definite advantage in that they are so simple to use. In most laboratories today, there is a need for greater efficiency, and through the use of photometry the results of certain tests can be determined not only simply but quickly.

To understand the use of photometry, one must first understand the fundamentals of color. A combination of all colors (red, orange, yellow, green, blue, and purple) is called "daylight," or "white light." Every color that is seen is light of a particular wavelength. If white light is diffracted or partially absorbed, it becomes visible as certain colors. The color seen depends on the wavelength of the color not absorbed. When light is not absorbed, it is transmitted. When white light is passed through a solution, part of the light is absorbed, and that remaining is transmitted. When a rainbow is seen, it simply means that there are droplets of moisture in the air and that these droplets have refracted certain rays of the sun and allowed others to pass through. The colors of the rainbow range from purple to red. These are called the colors of the visible spectrum. Colors which are visible to the human eye are the colors of the visible spectrum.

Every color is light of a particular wavelength. Wavelengths are measured in units called millimicrons ($m\mu$). There are many solutions which contain particles which have the properties of absorbing certain wavelengths and of transmitting others. Solutions appear to have characteristic colors. For instance, a solution of ink appears to be blue. This simply means that certain particles in the solution of ink have absorbed all the wavelengths, or colors, except blue; the blue is then the color which is seen. A solution looks green when all the colors except green are absorbed by particles in that solution. The visible-spectrum colors range from purple (with a wavelength of 400 mμ) to red (with a wavelength of 700 mμ). Below 400 mμ (ultraviolet) and above 700 mμ (infrared), the colors are not visible to the human eye.

The use of photometry, or colorimetry, as a means of quantitative measurement depends primarily on two factors, the color itself and the intensity of the color. Any substance to be measured by using photometry must be colored to begin with or must be capable of being colored. An example of a substance that is colored to begin with is hemoglobin (determined by use of photometry in the hematology laboratory). Sugar, or glucose specifically, is an example of a substance that is not colored to begin with but is capable of being colored with the use of certain specific reagents and reactions. Sugar content can therefore be measured by using photometry.

The measurement of a substance using photometry is based on the results of a reaction between the substance to be measured and a reagent, or chemical, used to produce color. The amount of color produced by a reaction between the substance to be measured and the reagent is dependent on the concentration of the substance (the amount of the substance present). Therefore, the intensity of the color is proportional to the concentration of the substance. The Beer-Lambert law (or Beer's law) states this relationship: color intensity at a constant depth is directly proportional to the concentration. The Beer-Lambert law is the basis for the use of photometry in quantitative measurement. Using this law, if you saw a solution with a very intense red color, you would be correct in assuming that this solution had a high concentration of the substance making the solution red. Another explanation of the Beer-Lambert law is that any increase in the concentration of the color-producing substance would increase the amount of color seen.

As the law states, the depth of the color must be constant. The depth of the solution is regulated by the test tube used to hold the solution being measured. An increase in depth of the solution (by using a test tube with a larger diameter) through which the light must pass is the same as placing more particles between the light and the eye, thereby creating an apparent increase in concentration, or intensity, of color. To avoid this alteration from the actual concentration, only tubes with a constant diameter can be used. The use of special tubes calibrated for photometry will be discussed under Calibration of Tubes for the Photometer.

When using photometry as a quantitative measurement tool, the undetermined colored substance is compared with a similar substance of known strength (a standard solution) on the principle that the intensity of the color is directly proportional to the concentration of the substance present. The device used to show the quantitative relationship between the colors of the undetermined solution and the standard solution is called a *photometer,* or *colorimeter.* Whenever the photometer is used, there must be a basis of comparison. This basis of comparison is the standard solution. A standard solution is one in which the exact amount of substance is known. Standard solutions will be further defined under Means of Ensuring Reliable Results.

There are many types of photometers in common use in the clinical laboratory. The principle of most of these machines is the same in that the amount of light transmitted by the standard solution is compared to the amount of light transmitted by the solution of unknown concentration. Precise, accurate methods are needed to accomplish the numerous chemistry determinations required of the modern laboratory. The photometer is one piece of equipment that is essential and can be considered to be of prime importance. Photometers are also known as *photoelectric colorimeters.* The many available photometers each have their own technical variations, but all operate according to the same general principles.

GENERAL PARTS ESSENTIAL TO ALL PHOTOMETERS

There are certain parts necessary to all photometers (Fig. 2-6). These are:

1. Light source. Each photometer must have a light source. This can be a light bulb constructed to give the optimum amount of light. The light source must be steady and constant; therefore, the use of a voltage regulator or electronic power supply is recommended. The light source may be movable or stationary.

2. Wavelength selector. Before the light from the light source reaches the sample of solution to be measured, the interfering wavelengths must be removed. In doing this the light is actually being reduced to a particular wavelength. Filters can be used to accomplish this. Some are very simple

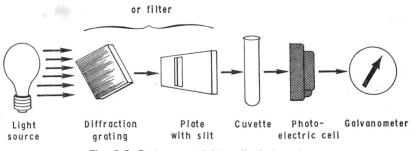

or filter

| Light source | Diffraction grating | Plate with slit | Cuvette | Photo-electric cell | Galvanometer |

Fig. 2-6. Parts essential to all photometers.

ones composed of one or two pieces of colored glass. Some are more complicated. The more complicated filters are found in the better photometers. The filter must transmit a color which the solution *can* absorb. A red filter transmits red, and a green filter transmits green. Filters are available to cover almost any point in the visible spectrum and have inscribed on them a particular number that indicates the wavelength of light which that filter transmits. For example, a filter inscribed with 540 mμ absorbs all light except that of wavelengths around 540 mμ. Since the filter must transmit a color which the solution can absorb, for a red solution the filter chosen should not be red (all colors *except* red are absorbed). The wavelength of light transmitted is, then, the important thing to consider in choosing the correct filter for a given procedure.

Light of a desired wavelength can also be provided by means other than by use of a filter. One of the more commonly used machines employs the use of a diffraction grating with a special plate and slit in it to reduce the spectrum to the desired wavelength. This consists of a highly polished surface with numerous lines on it which break up the white light into the spectrum. By moving the spectrum behind a slit (the light source must be movable), only one particular portion of the spectrum is allowed to pass through the narrow slit. The particular band of light, or wavelength, being transmitted through the slit is indicated on a viewing scale on the machine. Certain wavelengths are more desirable than others for a particular color and procedure. The wavelength chosen is determined by running an absorption curve and selecting the correct wavelength after inspecting the curve obtained. Only when new methods are being developed is it necessary to run an absorption curve.

3. Cuvettes, or photometer tubes. Any light (of the wavelength selected) coming from the filter or diffraction grating will next pass on to the solution in the cuvette. Calibrated cuvettes are tubes which have been optically matched so that the same solution in each will give the same reading on the photometer. In using calibrated cuvettes, the depth factor of the Beer-Lambert law is kept constant. The means by which these tubes can be obtained will be discussed under Calibration of Tubes for the Photometer. Depending on the concentration of the solution and thus the color of the solution, a certain amount of light will be absorbed by the solution, and the remainder will be transmitted. The light not absorbed by the solution is transmitted. This light next passes on to an electronic measuring device of some type.

4. Electronic measuring device. In the more common photometers the electronic measuring device consists of a photoelectric cell and a galvanometer. The amount of light transmitted by the solution in the cuvette is measured by a photoelectric cell. This cell is a most sensitive instrument, producing electrons in proportion to the amount of light hitting it. The electrons are passed on to a galvanometer, where they are measured. The galvanometer records the amount of current (in the form of electrons)

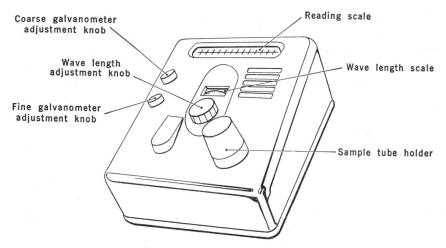

Coarse galvanometer
adjustment knob

Reading scale

Wave length
adjustment knob

Wave length scale

Fine galvanometer
adjustment knob

Sample tube holder

Fig. 2-7. Coleman Junior Spectrophotometer.

it receives from the photoelectric cell on a special viewing scale on the photometer. The results are reported in terms of percent transmission. In some cases, the readings are made in terms of optical density. The percent transmission (%T) is the percent of light that the solution transmits. This percent is dependent on the concentration of the solution and the depth of the solution. If the solution is very concentrated (the color appearing intense), a lesser amount of light will be transmitted than if the solution is dilute (pale). Therefore, the reading on the galvanometer viewing scale will be lower for a more concentrated solution than it will be for a dilute solution. This is the basis for the comparison of color intensity using the photometer.

There are several types of photometers available for use in the clinical laboratory. Some of these are Bausch and Lomb, Beckman, Coleman Junior, Evelyn, Klett-Summerson, and Leitz. For teaching purposes the Coleman Junior Spectrophotometer has proved to be very satisfactory (Fig. 2-7). As the name implies, a Spectrophotometer is really two instruments in a single case, a spectrometer (device for producing light of a specific wavelength, called a *monochromator*) and a photometer (device for measuring light intensity). Because of its common use, the operation of this specific machine is outlined below.

OPERATION OF THE COLEMAN JUNIOR SPECTROPHOTOMETER*

1. Mount the selected scale panel in the galvanometer viewing window. A general-purpose scale panel is usually used. These are several types

* From the "Operating Directions for the Coleman Model 6A and 6C Junior Spectrophotometer," Coleman Instruments Corporation, Maywood, Ill. September, 1966.

of scale panels available depending on the use to which the Spectrophotometer is to be put. The scale panel is calibrated both in percent transmission and optical density (absorbance).

2. Insert in the cuvette well the cuvette adapter of the proper size to accommodate the proper type of cuvette specified in the analytical procedure.

3. Turn on the switch located on the back of the instrument. Allow the instrument to warm up for 5 minutes.

4. Verify the galvanometer zero setting, and readjust if necessary. The indicator line on the galvanometer spot should register at zero on the percent transmission scale. The zero adjustment level for this instrument is located under the raised housing just to the left of the cuvette well. If the Spectrophotometer is not disturbed or its position altered, this galvanometer adjustment remains very stable.*

    a. To check the zero position, darken the photoelectric cell by inserting a cuvette adapter in the cuvette well turned 90 degrees from the calibration marker. In this position, the body of the adapter completely blocks the pathway of light. A piece of opaque paper may also be slipped in the adapter well; in this way the light pathway is also completely stopped.

    b. Cover the well with the light shield or other suitable cover.

    c. With a pencil point move the galvanometer adjusting the lever so that the indicator line on the galvanometer spot reads zero on the left zero index of the selected scale panel.

    d. Complete the adjustment by sliding the scale panel until the index is *exactly* at zero on the scale.

5. Adjust the wavelength knob so that the specific wavelength is set. Different procedures will need different wavelengths. The wavelength to be used will be specified in the procedure.

6. Cuvettes used for reading in the Spectrophotometer must be free from scratches. Before placing the cuvette in the adapter for reading, the cuvette must be free of finger marks and bubbles; the Spectrophotometer does not recognize the cause of light impediment and will respond alike to a scratched tube, lint, bubbles, finger marks, and the absorbance of the solution being examined. Therefore, wipe the cuvettes with a clean, dry, soft cloth or gauze before reading.

All cuvettes must contain a certain volume of solution, called the *minimum volume*. Various-sized cuvettes need various minimum volumes to ensure that the light passes through the solution rather than through the empty space in the tube.

7. Place the cuvette containing the reagent blank in the adapter first. The calibration mark (or trademark, if precalibrated Coleman cuvettes are used) must face the light source to ensure constancy of the light path. Adjust the galvanometer control knobs (labeled "GALV Coarse"

and "GALV Fine") until the galvanometer index on the viewing scale reads 100%T for the "blank" tube.

8. Remove the blank tube.

9. Place the next polished cuvette containing the solution to be read in the adapter well, again taking note of the calibration mark. Place this mark in a position facing the light source.

10. Record the galvanometer reading to the nearest $\frac{1}{4}$%T reading.

11. Remove the cuvette, and reinsert the blank tube.

12. Observe the reading for the blank tube on the galvanometer scale. It should still read 100%T. If it does read 100%T, remove the blank tube, and proceed with the next tube to be read. If the blank tube does not read exactly 100%T, adjust it to read 100%T with the GALV Coarse and Fine knobs. Then read the next tube. The blank tube should be reinserted between each reading, and it should always read 100%T.

13. Read all tubes, and record results to the nearest $\frac{1}{4}$%T reading. Parts of percent transmission readings are recorded using the numerator figure only. For example, if a reading is $75\frac{1}{2}$, the result is recorded as 75^2%T. For a reading of $75\frac{3}{4}$, the result is recorded as 75^3, and for a reading of $75\frac{1}{4}$, the result is recorded as 75^1.

14. When finished, return the galvanometer index to the original position by turning both the GALV Coarse and Fine knobs completely counterclockwise, and turn off the machine switch.

15. Clean up the area around the instrument, wipe up anything spilled on the machine, and cover the Spectrophotometer with the protective cover provided.

For operation of machines other than the Coleman Junior Spectrophotometer, the student is referred to the manuals supplied with each photometer by the manufacturer.

GENERAL CARE AND USE OF PHOTOMETERS

When using a photometer, error due to color in the reagents used must be eliminated. Since color is so important and since it is the color produced by the undetermined substance that is the desired one, any color due to the reagents themselves or due to interaction between reagents could cause confusion and error. By using a "blank" solution, correction can be made for any color due to reagents used. The blank solution contains all the same reagents as do the unknown and standard tubes with the exception of the substance being measured. The use of blank solutions will be discussed further under Means of Ensuring Reliable Results.

A photometer, as is the case with any expensive, delicate instrument, must be handled with care. The manufacturer supplies a manual of complete instructions on the care and use of a particular machine. Care should be taken not to spill reagents on the photometer. Spillage could damage the delicate instrument, especially the photoelectric cell. Any reagents spilled must be wiped up immediately. Photometers using filters should not be operated without the filter in place, as the unfiltered light from the light source may damage the photoelectric cell and the galvanometer. A photometer should be placed on a table with good support, where it will not be bumped and jarred.

In general, photometers employing filters are called *filter* photometers, and those with diffraction gratings are called spectrophotometers. Photometers utilize an electronic device to compare the actual color intensities of the solutions measured.

VISUAL COLORIMETRY

Before photometers became readily available to the laboratory for quantitative measurement, another type of color-comparing device was in common use. This device utilized the human eye to compare color intensity differences and was called a *visual colorimeter*. Visual colorimetry is now used only rarely and has been replaced by the photometer. In visual colorimetry, the human eye acts as the instrument for measuring color comparison (in the photometer, the photoelectric cell and galvanometer accomplish this).

The human eye is a poor instrument for measuring light intensity. It is difficult for the human eye to measure accurately shades of color or intensity. There is an error of 5 percent or greater even with experience and proper technique, which is one of the reasons why visual colorimetry is inadequate for today's laboratory procedures. Many times interfering spectrums will present an even greater error. Such interference often can be reduced or eliminated by the use of a filter.

The visual colorimeter has several other disadvantages. One of these is that more time is required to carry out the desired procedure. In the modern laboratory, many tests are run, and speed is important. The temperature of the surrounding area and the order of adding the reagents can also affect the visual colorimeter. In using visual colorimetry, there is a need for deep colors, which requires a larger quantity of the specimen and more reagents. It is not always possible to obtain enough specimen (blood, for example) to run the test satisfactorily with a visual colorimeter.

The names of some of the visual colorimeters used in years past are the Klett, Duboscq, and Dennison colorimeters.

CALIBRATION OF TUBES FOR THE PHOTOMETER

Essential in photometry is the use of calibrated tubes, or cuvettes. It is necessary that the depth of the tubes used in the photometer be constant (for the Beer-Lambert law to apply). Only through checking each tube used can its depth be made certain. Tubes (cuvettes) for the photometer can be purchased precalibrated, but these are expensive. Precalibrated tubes must also be checked before being put into actual use in the laboratory. Most laboratories, especially those involved with teaching, calibrate tubes for the photometer. As noted previously, these tubes have been optically matched so that the same solution in each will give the same percent transmission reading on the galvanometer viewing scale.

In calibrating tubes for use in photometry, the tube is carefully checked to see that the solution in that particular tube will read the same as the identical solution did in a previously calibrated tube. Different-sized tubes can be used, depending on the photometer. One of the more common sizes of tubes, especially for the Coleman Junior Spectrophotometer described earlier, is 19 by 105 mm. The Coleman Junior Spectrophotometer can be adapted to use several different-sized tubes in the same machine. For each size, a special cuvette adapter is used, enabling the tube to fit securely in the tube holder. Only when the tube fits securely will the readings obtained be precise and accurate.

Procedure

1. Use only clean, dry tubes for calibration purposes.

2. Filter a portion of the chosen colored solution to be placed in the tubes. One solution used frequently for calibration is 5% copper sulfate. Filter enough solution to fill the tubes to be calibrated. The tubes should be filled to approximately the same level.

3. Fill the uncalibrated tubes to approximately the same level with the filtered solution.

4. Polish the tubes with a gauze or tissue.

5. Calibrate the new tubes against previously calibrated tubes.

    a. Fill four or five calibrated tubes with the same filtered solution to approximately the same level. Polish the tubes thoroughly and read in the photometer, noting the readings in percent transmission for each (see Steps 6 to 9).

    b. Read the uncalibrated tubes in the same manner, following the directions given in the next steps.

6. Set the wavelength at 550 mμ (or other suitable wavelength chosen for this procedure).

7. Prepare the photometer for reading tubes by following the directions given for the particular machine being used.

8. Pick an arbitrary setting on the galvanometer reading scale against which to read the tubes. Usually a setting near the center of the viewing scale is chosen (50, 60, or 70% T, for example).

9. Read the previously calibrated tubes first, checking the arbitrary setting between each reading. Adjust and reread, if necessary. Record these readings. All the readings for the previously calibrated tubes should be within a $\frac{1}{2}$% T reading of each other on the galvanometer scale.

10. To calibrate the new tubes:

    a. Check the arbitrary center setting; adjust if necessary.

b. Place the polished uncalibrated tube in the tube holder; note the reading on the galvanometer viewing scale.

c. If the reading is the same as for the standard tubes read previously, mark the tube with a wax pencil at the place corresponding to the mark on the calibrated tubes (that is, the side of the tube facing the light source); this mark will later be permanently etched on the tube.

d. If the reading is not the same as for the precalibrated tubes, slowly rotate the tube in the holder until the same reading is obtained. Mark the tube with a wax pencil as in Step 10*c* above. If on complete rotation in the tube holder the reading is not obtained, the new tube cannot be used for this particular set of calibrated tubes. Set it aside to be calibrated for a different set of calibrated tubes.

e. Etch the tubes with a glass etcher, making a well-defined mark where the wax pencil mark was made. The tubes are now ready to be washed and used.

PIPETTING

The general discussion of laboratory glassware, including types used for measuring volume, has been covered in an earlier section of this chapter (see under Glassware). The importance of knowing the correct usage of these various pieces of glassware must be thoroughly appreciated by the student. The four basic pieces of volumetric glassware, volumetric flasks, graduated measuring cylinders, burets, and pipets, are each specialized types, and each has its own particular use in the laboratory.

Pipets used in volumetric measurement in the chemistry laboratory must be free from all grease and dirt. For that reason, a special cleaning solution is used for these pipets. One made from a combination of sulfuric acid and either sodium or potassium dichromate is commonly used. For a detailed description of this cleaning solution, see Cleaning Laboratory Glassware in Chapter 1. *Dont use sulfuric acid etc, — use detergent. pipet holder goes inside vat.*

Since the accuracy of chemical determinations depend to such a large extent on the equipment used and since pipets are a principal means of volume measurement, it is imperative that any pipets used in the clinical laboratory be of the finest quality and be manufactured and calibrated by a reputable company. Care and discretion should be used in selection of laboratory pipets.

There are several types of pipets used commonly in the laboratory. It is necessary that the student understand the uses of these different pipets and know how to handle them in a clinical determination. Practice, again, is the key to success in the use of laboratory pipets; only through repeated practice will the student become proficient in pipetting.

As already mentioned under Volumetric Glassware, there are two categories of pipets: to-contain and to-deliver. To-contain pipets are calibrated to contain a specified amount of liquid but are not necessarily calibrated to deliver that exact amount. A small amount of fluid will cling to the inside wall of the pipet, and for this reason when these pipets are used, they should be rinsed out with a diluting fluid to ensure that the entire contents of the pipet have been emptied. The to-deliver pipets are calibrated to deliver the amount of fluid designated on the pipet; this volume will flow out of the pipet by gravity when the pipet is held in a vertical position with the tip of the pipet against the side of the receiving vessel. A small amount of fluid will remain in the tip of the pipet; this amount is to be left in the tip as the calibrated portion has been delivered into the receiving vessel. There is another category of pipet, called *blowout*. The calibration of these pipets is similar to that of the to-deliver pipets, except that the drop remaining in the tip of the pipet must be blown out into the receiving vessel. If a pipet is to be blown out, an etched ring will be seen on the mouthpiece near the mouth hole.

TYPES OF PIPETS

Volumetric Pipets

A pipet that has been calibrated to deliver by drainage is known as a *volumetric* pipet, or *transfer* pipet. These pipets have a bulb midway between the mouthpiece and the delivery tip and always carry a calibration mark (Fig. 2-8). Volumetric pipets are suitable for all accurate measurements of volumes of 1 ml or more. They are calibrated to deliver the amount inscribed on them. This volume is measured from the calibration mark to the tip by draining freely. A 5-ml volumetric pipet will deliver a single measured volume of 5 ml, and a 2-ml volumetric pipet will deliver 2 ml. The tolerance of volumetric pipets varies with the size of the pipet. The allowable tolerance increases when the capacity of the pipet increases. A 10-ml volumetric pipet will have a greater tolerance than will a 2-ml volumetric pipet. The tolerance, or limit of error, for a 5-ml volumetric pipet is ±0.01 ml. When volumes of liquids are to be delivered with great accuracy, a volumetric pipet is used. Volumetric pipets are used to measure standard solutions, unknown blood and plasma filtrates, serum, plasma, urine, spinal fluid, and some reagents.

Each measurement using a volumetric pipet is handled individually, and the volumes can be whole milliliters only (1 ml, 2 ml, 5 ml, 10 ml, etc.). To transfer volumetrically 1 ml of a standard solution into a test tube, a 1-ml volumetric pipet is used. To transfer 5 ml of the same solution, a 5-ml volumetric pipet is used. After draining a volumetric pipet, there is a drop remaining on the *inside* of the delivery tip. The specific volume the pipet is calibrated to deliver is dependent on the fact

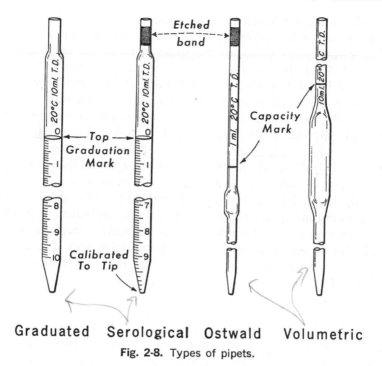

Fig. 2-8. Types of pipets.

that the inside drop is left in the tip of the pipet. In volumetric pipets, this drop is *not* to be blown out. Information designated on the pipet itself includes temperature of calibration (usually 20°C), capacity, manufacturer, and usage (T.D.). Technique in using these volumetric pipets correctly is of the utmost importance in overall laboratory performance, and a certain amount of skill is required (see General Pipetting Procedure).

Graduated Pipets

Another way to deliver a given amount of liquid is to deliver that amount of liquid contained between two calibration marks on a cylindrical tube, or pipet. Such a pipet is the *graduated,* or *measuring* pipet. Another name for this pipet is the *Mohr* (pronounced "more") pipet, named for its designer. These pipets have several graduation, or calibration, marks on them (Fig. 2-8). Many measurements in the laboratory do not need the precision of the volumetric pipet. Graduated pipets are used when great accuracy is not required. This does not mean that these pipets may be used with less care than the volumetric pipets. Graduated pipets are used primarily in measuring reagents, but they are not calibrated with sufficient tolerance to use in measuring standard solutions and filtrates.

A graduated pipet is a straight piece of glass tubing with a tapered end and graduation marks on the stem separating it into parts. Depending on the size used, graduated pipets can be used to measure parts of a milliliter or many milliliters by noting the marks on the stem. These pipets come in various sizes or capacities, some of these are 0.1 ml, 0.2 ml, 1 ml, 2 ml, 5 ml, 10 ml, and 25 ml. If 4 ml of deionized water is to be measured into a test tube, a 5-ml graduated pipet would be the best choice. Since graduated pipets require draining between two marks, one more possibility of error is introduced, as compared with the volumetric pipets with only one calibration mark. This makes the graduated pipet less precise in its measurements. Because of this relatively poor precision, the graduated pipet is used where speed is more important than precision.

The volume of the space between the last calibration mark and the delivery tip is not known. In the graduated pipets, this space cannot be used for measuring fluids. Graduated pipets are calibrated in much the same manner as are the volumetric pipets; however, they are not constructed with as strict specifications or capacity tolerances. The allowable tolerance for a 5-ml graduated pipet is ±0.02 ml. The graduated pipets are calibrated to deliver.

To-contain Pipets   serological type

The *to-contain* pipet, when use properly, is one of the more precise pipets used in the clinical laboratory. This type of pipet is calibrated to contain a specified amount of liquid. For example, if a pipet *contains* only 0.1 ml and 0.1 ml of blood is needed for a chemistry determination, then none of the blood can be left on the inside of the pipet. The *entire* contents of that pipet must be emptied. If this pipet is *rinsed well* with a diluting solution, then all the blood or similar specimen will be removed from the pipet. The correct way to use a to-contain pipet is to rinse it with a suitable diluent. A to-contain pipet cannot be used properly unless the receiving vessel contains a diluent; that is, a to-contain pipet should not be used to deliver a specimen into an empty receiving vessel (no diluent would be present with which to rinse out the inside of the pipet). Since all the liquid in a to-contain pipet is rinsed out and used, there is need for only one graduation mark. Examples of to-contain pipets are 0.1-ml T.C. pipets for measuring blood in the chemistry laboratory and the hemoglobin pipets used in the hematology laboratory.

Ostwald Pipets   a T.C. type pipet

specifically designed volumetric pipet.

There is a special type of pipet that has been designed for use in measuring viscous fluids such as blood. This pipet is known as the *Ostwald* pipet (or Ostwald-Folin pipet). When blood is to be measured in the chemistry laboratory, the Ostwald pipet is used. This pipet is similar in appearance to the volumetric pipet, except that the bulb is closer to the delivery tip (Fig. 2-8). Ostwald pipets are usually calibrated to be blown out, and, therefore, an etched ring or band will be seen near the mouth hole. To minimize the effects of viscosity the Ostwald pipet is designed with a large oval bulb and a short delivery tip.

Ostwald pipets come in several sizes. The most common sizes are 0.5 ml, 1 ml, and 2 ml. When using an Ostwald pipet to measure blood, the blood should be allowed to drain as slowly as possible, so that no residual film is left on the sides of the pipet. Contrary to the usual reading of the bottom of the meniscus for other liquids being measured by pipets, when pipetting blood using the Ostwald pipet, the top of the meniscus is read (blood is not transparent, and the bottom of the meniscus cannot be seen clearly).

Serologic Pipets

Another pipet used in the laboratory, but not often in the chemistry laboratory, is called a *serologic* pipet. It is much like the graduated pipet in appearance (Fig. 2-8). The orifice, or tip opening, of the serologic pipet is larger than in other pipets. The rate of fall of liquid is much too fast for great accuracy or precision. For chemistry uses, it would be necessary to retard the flow of liquid from the delivery tip of the serologic pipet. The serologic pipet is graduated to the end of the delivery tip and has an etched band on the mouthpiece. It is, therefore, designed to be blown out. The serologic pipet is less precise than any of the pipets discussed thus far. It is designed for use in serology work where relative values are sought. It is best not to use the serologic pipet for chemistry purposes. Used for screening, but not quantitative work

Stopcock Pipets

Another type of pipet is the *stopcock* pipet. This is a special pipet designed for delivering blood into a Van Slyke machine, a machine used for the determination and analysis of gases such as oxygen and carbon dioxide. The stopcock pipet can be used to deliver anything that is not to be exposed to the air. The stopcock pipet resembles a small volumetric pipet with a stopcock attached near the delivery tip for better control of delivery of the blood into the machine. These pipets have two calibration marks, one on either side of the bulb. Don't do this anymore.

We titrate instead,

GENERAL PIPETTING PROCEDURE

With few exceptions, the same general steps (Fig. 2-9) apply to pipetting with any type of pipet. These are:

1. Check the pipet to ascertain its correct size, being careful also to check for broken delivery tips or mouthpieces.

2. Hold the pipet lightly between the thumb and the last three fingers, leaving the index finger free.

3. Place the tip of the pipet well below the surface of the liquid to be pipetted.

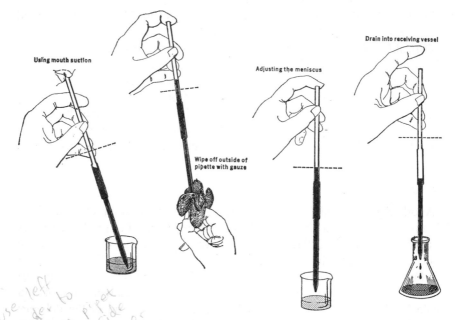

Fig. 2-9. Pipetting technique.

4. Using mouth suction, carefully draw the liquid up into the pipet until the level of liquid is well above the calibration mark (approximately 1 to 2 in. above the mark).

Note: Do not use mouth suction to pipette any solution suspected of high potency. Use another suction apparatus (water or pump, for example) for measuring these solutions. If a reagent is pipetted into the mouth, do not swallow it, but spit it out immediately. Rinse the mouth many times with water; consult an instructor for any further treatment necessary.

5. Quickly remove your mouth from the mouth hole of the pipet, and close the opening at the top of the pipet with the index finger.

6. Wipe the outside of the pipet dry with a piece of gauze or tissue.

7. Hold the pipet in a vertical position with the delivery tip against the inside of the original vessel. Carefully allow the liquid in the pipet to drain by gravity until the *bottom of the meniscus* is exactly at the calibration mark. To do this, the index finger should not be removed entirely from the mouth-hole end of the pipet but merely moved somewhat to allow a slow drainage to take place.

8. While still holding the pipet in a vertical position, touch the tip of the pipet to the inside wall of the receiving vessel. Remove the index finger from the top of the pipet to permit free drainage. Remember, in to-deliver pipets, a small amount of fluid will remain in the delivery tip.

9. To be sure that the drainage is as complete as possible, touch the

delivery tip of the pipet to another area on the inside wall of the receiving vessel.

10. Remove the pipet from the receiving vessel, and place it in the appropriate place for washing.

GENERAL CONSIDERATIONS IN PIPETTING

After the pipet has been filled above the top graduation mark, removed from the vessel, and held in a vertical position, the meniscus must be adjusted. The pipet should be held in such a way that the calibration mark is at eye level. The delivery tip is touched to the inside *wall* of the original vessel, not the liquid, and the meniscus of the liquid in the pipet is eased, or adjusted, down to the calibration mark.

To read the meniscus properly using clear solutions, the bottom of the meniscus is read. For ~~colored or viscous~~ blood solutions, the top of the meniscus is read. All readings must be made with the eye at the same level as the meniscus.

Before the measured liquid in the pipet is allowed to drain into the receiving vessel, any liquid adhering to the outside of the pipet must be wiped off with a clean piece of gauze or tissue. If this is not done, any drops present on the outside of the pipet might drain into the receiving vessel along with the measured volume. This would make the volume greater than the one specified, and error would result.

TITRATION

The final method of quantitative analysis to be discussed is the technique known as *titration*. Titration is a method of measuring the concentration of one solution by comparing it with a measured volume of a solution whose concentration is known. This technique is often used to determine the concentration of an unknown acid or an unknown base by means of comparison with a known base or a known acid. In this case the quantity of hydronium ions which react with hydroxyl ions with the formation of water is measured. However, there are numerous reactions, other than the neutralization reaction between acid and base, which make use of titration in order to determine the concentration of a solution. For example, in the chloride determination, which will be described later in this chapter (see under Plasma Chloride), a known amount and concentration of mercury ions are titrated with an unknown concentration and known amount of chloride ions; the formation of mercury chloride is the end product in this case.

In any titration procedure there are certain requirements that must always be present: (1) a standard solution of known concentration, (2) an accurately measured volume of the standard solution, (3) an indicator to show when the reaction has reached completion, and (4) a buret (or similar device) to measure the volume of a solution required to reach the end point. It is essential that chemically clean, well-calibrated volumetric equipment be used throughout the procedure to ensure reliable results.

When titration is used to determine concentration, the concentration is traditionally expressed in terms of normality. Normality is employed because it is a unit which provides a basis for direct comparison of strength for all solutions. Normality is the number of gram equivalents per liter of solution. As stated in Chapter 1, a gram equivalent is the amount of a compound which will liberate, combine with, or replace one gram atom of hydrogen. Therefore, 1 equiv of any compound will react with exactly 1 equiv of any other compound. For example, 1 equiv of any acid will exactly neutralize 1 equiv of any base.

The device that is most often employed to measure the volume required to achieve completion of the particular reaction in a given titration procedure is the buret. The buret is basically a graduated pipet with a stopcock near the delivery tip to facilitate better control and delivery of the solution (Fig. 2-1). Burets may be obtained in many different capacities and tolerances. The particular buret capacity and tolerance used in a given procedure will be determined by the degree of accuracy that is desired. To assure that the particular buret which is used is employed at maximum accuracy, a very specific technique or procedure must be followed. Mastery of this technique will come only with practice.

Procedure

1. By means of the buret clamp fasten the buret, which must be clean and free from chips or cracks, to the buret stand which will support it during the titration procedure. Fasten the clamp to the stand about halfway up the rod.

2. Lightly grease the buret stopcock. The stopcock should turn easily and smoothly, but an excess of lubricant will plug the stopcock capillary bore, preventing emptying of the buret. To grease a clean stopcock properly, apply a bit of grease with the fingertip down the two sides of the stopcock away from the capillary bore. Then insert the stopcock in the buret and rotate it until a smooth covering of the whole stopcock is obtained. If the buret is equipped with a Teflon plug, the stopcock need not be lubricated.

3. Rinse the buret with the titrant. In the case of an acid-base titration using phenolphthalein as the indicator, the titrant (or solution which is to be added and measured by means of the buret) will always be the base. In rinsing the buret, fill it completely with the titrant, and then let it drain. Discard the rinse solution. Fill the buret slowly and carefully in order to prevent air bubbles from forming in the narrow buret tube. It is essential that the buret be absolutely clean if the results are to be

accurate. A clean buret will drain without solution clinging to the sides of the buret tube; if the buret is dirty, there will be droplets of liquid clinging to the sides. After rinsing the buret several times with the titrant solution, fill the buret past the zero mark, and then bring the meniscus exactly to the zero mark by draining, using the stopcock to control the flow.

4. Into an erlenmeyer flask, pipet the stated amount of the second solution to be employed in the titration. Pipet this solution with a volumetric pipet using great care to ensure maximum accuracy.

5. Add the required amount of the indicator solution employed to show when the titration reaction has reached completion. (At this point, approximately 5 to 10 ml of water is often added to the erlenmeyer flask in order to dilute the indicator and make the end point more visible. The volume of this diluent is not critical, since it does not enter into the reaction or affect the volumes of the solutions which are being titrated.)

6. Titrate each flask in the following manner:

   a. Inspect the buret to be sure that there are no air bubbles trapped in the capillary tube or tip. Air bubbles will add to the apparent volume required to reach the end point, with erroneous results. If bubbles are present, drain the buret and refill it with the titrant until no bubbles are present.

   b. Inspect to see that the meniscus is exactly at zero, or record the actual buret reading immediately before beginning the titration.

   c. Add the solution in the buret to the flask by rotating the stopcock carefully. A right-handed technician encircles the buret stopcock with the left hand, using the right hand to swirl the flask during the titration (Fig. 2-10). This will be awkward at first but when mastered will become natural.

   d. The titrant may be added fairly rapidly at first, but as the reaction nears completion, the titrant is added drop by drop and finally by only portions of drops (split drops). Clues as to when the reaction is near completion depend on the particular reaction and indicator being employed. In the case of an acid-base titration using phenolphthalein as the indicator there is a change from a colorless to a red solution. The phenolphthalein is colorless in acid solutions and red in alkaline solutions. In the neutralization reaction itself hydronium ions react with hydroxyl ions to form water. The reaction begins with an excess of hydronium ions in the erlenmeyer flask, and the titration is performed until all hydronium ions have been neutralized by the hydroxyl ions which are added by means of the buret. The titration should be stopped at the actual point of neutralization, or as close to it as possible.

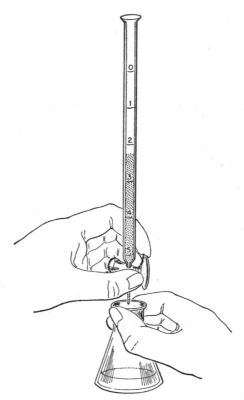

Fig. 2-10. Method of titration.

In actual practice, a pink color will appear when the alkali is added to the acid. This color will disappear on shaking. As the titration nears completion, the pink color will remain for a longer time. The base is then added slowly, by split drops, until a faint pink color remains. When the pink color no longer disappears but remains for over 30 seconds, the end point (or neutralization) has been achieved. It is essential that any titration, using any indicator, be stopped at the actual end point which is the first faint, but permanent, color change, or the results will be inaccurate.

e. Immediately upon reaching the end point, record the buret reading. Be sure to record a figure which is significant considering the tolerance of the particular buret being used.

7. Clean the buret by rinsing thoroughly with tap water and then with deionized water. Remove any grease from the stopcock with ether. The buret should not be left containing the titrant. Alkali will "freeze" the

stopcock to the buret, and the concentration of the titrant will increase because of evaporation.

8. Use the buret readings obtained in the titration procedure to determine the concentration of the unknown solution.

GENERAL CONSIDERATIONS AND CALCULATIONS

Chemically clean, well-calibrated volumetric equipment, including flasks, pipets, and burets, must be used in any titration procedure. Accurately prepared standard solutions are essential for accurate results. These are weighed analytically and diluted volumetrically. Indicators must be employed to show when the particular reaction has reached completion. These are often color indicators which change from colorless to a faint permanent color when the reaction has reached completion. However, such instruments as pH meters may also be employed where the end point is a particular hydronium ion concentration as recorded on the pH meter.

In acid-base titrations in the clinical laboratory, the most commonly used alkali is 0.1 N sodium hydroxide. This is relatively stable and can be used to determine the concentration of an acid. However, the sodium hydroxide is not absolutely stable and should be checked daily against a standard acid to be considered reliable.

The acids most commonly used in titration are hydrochloric acid, sulfuric acid, and nitric acid. A 0.1 N solution of hydrochloric acid made from constant boiling hydrochloric acid may be used as the reference, or primary standard, in the clinical laboratory. The acid solution is made from constant boiling hydrochloric acid obtained by a process of distillation and collection of the constant boiling mixture. The constant boiling acid is then weighed on an analytical balance and diluted volumetrically. With preparation in this manner, using constant boiling acid weighed analytically, the primary standard is accurate to within 0.0000 ± 5 N.[2]

In order to find the concentration of a solution, the following information must be available: a standard solution of known concentration, the volume of the standard solution, and the volume of the undetermined solution required to reach completion of the given reaction. As mentioned previously, the concentration is usually expressed in terms of normality, which permits a basis of direct comparison. Normality equals the number of gram equivalents per liter of solution, or milliequivalents per milliliter of solution. However, in practice, 1 liter of a given solution is rarely used; rather, parts of 1 liter are used. Therefore, the number of equivalents is actually the normality of the solution times the particular volume that is used in the titration procedure. All the ingredients required for the equation to determine the concentration of a solution in any titration procedure are now present. If the equivalents of solution 1 are equal to the equivalents of solution 2 and if the equivalents of a particular solution are actually the normality of the solution times the volume, it follows that the normality of solution 1 times the volume of solution 1 is equal to the normality of solution 2 times the volume of solution 2. Or in equation form:

Equivalents of solution 1 = equivalents of solution 2

or
$$N_1 \times V_1 = N_2 \times V_2$$

In the case of a typical acid-base titration assume that 2 ml of a standard 0.1000 N HCl solution required 1.50 ml of NaOH, added by means of a buret, to reach the first permanent pink color. What is the normality of the NaOH?

$$N_{(acid)} \times V_{(acid)} = N_{(base)} \times V_{(base)}$$
$$0.1000\ N \times 2\ ml = N_{(base)} \times 1.50\ ml$$
$$N_{(base)} = \frac{0.1000\ N \times 2\ ml}{1.50\ ml} = 0.1333$$

That is, the normality of the NaOH is 0.1333.

The titration technique has numerous uses in the clinical laboratory. It is the means whereby the concentration of several new reagents are checked before being put into use in the clinical laboratory. When weaker acids or bases are prepared from more concentrated solutions, the actual normality of the new solution must be determined by means of titration. In addition, titration is the basis for several chemical determinations which are performed in the clinical laboratory.

COLLECTION, PRESERVATION, AND PREPARATION OF SPECIMENS

Accurate chemical analysis of biologic fluids depends upon proper collection, preservation, and preparation of the sample, in addition to the actual technique and method of analysis used. The most quantitatively perfect determination is of no use if the specimen is not properly handled in the initial steps of the procedure. Each chemical method has unique problems of its own, but, in general, the collection, means of preservation, the initial preparation of samples to be used follow a similar pattern, regardless of what the final analysis is to be.

COLLECTION OF WHOLE BLOOD, PLASMA, AND SERUM

The majority of chemical determinations are done on whole blood, plasma, or serum. The plasma is the liquid portion of the circulating blood. Plasma contains fibrinogen. Serum is plasma with the fibrinogen removed, which is usually accomplished by the clotting mechanism.

There are several general precautions to observe when collecting blood samples for the laboratory. Some of these are:

1. Avoid prolonged stoppage of the circulation (stasis). Do not leave a tourniquet on for long periods of time. Prolonged stasis results in gross alterations in the blood constituents. Stasis should be used for a *minimum* of time.

2. Blood should not be taken while intravenous solutions are being administered.

3. Syringes, if used, should be chemically clean and dry. If any moisture is present, hemolysis or contamination of the blood will occur.

4. Blood should be placed in the appropriate labeled container for the test to be done.

For more information on the actual venipuncture itself, see Collection of Samples in Chapter 3.

Through numerous studies, it has been found that the average meal has no significant effect on the concentration of most blood constituents, with two exceptions: tests for glucose and phosphorus must be run on specimens drawn while the subject is fasting. Fasting specimens are unnecessary for tests other than for glucose or phosphorus.

PRESERVATION OF THE SAMPLE—USE OF ANTICOAGULANTS

Anticoagulants are used to prevent the blood from clotting. They are therefore used when whole blood or plasma is needed for the determination ordered. Several types of anticoagulants are available for various purposes. These anticoagulants are either dry powders or liquids. Some of the more commonly used anticoagulants are:

1. Sodium fluoride. This is a dry powder, used primarily for blood glucose specimens, since it is an enzyme poison (preventing glycolysis, or destruction of the glucose) as well as an anticoagulant. More information on the use of this anticoagulant will be found under Blood Glucose.

2. Potassium oxalate. This is a dry powder, used commonly in the chemistry laboratory for the determination of blood urea nitrogen (BUN), carbon dioxide, chloride, creatinine, and many other procedures. It is the oxalate in the anticoagulant which precipitates the calcium from the blood, thus preventing the clotting mechanism from progressing. When calcium ions are combined with oxalate and not available to participate in the clotting mechanism, the blood does not clot.

3. Ammonium and potassium oxalate. Also called *balanced oxalate,* or *double oxalate* by some, this combination is a dry powder. It is used mainly for hematology work and not used in chemistry as a rule, because the presence of ammonium in the anticoagulant interferes with some of the chemistry determinations.

4. Sequestrene (EDTA). This is a liquid anticoagulant, used primarily in the hematology laboratory. It is good for hematology work because it preserves the cell's morphologic features very well.

5. Sodium citrate. This is a liquid anticoagulant used for prothrombin

time tests; it also prevents hemolysis, which is an important factor in the prothrombin test.

6. Heparin. This liquid anticoagulant is theoretically the best anticoagulant, because it is a normal constituent of blood and introduces no foreign contaminants to the blood specimen. It is, however, expensive and has only a temporary effect as an anticoagulant.

If no anticoagulant is used, serum is obtained. After being placed in the tube, the blood is allowed to clot. The serum is then removed from the clot by centrifugation and placed in a clean, dry tube. Serum can be used for tests for sodium, potassium, calcium, phosphorus, acid and alkaline phosphatase, cholesterol, uric acid, and liver function.

It is important to remove the plasma or serum from the remaining blood cells, or clot, as soon as possible. After the anticoagulant is mixed with the blood sample, the cells are removed by centrifugation. It is especially important to remove the plasma quickly from the cell layer when potassium oxalate has been used as the anticoagulant, because the salt (potassium oxalate) shrinks the red blood cell, and the intracellular water diffuses into the plasma (fluid inside the red cell leaves the cell and thus causes shrinkage).

Some chemical constituents are subject to rapid change after being removed from the vein. The best policy is to perform tests on fresh specimens. On occasion, steps must be taken to preserve the specimen until the test can be run. There are ways to retard alterations. One example would be the use of sodium fluoride for the preservation of the glucose concentration. Sodium fluoride prevents glycolysis from taking place. Refrigeration is a simple and reliable method to retard alterations. Refrigeration retards bacteriologic action and glycolysis. Some changes still take place, even while the specimen is in the refrigerator. Refrigerated specimens must be brought to room temperature before any chemical analysis takes place. Removing cells from plasma and serum is another means of preventing some changes from occurring. Serum or plasma may be preserved by freezing. Whole blood cannot be frozen satisfactorily, because freezing ruptures the red cells. Freezing preserves enzyme activities in serum and plasma. When serum or plasma freezes, it does so in layers of concentration; for this reason these specimens must be well mixed before being used in a chemical determination.

Preservation should always be the exception rather than the rule. A laboratory test run on a fresh sample is best.

APPEARANCE OF SPECIMENS

Any person working with specimens in the laboratory must be able to recognize the appearance of normal plasma or serum as opposed to abnormal. Normally, serum or plasma is straw-colored. However, varying shades of yellow are also normally seen. There are several instances where abnormal-appearing serum and plasma are clinically indicative of serious disorders and also instances where the use of these abnormal specimens can interfere with the chemical determinations being run.

Hemolysis in specimens is perhaps the most common of the abnormal appearances to be considered in this section. A specimen which is hemolyzed appears red, usually clear red. The red blood cells have, for some reason, been lysed and the hemoglobin released into the remaining portion of the blood. Many times the fault producing hemolyzed specimens lies in the technique used for the venipuncture. A poor venipuncture, with excessive trauma to the blood vessel, can result in a hemolyzed specimen. Using dirty tubes or tubes not entirely dry can also result in hemolysis of the blood placed in those tubes. In these cases, repeating the venipuncture and using clean, dry equipment will produce a normal-appearing specimen and one which can adequately be used for chemical determinations. Hemolysis of blood can also be attributed to freezing, prolonged exposure to warmth, unnecessary forceful spraying of blood from the needle of a syringe when transferring it to a specimen tube, or allowing the serum or plasma to remain too long on the cells before removing the serum or plasma to another tube. Hemolyzed serum or plasma is unfit as a specimen for several chemistry determinations. The procedure to be run should always be checked first to see if abnormal-appearing specimens can be used.

Jaundiced serum or plasma is another specimen with an abnormal-appearing hue. When serum or plasma takes on a brownish yellow color, there is most likely an increase in the presence of bile pigments, namely, bilirubin. In cases of obstruction of the bile duct or impairment of the liver, there is an accumulation of bile pigments in the blood, and the skin becomes yellow. When this condition occurs, the skin of the patient is said to be *jaundiced*. The serum or plasma can also be jaundiced, or yellow. Anyone performing clinical laboratory determinations should note any abnormal appearance of serum or plasma and record it on the report slip. Another term for jaundiced is *icteric*.

When the blood, serum, or plasma takes on a milky white appearance, the specimen is said to be *lipemic*. The presence of lipids, or fats, in the serum causes this abnormal appearance in the specimen. Many times if the blood specimen were drawn from the patient soon after a meal, the specimen would appear lipemic. Lipemic specimens, for the most part, do not cause interference in chemical determinations.

PREPARATION OF A PROTEIN-FREE FILTRATE

Before most chemical determinations can be carried out, the protein in the specimen must be removed. If not removed, the protein would interfere with the final results of the test run. There are several methods for removing protein, and each chemical procedure will call for a specific agent or method. In general, each agent removes the protein by making it insoluble. The protein precipitates out and leaves behind a protein-free solution. There are three main categories of protein-precipitating agents: (1) salts of heavy metals, (2) acids, and (3) alcohols. Examples of these agents are:

1. Salts of heavy metals—sodium sulfate or ammonium sulfate
2. Acids—trichloroacetic acid, tungstic acid, or picric acid
3. Alcohols—ethyl alcohol or methyl alcohol

One of the most common methods for precipitating protein is by making a Folin-Wu filtrate.[3] The original method devised by Folin and Wu calls for 1 ml of blood, 7 ml of water, 1 ml of $\frac{2}{3}$ N H_2SO_4, and 1 ml of 10% sodium tungstate (Na_2WO_4). The modification of the original Folin-Wu filtrate devised by Hayden is more commonly used than the original procedure. The Hayden modification is described below.

Procedure for Hayden Modification of the Folin-Wu Filtrate

1. Into a test tube pipet 8 ml of 0.083 N H_2SO_4.
2. Using an Ostwald pipet, pipet 1 ml of well-mixed blood into the test tube. Blow out the last drop from the pipet. If serum or plasma is to be used, choose a volumetric pipet for measuring the sample into the test tube. Use a centrifuge tube, which is one specifically constructed to withstand centrifugal force.
3. Place rubber stoppers in the tube and mix by gentle inversion four or five times. In this initial step, the hemoglobin is converted to acid hematin (a dark brown color is seen). Thorough mixing is important after each new chemical reagent is added.
4. Into the test tube, pipet 1 ml of 10% sodium tungstate (for this addition a graduated pipet may be used) to complete the precipitation of the protein.
5. Stopper the tube again, and mix well. Shake the tube until a "metallic click" is heard. It is during this step that the actual precipitation of protein is accomplished; thorough shaking is of primary importance.
6. Remove the insoluble protein by filtration or centrifugation. For whole blood filtration is the means usually employed, while for serum or plasma centrifugation is used.
   a. Filtration method. Place filter paper into a funnel and a clean, dry test tube under the funnel. Pour the mixture into the filter paper, being careful that none of it spills down the sides of the funnel. Allow *all* of the filtrate to collect in the test tube under the funnel before any is used for analysis. Before pipetting any of the filtrate, mix it well. After filtration of the mixture, the fluid collected in the test tube is called the *filtrate*. This solution should be water-clear and colorless.

b. Centrifugation method. Place the tube in the centrifuge, being certain to balance the tube with another like tube. Centrifuge for at least 5 minutes at 3,000 rpm. After centrifuging, the protein will be packed at the bottom of the tube, and the clear supernatant solution at the top is free of protein and can be pipetted for eventual analysis. This solution too should be clear and colorless in order to be used for chemical analysis.

The Hayden modification of the Folin-Wu filtrate yields a nearly neutral filtrate. The acid is used up in the protein precipitation. If the solution is too acid or too alkaline, the protein will not be completely precipitated. The reaction occurring in this procedure is made up of two steps:

1. $Na_2WO_4 + H_2SO_4 \dashrightarrow Na_2SO_4 + H_2WO_4$ (tungstic acid)
2. H_2WO_4 + protein (in blood, serum, plasma, etc.) $\dashrightarrow$
   protein tungstate (insoluble)

Quantitative Analysis of the Protein-free Filtrate

The protein-free filtrate can be analyzed quantitatively by photometric or volumetric methods. The directions for specific procedure used will list the agents to be employed for the removal of protein and will state how to analyze the resulting protein-free filtrate.

MEANS OF ENSURING RELIABLE RESULTS

It is the responsibility of the laboratory to the patient and physician to ensure that the results reported are reliable and accurate.

In the chemistry laboratory, it is impossible to obtain exactly the same results each time a determination is performed on a given specimen. This variation is due to limitations in the procedure itself and the sampling mechanism used. The physician does, however, use the results of the chemical determination to diagnose and follow the course of a disease under treatment; therefore the laboratory must be sure that there is a sufficient amount of accuracy for the results to have meaning.

A laboratory has several ways by which it can control the reliability of its reports. As already mentioned, one of the difficulties in guaranteeing reliable results is that the amount of sample taken from the patient is limited. Of the many thousands of milliliters of blood available only a small amount is taken (5 to 10 ml). In controlling the precision and accuracy of chemical determinations, it is necessary to reject those results in which there is evidence of more than the permitted amount of error.

When chemical determinations are performed, often the term *batch* is used. A batch, or series, is a collection of any number of specimens to be measured plus any of or all the following aids for ensuring reliable results:

1. Standard solutions
2. Blanks
3. Control specimens
4. Duplicates
5. Recoveries

STANDARD SOLUTIONS

In order to determine the concentration of a substance in a given specimen, there must be a basis of comparison. Most commonly, for solutions capable of being colored, in the chemistry laboratory a photometer is used in making this comparison (see under Photometry). The buret too, discussed previously, is used in the clinical laboratory for comparison purposes, in titration or volumetric analysis (see under Titration).

A standard solution is one which contains a known, exact amount of the substance being measured in the sample. The standard solution is measured accurately and then treated as if it were a specimen with contents to be determined. Standard solutions are prepared from high-quality chemicals which have been dried and placed in a dessicator. The standard chemical is weighed on the analytical balance and diluted volumetrically. This standard solution is usually most stable in a concentrated form, in which case it is usually referred to as a *stock* standard. Working standards (a more dilute form of the stock standard) are prepared from the stock, and sometimes an intermediate form is prepared. The working standard is the one employed in the actual determination. Stock standards are usually stored in the refrigerator. The accuracy of the procedure is absolutely dependent on the standard solution used; therefore extreme care must be taken whenever these solutions are prepared or used in a clinical laboratory.

In order to use the standard solution as a basis of comparison in quantitative analysis employing the photometer, a series of calibrated colorimeter tubes (or cuvettes) are prepared. Each tube has a varying amount of the known standard solution. In this way, a series of tubes is available containing known varying amounts of the standard. Standard tubes are carried through the same developmental steps, from the filtrate stage, usually, as tubes containing specimens to be measured. This set of standard tubes is read in the photometer and the galvanometer readings recorded. These readings can be recorded in percent transmission or in optical density (see under Photometry).

STANDARDIZATION OF A PROCEDURE AND USE OF A STANDARD CURVE

Once the series of standard tubes has been read in the photometer, the galvanometer readings and standard concentrations are plotted on graph paper. This is the first step in the use of a standard curve, a most essential tool in the majority of chemistry determinations.

Semilogarithmic graph paper is the type most commonly used to plot the readings from the photometer. The horizontal axis of this graph paper is on a linear scale, and the vertical axis is on a logarithmic scale. The concentration of the standard tubes is plotted on the horizontal axis, or linear scale. The readings from the photometer are plotted along the vertical axis, or logarithmic scale. In most cases, the percent transmission readings are the ones used (as opposed to optical density readings). These readings can be plotted directly on the logarithmic scale, as the concentration is proportional to the logarithm of the galvanometer readings. In this way percent transmission readings are converted to the appropriate number on a logarithmic scale. Using semilogarithmic graph paper is simple and convenient for most laboratory purposes. When plotting percent readings versus concentrations, using semilogarithmic graph paper, the proportional relationship is direct, and a straight-line graph is obtained when the individual standard points are connected. Criteria of a good standard curve are that the line is straight, that the line connects all points, and that the lines goes through the origin, or intersect, of the two axes. The origin, or intersect, of the graph paper is the point on the vertical and horizontal axes where there is 100% T and zero concentration.

Another type of graph paper, called *linear graph paper,* is available for plotting standard curves. This graph paper has linear scales both horizontally and vertically. If linear graph paper is used to construct a standard curve, the percent transmission readings must first be converted to logarithmic values and the logarithmic values plotted on the vertical axis. If percent transmission readings are converted to optical densities or if the galvanometer scale is calibrated in optical density units, the optical density readings can be plotted directly against the concentration. Again a straight-line graph must be obtained. To eliminate the conversion of percent transmission to optical density in order to obtain the necessary straight-line graph, the use of semilogarithmic graph paper is suggested.

When plotting on graph paper, whether it be concentrations or galvanometer readings, care must be taken to note the intervals on the graph paper. Many errors result from carelessness in the initial plotting of points on the graph paper.

When a graph is prepared, the axis must also be properly labeled. Additional information usually recorded on the paper includes the following: the name of the person constructing the graph, the procedure for which the graph was prepared, the date, the photometer used, and the wavelength setting used.

Once the standard curve has been constructed, it is used to calculate the concentration of any unknowns which were included in the same batch

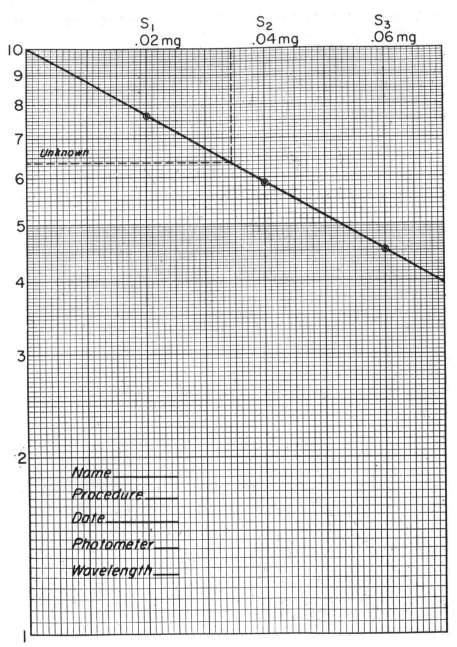

Fig. 2-11. Construction of a standard curve.

as were the standards used to construct the graph. In order to find the concentration of a solution, there must be some way of comparing it with a solution of known concentration. An example of construction and use of a standard curve follows (Fig. 2-11):

Three standard solutions are prepared with the following concentrations of standard: standard 1 (S_1) = 0.02 mg, standard 2 (S_2) = 0.04 mg, and standard 3 (S_3) = 0.06 mg. These concentrations are plotted on the linear, horizontal scale of the graph paper. The three standard tubes are read in a photometer, giving these readings in percent transmission: $S_1 = 76^2$, $S_2 = 58^3$, and $S_3 = 45^1$. The percent transmission readings are plotted under their respective concentrations on the logarithmic, vertical scale of the paper. The points are connected using a ruler. An undetermined substance gives a reading of 63^2 %T. Using the example graph in Fig. 2-11, the 63^2 point on the vertical scale is found, followed horizontally to the graph line just drawn, and then followed vertically to the concentration scale. The degree of accuracy to which an unknown concentration can be read depends upon the concentration of the standards used. In this example, the unknown concentration is 0.0343 mg (the fourth decimal place is an approximate figure).

Using standard solutions to standardize the analyses of each batch, rather than relying on a permanently established calibration curve, allows the clinical laboratory to produce more reliable results. The use of standard solutions compensates for variables present, such as time, temperature, and age of reagents. It is always best to use several varying amounts of the desired standard solution, not just one. In order to use the photometer to give any reliable information about the concentration of a substance, standards must be used as a basis of comparison.

Standard solutions are also used in quantitative analytical procedures not employing the photometer. For example, whenever titration is used to measure concentration, a standard solution must be employed. There must be some basis of comparison in this technique also.

BLANKS

For every procedure using the photometer, a blank must be included in the batch. The blank contains reagents used in the procedure, but it does not contain the substance to be measured. It is treated with the same reagents and processed along with the undetermined specimens and the standards. The blank solution is set to read 100%T on the galvanometer viewing scale. In other words, the blank tube is set so as to transmit 100 percent of the light. The other tubes in the same batch (undetermined specimens and standards, for example) transmit only a fraction of this light, because they contain particles which absorb light (particles of unknown substance present), and thus only part of the 100 percent is transmitted. Using a blank solution corrects for any color which may be present because of reagents used or an interaction between those reagents.

CONTROL SPECIMENS

Some type of control system for the clinical laboratory is essential, a fact that has been proved by numerous laboratory accuracy surveys. The use of control solutions in clinical chemistry determinations is absolutely necessary, so that the physician can more accurately rely on the results obtained. An accurately measured portion of the proper control solution is included in each batch of chemistry determinations and is subjected to the same set of experimental conditions and reagents as the specimens to be determined. Various types of control solutions are used; these systems have been developed not only to guarantee reliable results but, at the same time, to permit the use of only a small amount of the specimen or solution.

Since the "true" value of the control solution is known, it is used to judge the reliability of the results obtained on the specimens of unknown values run in the same batch. If the control value obtained in the procedure is not within the allowable limits for that procedure, one must assume that the values found for specimens being measured are also incorrect. After the procedure has been reviewed for any indication of error and the error found and corrected, the batch must be run again until the control value is acceptable. The use of control specimens checks for deterioration of reagents or standard solutions used in the procedure, for error in basic technique, or for machine failure. Control solutions will also aid in detecting certain errors or mistakes on the part of the laboratory personnel performing the tests.

Types of control specimens can be divided into two main categories: those prepared commercially and those prepared by the individual laboratory.

Commercially prepared controls can be purchased from the manufacturer. These control solutions are obtained in small samples, called *aliquots,* prepared originally from a large pooled supply of serum or plasma. The manufacturer prepares the control and establishes the "true" values for the various constituents a laboratory wishes to measure. One type of control specimen may often be used for several different procedures. The manufacturer has established different acceptable values for each procedure for which it can be used. There are commercial controls available for all the common constituents of the blood and for many of the less common ones also.

Control solutions can also be prepared by the individual laboratory. Excess serum or plasma is saved at the end of each day and frozen. After a pool of the serum or plasma has accumulated that amounts to about 2 or 3 liters, the control specimens for daily use can be made.

Only normal serum or plasma is saved (not lipemic or hemolyzed, for example). Beef serum can also be used. When enough serum has been saved, it is thawed and mixed thoroughly. After thorough mixing, the pool is divided into aliquots of a convenient amount. Aliquots of 2 to 3 ml in a small tube or vial are satisfactory. These samples are then stored in a freezer.

An aliquot of the pooled serum or a commercial control specimen is processed along with the regular batch of tests for 15 to 25 days. This number of repetitive tests on the aliquots of pooled control establishes a normal average value. The average value (mean) and acceptable limits (based on standard deviation) are calculated using certain statistical formulas. Once the range of acceptable results has been established, one of these control samples is included with each batch of determinations run. If the control value is not within the limits established and the procedure must therefore be repeated, no determination results are given out until the control value checks out.

It is conventional in most laboratories to plot the daily control specimen values on a quality control chart. This serves as a visual representation of the information derived from using control specimens.

Control charts may be constructed in such a way as to represent checks on the limits of accuracy or precision. Charts representing daily precision require the plotting of the average value of duplicate control specimen determinations. When a check for accuracy of the method is desired, controls are run singly, and the value is plotted on the control chart.

It is possible to observe trends leading toward trouble by plotting the control values daily on a control chart. This observation can assist in preventing possible difficulties and can aid in troubleshooting. Such visual representation is particularly useful for observing these trends before the control specimen values are actually out of the established acceptable limits.

DUPLICATE DETERMINATIONS

In each batch of determinations, one of the specimens to be measured is run in duplicate. This specimen is chosen at random from those to be run. The use of duplicates checks the manual technique used, that is, the precision, or repeatability, of the method. Duplicates do not measure accuracy. It is possible to have grossly inaccurate results which duplicate perfectly. Duplicate determinations are also a means of quality control.

RECOVERY SOLUTIONS

The use of a recovery solution tells just how accurate the method or procedure really is. To any specimen in the batch (or to a control solution), in addition to the regular specimens, a measured amount of the pure substance being analyzed is added. Theoretically, the amount of substance added should be recovered at the end of the determination if the method is an accurate one. Some chemistry procedures require the use of a recovery solution routinely, while others are checked at the time when the method is set up (or evaluated). One method to be discussed in this chapter, the blood urea nitrogen determination, requires a recovery solution as a part of the regular batch. Recovery solutions are another means of quality control.

PLASMA CHLORIDE titration

One of the few procedures in the chemistry laboratory which employs the use of titration as a means of quantitative measurement is the one for chloride. Because titration is an important technique in the clinical laboratory, the plasma chloride procedure will be described in some detail.

Chloride is one of the negatively charged constituents (anions) of the extracellular fluid. It is found in serum, plasma, cerebrospinal fluid, tissue fluid, and urine. There is very little chloride inside the cells of the body, with the exception of the red cells, where there is some chloride. The chief extracellular anions are chloride and bicarbonate, and there is a reciprocal relationship between them. That is, when there is a decrease in the amount of one, there is an increase in the amount of the other. In the blood, two-thirds of the chloride is found in the plasma and only one-third in the red cells. Since there is this difference in chloride concentration in the red cell and plasma, the test for chloride is routinely performed on plasma (or serum) and not on whole blood. Physiologically, only the concentration of chloride in the extracellular fluid is important. This is another reason why plasma or serum is chosen as the specimen for this determination.

Chloride functions in two important ways in the body: it assists in maintaining the acid-base balance, and it regulates the fluid content of the body and its influence on the kidney. Both functions are extremely important.

In the maintenance of acid-base balance, chloride assists in the interchange of bicarbonate from the cells to the plasma. In carbon dioxide transport, a series of reactions called the *chloride shift* takes place. Whenever bicarbonate goes from the red cell to the plasma (as it must do during carbon dioxide transport), the bicarbonate anions are replaced by an equivalent amount of chloride anions.

An example of the chloride shift in the laboratory is the replacement action that occurs when a specimen for a chloride determination is allowed to stand for a while before the cells and plasma are separated. When whole blood comes into contact with air, carbon dioxide (thus bicarbonate) escapes from the blood. As carbon dioxide leaves the plasma, chloride diffuses (or shifts) out of the red cells to replace it. The contact between whole blood and air, therefore, has the effect of lowering the plasma carbon dioxide and raising the plasma chloride. Specimens of whole blood left in contact with air will, therefore, result in falsely high plasma or serum chloride values.[4]

Under Collection, Preservation, and Preparation of Specimens, the concept of proper handling of blood specimens was discussed. The cells must be removed from the plasma by centrifugation as quickly as possible. Once separated from the cells, the serum or plasma chloride concentration is very stable.

The other important function of chloride is to regulate the fluid content of the body and its influence on the kidney. The kidney maintains the electrolyte concentration of the plasma within very narrow limits. This regulation is necessary for life. Renal function is set to regulate the composition of the extracellular fluid first and then the volume. Consequently, if the body loses salt (sodium chloride, an electrolyte), it loses water.

The electrolytes are the major charged particles present in the extracellular fluid. The chief negatively charged constituents (anions) consist of chloride and bicarbonate. The chief positively charged constituents (cations) consist of sodium and potassium. There are other electrolytes, but the major ones mentioned are the ones most likely to show variation in electrolyte problems. Collectively, the four charged particles, chloride, bicarbonate, sodium, and potassium, make up the electrolytes. It is essential that the positively charged particles balance, or electrically neutralize, the negatively charged particles. When this balance is not achieved, electrolyte imbalance occurs, and this results in an extremely dangerous situation for the patient. Death can result. Therefore, to assess electrolyte balance, the laboratory must often run electrolyte determinations. A set of electrolyte determinations consists of tests for chloride, bicarbonate, sodium, and potassium. These determinations are often run as emergency procedures, for electrolyte imbalance cannot be tolerated by the patient for any period of time. Treatment to remedy the imbalance must be started as quickly as possible.

SPECIMENS

As discussed earlier, the distribution of chloride is one-third in the red cells and two-thirds in the plasma. For this reason, plasma or serum are ordinarily used for analysis of chloride level. After venipuncture, the blood is placed in a properly labeled tube. The anticoagulant used most frequently is potassium oxalate. Heparin is a very good anticoagulant for this purpose, but it is very expensive and therefore not used as a rule. Sodium fluoride cannot be used for the chloride determination, because the fluoride is a halogen (as is chloride), and both react in the same manner in the analysis. The results using sodium fluoride as the anticoagulant would give a falsely high chloride value because of the additional fluoride that is being measured. If serum is used, the blood is placed in a labeled tube containing no anticoagulant and is allowed to clot. The serum or plasma should be removed from the red cells as soon as possible after the blood is drawn to prevent the chloride shift from occurring. The serum or plasma can be refrigerated until used, if necessary.

METHODS FOR QUANTITATIVE DETERMINATION

After properly obtaining the serum or plasma, the quantitative determination of the chloride level can begin. Most analyses for chloride employ some type of a titration procedure. Various methods for the detection of chloride are used; some of these are the Cavett and Bolderidge method, Volhard method, Whitehorn method, and Schales and Schales method. The procedure to be discussed in this section is the Schales and Schales method.[5]

SCHALES AND SCHALES CHLORIDE METHOD

Principle

The interfering proteins are first removed by precipitation with tungstic acid (the modified Folin-Wu filtrate). Proteins, if present, will interfere with color detection and with the reaction taking place. Titration is the next step. The chloride in the protein-free filtrate is titrated with mercuric nitrate using diphenylcarbazone to indicate when the end point has been reached. When all the chloride in the filtrate has reacted with the mercuric nitrate, the diphenylcarbazone indicator will change color. The color change is from an orange-red to a faint blue-violet.

In the titration with mercuric nitrate, the reaction taking place is

$$2NaCl + Hg(NO_3)_2 \dashrightarrow 2NaNO_3 + HgCl_2$$

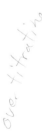

When all the chloride ions have reacted with the mercuric nitrate, the first excess of mercuric ions react with the indicator to form a faint blue-violet-colored complex salt. The reaction is complete when the end point is reached, that is, when the first blue-violet color is produced by the addition of a drop or split drop of mercuric nitrate. The first, faintest, permanent blue-violet color is the end point. It is most important to use caution in titrating, as even a fraction of a milliliter of overtitration will result in grossly inaccurate results.

Reagents

For the preparation of the protein-free filtrate:
1. 0.083 N sulfuric acid.
2. Ten percent sodium tungstate. Ten grams of $Na_2WO_4 \cdot H_2O$ is dissolved and diluted to 100 ml with deionized water.
For titration of chloride in the filtrate:
1. Mercuric nitrate. Weigh 3.0 g of $Hg(NO_3)_2$, and dissolve it in 200

ml of deionized water and 20 ml of 2 N HNO$_3$. Quantitatively transfer the solution to a 1-liter volumetric flask, and dilute it to the calibration mark. Mix well.

The mercuric nitrate solution is used in the buret for titrating the chloride ions. It is necessary to know the concentration of the mercuric nitrate if the concentration of the chloride is to be determined. It is difficult to weigh mercuric nitrate accurately, since it takes up water readily. Therefore, it is weighed approximately and checked as to its concentration against a known, stable, standard solution of sodium chloride each time a batch of chlorides is run. The addition of a specific amount of nitric acid in the initial preparation of the reagent serves to sharpen the end-point reaction. If more or less nitric acid is added, the end-point color will not be as sharp.

2. Standard sodium chloride. Weigh 584.5 mg of NaCl analytically; dissolve and dilute it to 1 liter in a volumetric flask.

This reagent is used to find the concentration (normality) of the mercuric nitrate solution. This standard can be weighed accurately on the analytical balance. Chemically pure (C.P.) sodium chloride is dried at 120°C and stored in a dessicator. This is the chemical that should be used to prepare the standard solution. The concentration for the sodium chloride expressed in normality terms is 0.01 N. The concentration can also be expressed as 0.01 equiv/liter, or 0.01 meq/ml.

3. Diphenylcarbazone indicator. Dissolve 100 mg of diphenylcarbazone (Eastman Kodak number 4459) in 100 ml of 95% alcohol.

This reagent must be stored in the dark, preferably in the refrigerator. In the daylight, the orange-red solution turns yellow in a few days and cannot be used. Even in the dark, its color changes slowly to cherry red. Because it is unstable to this degree, this reagent is prepared fresh each month. If the indicator is cherry red, it is no longer suitable for use in this procedure.

Procedure

Results for this procedure are precise within 1 percent. This method is applicable to the determination of chloride in a variety of biologic fluids (serum, plasma, urine, and cerebrospinal fluid).

Preparation of Protein-free Filtrates

1. Prepare duplicate Folin-Wu filtrates from serum, plasma, or control specimens by pipetting the following into centrifuge tubes:

8 ml of 0.083 N H$_2$SO$_4$.

1 ml of plasma, serum, or control. Cork and mix well.

1 ml of 10% Na$_2$WO$_4$. Cork and mix well.

2. Centrifuge for 5 minutes at 2,000 to 3,000 rpm.

3. From the centrifuge tube, pipet 2 ml of the clear, supernatant filtrate into a labeled 25-ml erlenmeyer flask. Pipet a duplicate aliquot into an-

other labeled 25-ml erlenmeyer flask. Each filtrate is always pipetted in duplicate.

Titration of Standard Sodium Chloride to Determine Normality of Mercuric Nitrate Solution

1. Into duplicate 25-ml erlenmeyer flasks pipet aliquot 2-ml samples of the NaCl standard solution. To each of the flasks add 0.06 ml of diphenylcarbazone indicator *just before* titration (indicator is made up in alcohol and will evaporate if exposed to room temperature for too long a time).

2. From a buret containing $Hg(NO_3)_2$, add reagent until the blue-violet end point is reached. As the end point is approached, add the $Hg(NO_3)_2$ in split drops.

3. Titrate each of the 2-ml samples of standard solution, and record the amount of reagent needed to reach the end points. The duplicate titrations must agree within the allowable range established. This range will depend on the size of the buret used. For a 5-ml buret with 0.02-ml calibrated divisions, the titrations of duplicate solutions must agree within 0.02 ml. If this agreement is not achieved, additional samples must be pipetted and titrated until the duplicates do agree.

Titration of Chloride in the Filtrate

1. To each of the flasks containing the 2 ml of filtrate of unknown value, add 0.06 ml diphenylcarbazone just before titrating.

2. Titrate with the mercuric nitrate in the buret until the blue-violet end point is reached. Again the final end point is approached by addition of split drops from the buret. Record the buret readings. Duplicate titrations must agree within the established amount to be considered accurate.

Calculations

When titration has been completed, calculation of the results to be reported to the physician is necessary. The usual way of reporting chloride results is in units of milliequivalents per liter (meq/liter). These units are used because the major functions of chloride in the body are associated with osmotic pressure regulation and acid-base balance.

1. *To calculate the normality of standard sodium chloride solution:*
The standard NaCl was weighed analytically and diluted volumetrically: 584.5 mg of NaCl was diluted to 1 liter with deionized water; this is the same as 0.5845 g/liter. A 1 N NaCl solution would contain 58.45 g/liter, or 58.45 mg/ml. For the standard solution used in this procedure

$$\frac{58.45 \text{ g}}{1\ N} = \frac{0.5845 \text{ g}}{x\ N}$$

$$x = 0.01\ N \text{ for standard NaCl}$$

0.01 N NaCl is the same as 0.01 equiv/liter, or 0.01 meq/ml, so 1 ml of the standard NaCl solution contains 0.01 meq of NaCl.

2. *To calculate the normality of the mercuric nitrate solution:*

Two milliliters of the standard NaCl is titrated with the mercuric nitrate reagent, and the volume of mercuric nitrate (in milliliters) required to reach the end point is recorded. Using the following equation, the normality of the mercuric nitrate can be calculated:

$$N_{std\ NaCl} \times V_{std\ NaCl} = N_{Hg(NO_3)_2} \times V_{Hg(NO_3)_2}$$
$$0.01 \times 2\ ml = x \times ml\ used\ for\ titration$$
$$x = normality\ of\ mercuric\ nitrate\ solution$$

where N = normality
V = volume

3. *To calculate the normality of unknown serum or plasma:*
The filtrate was prepared in the following way:

1 ml of serum or plasma
8 ml of 0.083 N H_2SO_4
1 ml of 10% Na_2WO_4

In the final filtrate, there is 1 ml of serum in a total volume of 10 ml, or 0.1 ml of serum in 1 ml of filtrate. The measured 2-ml aliquot titrated, therefore, contains 0.2 ml of serum or plasma. The following equation is used to calculate the normality of the unknown:

$$N_{Hg(NO_3)_2} \times V_{Hg(NO_3)_2} = N_{serum} \times V_{serum}$$
normality from Step 2 $\times$ buret reading = $x \times 0.2$ ml
$$x = normality\ of\ serum\ or\ plasma$$
$$(meq/ml\ or\ equiv/liter)$$

4. *To calculate the chloride value in terms of milliequivalents per liter (desired units for report to physician):*

One equivalent equals 1,000 milliequivalents. Therefore multiplying the result obtained in Step 3 by 1,000 converts the value to the desired units, milliequivalents per liter. Results are rounded off and reported to the nearest whole number.

Technical Factors and Sources of Error

Pipetting errors can cause inaccurate results. This is probably the major cause of error. Pipetting is involved in the preparation of the protein-free filtrates, transfer of the filtrate to the erlenmeyer flask for titration, and measuring of standard solutions and diphenylcarbazone indicator. In any of these steps, a pipetting error can cause the entire determination to be in error.

Poor titration techniques are also a cause of error. Improper handling of the buret or carelessness in detecting the end point are common causes of errors.

All reagents used in the chloride determination must be free from any outside chloride contamination. No anticoagulant containing a halogen (chloride, bromide, fluoride, or iodide) can be used in the determination without falsely high results. Glassware and pipets must be chemically clean. Sources of chloride contamination in the laboratory are many (including significant amounts in tap water). For this reason, all glassware must be rinsed well with deionized water, and all reagents must be prepared using deionized water.

Reporting Results and Recording Laboratory Data

The usual way of reporting chloride results to the physician is in terms of milliequivalents per liter. This result is reported to the nearest whole number. Laboratory records, however, are recorded in milliequivalents per liter to the nearest 0.1. Results are reported to the physician only when the control specimen value checks out.

Normal Values

For serum and plasma: 100 to 106 meq/liter
For cerebrospinal fluid: 110 to 130 meq/liter

BLOOD GLUCOSE

One of the most commonly performed chemistry determinations is the test for blood glucose. Although several different methods are used to measure quantitatively the amount of glucose in a blood specimen, in almost all these methods the photometer is used. Because the test is so common and because the techniques involved in most of the methods are basic to so many other types of laboratory procedures, the blood glucose determination will be discussed in some detail.

Carbohydrates are organic compounds containing carbon, hydrogen, and oxygen. They serve as the principal source of energy for the life processes carried on by the body. The carbohydrates include the sugars and compounds that yield sugar on hydrolysis. Glucose, also known as dextrose, is the common sugar of the body and of the blood. It is the one usually given when an intravenous solution of sugar is desired.

Under ordinary conditions, the concentration of sugar in the blood is kept within a narrow range by an elaborate system of mechanisms. Some of the mechanisms used by the body to keep the glucose within this range are the ability of the intestine to absorb glucose, the ability of the liver to store and break down glycogen (the form in which the glucose is stored in the body), the mass of skeletal muscles, and the production and release of insulin by the pancreas.

Most of the common methods for determination of blood glucose make use of the fact that glucose contains an aldehyde group and thus has

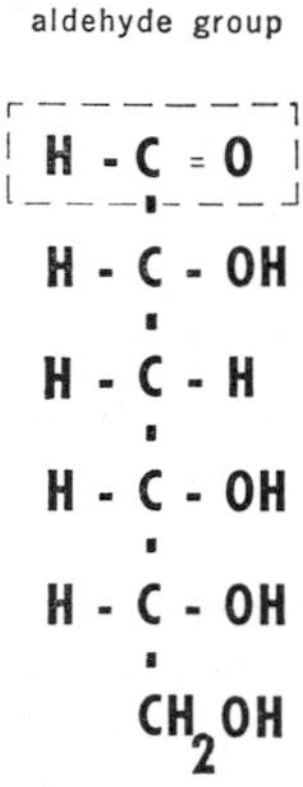

aldehyde group

$$H - C = O$$
$$H - C - OH$$
$$H - C - H$$
$$H - C - OH$$
$$H - C - OH$$
$$CH_2OH$$

Fig. 2-12. Glucose molecule.

reducing properties (Fig. 2-12). Other substances in blood also have re-ducing properties. Some of these nonglucose reducing substances (NGRS) are proteins, uric acid, creatine, and creatinine. The many different meth-ods devised for the determination of blood glucose differ primarily in the manner in which they handle the nonglucose reducing substances. When the nonglucose reducing substances are removed as part of a glucose determination, the resulting value is called the "true glucose" value.

SPECIMENS

The amount of glucose in the blood increases following a meal. It is therefore important that the test be run only on fasting blood specimens. A random sample of blood is of little value for a glucose determination. The blood should be drawn sufficiently long after the last meal, so that the food is completely digested and absorbed and any excess stored. The specimen for a blood glucose test is usually drawn in the morning before breakfast and is called a *fasting blood sugar,* or FBS. The term "fasting" in this case means that the patient has had not only no breakfast but also no cream or sugar, no tea or cola drink, no drugs that might affect the blood glucose level, and no emotional disturbances that might cause liberation of glucose into the blood.

Routine blood sugar determinations are made on specimens of whole blood. When plasma or serum is used, the sugar concentration will average approximately 20 mg/100 ml higher than for whole blood. If plasma or serum is used in place of whole blood, this fact should be noted on the report slip sent out with the result.

As mentioned previously, glucose, being a carbohydrate, is utilized by many body tissues to form energy. It is constantly being removed and added to the blood. The glucose not being used is stored in the liver as glycogen. There are many enzymes present in the blood, particularly in the red cells, which use glucose. As whole blood is allowed to stand at room temperature in a test tube outside the body, these enzymes continue their destructive action, and the glucose disappears. This action is called *glycolysis*. Steps must be taken to prevent glycolysis from taking place in order to provide a reliable specimen on which to perform the test. Blood samples for glucose analysis should be delivered to the laboratory as soon as possible after being drawn from the patient. A protein-free filtrate should be prepared as soon as possible. In the filtrate stage, the concentration of glucose is kept relatively stable.

Using a special anticoagulant for blood glucose specimens seems to be the best way to preserve the concentration of glucose. The anticoagulant used is sodium fluoride. Sodium fluoride acts in two ways to preserve the glucose concentration: it acts as an anticoagulant by tying up the calcium and thus preventing the clotting mechanism from taking place, and it is an enzyme poison. The fluoride is the enzyme inhibitor; it poisons the enzymes so that they cannot destroy the glucose. In this way, glycolysis is prevented. When the blood sample is placed in the sodium fluoride tubes, thorough mixing must take place in order to ensure the proper effect. If sodium fluoride is used as the anticoagulant, it must be remembered that this same specimen cannot be used for any urea nitrogen method using urease (see under Urea Nitrogen). Urease is an enzyme and will also be destroyed by the fluoride.

If an anticoagulant other than sodium fluoride is used, such as potassium oxalate, the filtrate must be set up within 30 minutes after the blood has been drawn. If more than 30 minutes elapses, glycolysis will already have set in, and the glucose will disappear at a steady rate. The result for the glucose concentration will be invalid if such a specimen is used in the determination.

Refrigeration of the specimen can retard glycolysis, but even during refrigeration some glycolysis can occur.

METHODS FOR QUANTITATIVE DETERMINATION

As stated previously, most of the determinations for blood glucose depend on the fact that glucose contains an aldehyde group as part of its chemical structure, and the presence of this aldehyde gives glucose its reducing properties (Fig. 2-12). Of the many methods available for the determination of blood glucose, one reduction method employs potassium ferricyanide, and another uses alkaline copper solutions. In either case, the glucose acts to reduce the reagent to a lower oxidation product. This product is then analyzed by colorimetric means. A few glucose methods depend upon the direct reaction of glucose with certain organic reagents.

Another group of methods uses the enzyme glucose oxidase. This enzyme acts specifically on glucose and catalyzes the oxidation of glucose to gluconic acid and hydrogen peroxide. A peroxidase reagent is then added which serves to oxidize toluidine blue O to give a blue-colored compound.[6]

NELSON-SOMOGYI METHOD

The Nelson-Somogyi method[7-9] is a method widely used in clinical laboratories. It employs the reduction of an alkaline copper solution.

Principle

This method makes use of the fact that glucose contains an aldehyde group and thus has reducing properties. Blood proteins also contain reducing substances and therefore must be removed before the glucose can be measured. Before beginning the determination, the protein is removed by preparation of a protein-free filtrate. Protein, if present, will interfere with the reaction. There are many ways of precipitating protein; the Nelson-Somogyi method calls for the use of barium hydroxide and zinc sulfate, forming zinc hydroxide and barium sulfate. This method produces filtrates which are almost free from reducing substances other than glucose. Uric acid and protein are completely removed in this procedure. Thus, this filtrate gives a nearly true glucose value. Filter paper used in this precipitation step must be checked and must be free from outside contamination.

The Nelson-Somogyi method is accurate, simple, and convenient. It can be used with specimens of whole blood, serum, plasma, or cerebrospinal fluid.

After the protein-free filtrate has been prepared, the reduction step takes place. In a hot alkaline solution, the glucose present in the filtrate reduces cupric (Cu II) salts to cuprous (Cu I) salts. The amount of cuprous salts formed will be in direct relationship to the amount of glucose present in the specimen. The necessary heat is provided by a boiling-water bath. The alkalinity is provided in the copper reagent, which is prepared fresh daily in a working reagent form.

Arsenomolybdic acid is employed as a color-producing reagent. The acid is partially reduced by the cuprous salts, formed in the reduction step, to lower oxidation products of a blue color. The amount of blue present is measured in a photometer. The intensity of this blue is a measure of the amount of copper reduced to the cuprous state and, therefore, of the amount of glucose originally present in the blood specimen. The intensities of the colors of the specimens to be measured are compared in a photometer with the color formed in a series of standard tubes.

The reactions taking place in the Nelson-Somogyi method are given below in equation form:

1. Glucose (in filtrate) + Cu II $\xrightarrow[\text{solution}]{\text{hot, alkaline}}$ Cu I + oxidized glucose

2. Cu I + arsenomolybdic acid → Cu II + reduced arsenomolybdate

    (blue, stable color)

Reagents

For the preparation of the protein-free filtrate:

1. Five percent zinc sulfate. Dissolve 100 g of $ZnSO_4 \cdot 7H_2O$, and dilute to 2,000 ml in a graduated cylinder using deionized water.

2. 0.3 N barium hydroxide. Dissolve 90 g of $Ba(OH)_2 \cdot 8H_2O$ in water, and dilute to 2,000 ml in a graduated cylinder. Filter if cloudy. Store in tight polyethylene containers filled to capacity.

Concentrations of the solutions of zinc sulfate and barium hydroxide are not as important as the fact that they exactly neutralize each other. To titrate, measure 10 ml of zinc sulfate solution into a 250-ml flask, and add 50 ml water and 4 drops of 1% phenolphthalein. Add barium hydroxide dropwise from the buret using continual agitation until the end point is reached. If the barium hydroxide is added too rapidly, a false end point will be reached. Dilute the stronger solution so that 10 ml of zinc solution requires 10 ml of barium solution ±0.05 ml.

For the reduction process:

1. Copper reagent, solution A. Dissolve 50 g of Na_2CO_3 (anhydrous), 50 g of Rochelle salts (potassium sodium tartrate), 40 g of $NaHCO_3$, and 400 g of Na_2SO_4 (anhydrous) in about 1,600 ml of deionized water, and dilute to 2 liters. Filter if necessary. Store this solution where the temperature will not fall below 20°C. A sediment may form after a few days. This may be filtered off without detriment to the reagent.

2. Copper reagent, solution B. Dissolve 150 g of $CuSO_4 \cdot 5H_2O$ in a liter of deionized water. Add 0.5 ml of concentrated H_2SO_4.

3. Alkaline copper reagent. This must be prepared fresh each day. Measure 4 ml of solution B into a 100-ml volumetric flask, and dilute to 100 ml with solution A. Mix well.

This reagent provides the copper ions necessary for the glucose to reduce. It contains sodium carbonate to provide the proper alkalinity and Rochelle salts to keep the copper in solution.

4. Glucose stock standard (10 mg of glucose/ml). Dissolve 1 g of standard, pure, anhydrous glucose in a small amount of deionized water, and dilute to 100 ml with saturated benzoic acid. A saturated solution of benzoic acid can be prepared by dissolving 10 g of benzoic acid in a liter of heated deionized water. Some crystals of benzoic acid should remain to ensure that the solution is saturated.

5. Glucose intermediate standard (0.5 mg of glucose/ml). Dilute 5 ml of glucose stock standard to 100 ml with saturated benzoic acid. Prepare this solution once a week.

6. Glucose working standards. These must be prepared daily. Prepare four working standards by pipetting 1 ml, 2 ml, 3 ml, and 4 ml of intermediate glucose standard into 10-ml volumetric flasks. Dilute to volume with deionized water. The concentrations of these working standards are

0.05 mg of glucose/ml (S_1), 0.10 mg of glucose/ml (S_2), 0.15 mg of glucose/ml (S_3), and 0.20 mg of glucose/ml (S_4).

The working standards are used to construct the standard curve from which the unknown values are calculated. The working standards deteriorate and cannot be used for more than 1 day.

7. Control solution. This is commercially obtained or made by the laboratory by pooling glucose filtrates over a period of time, freezing, thawing, and mixing, dividing into 5-ml aliquots, and using as a control after establishing the control limit of values.

For the color development stage:

Arsenomolybdate color reagent. Dissolve 100 g of ammonium molybdate in 1,800 ml of deionized water, add 84 ml of concentrated H_2SO_4, and mix. Add 12 g of $Na_2HAsO_4 \cdot 7H_2O$ dissolved in 100 ml of water. Mix, and place in an incubator at 37°C for 24 to 48 hours. Store in a glass-stoppered brown bottle. This reagent is stable indefinitely.

Procedure

Results with the Nelson-Somogyi method are precise within 5%. This method can be used for spinal fluid glucose determinations as well as for whole blood, serum, or plasma. Whole blood, however, is the specimen of choice.

Preparation of Protein-free Filtrates

1. Prepare a barium hydroxide–zinc sulfate filtrate by pipetting the following into a clean, dry test tube:

7.5 ml deionized water.

0.5 ml blood. Cork and mix well.

1.0 ml $Ba(OH)_2$. Cork and mix.

1.0 ml $ZnSO_4$. Cork and mix thoroughly.

2. Mix after each addition, and filter through filter paper into a labeled test tube. Other dilutions may be made, where necessary. The filtrate should be clear and colorless.

Preparation of Reagents

These are to be made fresh daily.

1. Alkaline copper reagent
2. Working glucose standards (S_1, S_2, S_3, and S_4)

Reduction of Copper II to Copper I by Glucose

1. Pipet 1 ml of filtrates, controls, and working standards into Folin-Wu tubes. Pipet 1 ml of deionized water into one tube to serve as a blank. Folin-Wu tubes are specially constructed tubes with a constriction near the bulb end to prevent air from getting into the contents of the tube. Any oxygen present in the air would tend to reoxidize the copper as

it is being reduced by the glucose. Into these special tubes are pipetted the filtrates, control, and standards, plus the alkaline copper reagent. The reduction process takes place in the Folin-Wu tube. The fluid level in the tubes must be below the constriction in the tube and below the boiling-water level.

2. Add 1 ml of alkaline copper reagent, and mix well by hitting the tubes against the hand.

3. Place the tubes in a boiling-water bath for 20 minutes. During the boiling process, the copper is reduced, with the aid of heat and alkalinity, by glucose from its cupric form to cuprous oxide. This settles as a fine yellow or orange precipitate.

4. Remove the tubes from the boiling-water bath after 20 minutes, and immediately place them in a cold-water bath for 1 minute. The timing of boiling and cooling is critical and must be watched carefully. If over-cooled, copper I will reoxidize to copper II by action of oxygen in the air.

Color Development

1. Add 1 ml of arsenomolybdate color reagent to all tubes, and mix by hitting against the hand. The color develops very rapidly and will be completed by the time mixing and evolution of carbon dioxide are completed (carbon dioxide evolves as the color develops). The mixture will appear to foam during this process. Vigorous agitation is necessary to ensure complete reaction. The arsenomolybdate should be added to the Folin-Wu tubes as soon as possible.

2. A deep blue color is the result of reduction of arsenomolybdate. This color is stable indefinitely. The intensity of the blue color is directly proportional to the amount of glucose originally present in the specimen.

3. Dilute the Folin-Wu tubes to 25 ml (these tubes have a calibration mark on them to assist in the dilution step) with deionized water. Cork and mix thoroughly. Transfer to labeled calibrated cuvettes for reading in the photometer.

Reading Tubes in the Photometer

1. Polish the cuvettes.

2. Read in the photometer using a wavelength setting of 505 mμ.

3. The color is very stable, and the tubes, therefore, may be read in the photometer at any time.

4. Enter galvanometer readings for standards, controls, and unknowns on a work sheet. Prepare a standard graph, and calculate the milligrams of glucose per 100 ml of blood.

Calculations

Blood glucose results are reported in units of milligrams of glucose per 100 ml of blood, or mg%. These units are used to report many of the common chemistry values determined by the laboratory. The calculating of glucose results, like other results, is a stepwise procedure:

1. *To determine how much of the specimen was actually used in the procedure:*

In this procedure, 0.5 ml of blood is used to prepare the protein-free filtrate. This 0.5 ml is diluted to a total of 10 ml by the addition of 7.5 ml of water, 1.0 ml of barium hydroxide, and 1.0 ml of zinc sulfate. Of the resulting protein-free filtrate, 1 ml is pipetted into the Folin-Wu tube for the reduction process. These factors must be taken into consideration in the final calculation. The 1 ml of filtrate used in the Folin-Wu tube is the actual amount of specimen treated in the determination steps: copper reduction, color development, and analysis in the photometer. Using the following formula, the amount of blood actually being measured in the photometer cuvette and the amount which the percent transmission reading represents is found:

$$\frac{0.5 \text{ ml blood}}{10 \text{ ml filtrate}} = \frac{x \text{ ml blood}}{1 \text{ ml filtrate}}$$

$$x = 0.05 \text{ ml blood/ml filtrate}$$

The final result is reported in units of glucose present in 100 ml of blood, however, so that another step is necessary in these calculations.

2. *To determine how many milligrams of glucose is present in 100 ml of blood (units known as mg%):*

The value read from the standard graph is the milligrams of glucose in 1 ml of filtrate or in 0.05 ml of blood. Using the following formula the glucose value in mg% may be found:

mg glucose/0.05 ml blood (read from standard graph)

$$\times \frac{100 \text{ ml blood}}{0.05 \text{ ml blood}} = \text{mg}\%$$

If any other dilutions have been made during the procedure, this must be taken into consideration in the calculations. In cases of high blood glucose values, dilutions are often made.

Technical Factors and Sources of Error

Causes of poor duplicates or inaccurate results are many. Pipetting errors in preparing the filtrates, in pipetting the standards, controls, and filtrates, or in preparing the reagents are one major cause of inaccurate results. Adequate mixing is another important step; if mixing is not done correctly, this can lead to difficulties. Whenever a reagent is added to another mixture (copper reagent or arsenomolybdate reagent, for example), adequate mixing of the contents of the tube is essential. If the photometer is not used correctly or if the blank tube is not adjusted properly at the beginning of the readings, the end results will be inaccurate.

Sodium fluoride is recommended as the anticoagulant of choice for blood glucose determinations. If another type of anticoagulant is used, the protein-free filtrate must be set up within 30 minutes after the blood has been drawn.

It is important that the timing during reduction of copper in the water bath be watched carefully. It is also important that the water be actually boiling in order to ensure complete reduction. The cold-water bath is also essential, as it stops the reaction.

The standards used for the procedure must be in good condition. The standards must be run at the same time as the rest of the batch, and if another batch is run later in the day, new standards must be run.

For any specimen with a glucose concentration that is higher than that of the most concentrated standard, special steps must be followed. The value of such a specimen cannot be read from the standard graph for this batch. If this be the case, a dilution of the filtrate is made. For a 1:2 dilution, use 1 ml of filtrate and 1 ml of deionized water. For a 1:5 dilution, use 1 ml of filtrate and 4 ml of deionized water. The dilution made will depend on the concentration of glucose present in the specimen. One milliliter of this dilution is pipetted into a Folin-Wu tube, and this is run, along with a blank, standards, and controls, in the regular manner. The standard graph is prepared and the unknown value read from it. The additional dilution factor must be applied in the final calculation of the glucose value. Making a dilution of the colored solution in the cuvette is not enough. A filtrate dilution must be made. In cases of high blood glucose levels, there is not enough copper present in the copper reagent to be completely reduced by the amount of glucose present in the specimen. To allow for this possibility, a diluted filtrate is recommended.

Reporting Results and Recording Laboratory Data

The usual way of reporting glucose results is in milligrams percent. This result is reported to the nearest whole number. The laboratory retains the standard graphs, along with the galvanometer readings obtained for a particular procedure for a period of time. The actual results are kept by the laboratory indefinitely as a permanent record. The results are reported to the physician only when the control values check out.

Normal Values

For blood glucose: 65 to 90 mg%
For cerebrospinal fluid glucose: 40 to 75 mg%

CLINICAL SIGNIFICANCE

Glucose is one of the few chemical constituents of the blood that can change rapidly and dramatically in concentration. There are many diseases which cause a change in glucose metabolism, but the most frequent cause of an increase in the blood glucose is diabetes mellitus.

In diabetes mellitus, the ability of the body to oxidize sugar is reduced. Diabetes mellitus is also associated with a relative or absolute deficiency of insulin. The control of the disease is by evaluation of the effect of various dosages of insulin and composition of diet on the blood glucose level. The result of uncontrolled diabetes mellitus is a high blood glucose level with glucose subsequently appearing in the urine. In a diabetic patient, the glucose concentration can attain a very high or a very low level. At either of these stages, the patient may be in a state of unconsciousness. It is therefore necessary for the physician to know whether this coma is due to a high glucose concentration (called *diabetic coma*) or a low glucose concentration (called *insulin shock*). It is the responsibility of the laboratory to get the result of the glucose determination to the physician as soon as possible, so that the correct treatment can be started. In this type of emergency glucose determination, the test must be run rapidly but with the utmost accuracy, as error or delay may have a serious effect.

The detection of a low blood glucose level is important to the physician in cases of liver disease and tumor of the pancreas. There are numerous cases of high blood glucose value due to conditions other than diabetes mellitus. Some of these are traumatic injury to the brain, febrile disease, certain liver diseases, and hyperthyroidism.

UREA NITROGEN

One of the most important chemical tests done to detect cases of kidney damage and kidney disease is the test for urea nitrogen. This test is performed routinely in all laboratories and is one which any student in clinical laboratory procedures should learn how to run accurately. The techniques involved in performing the blood urea nitrogen test are quite basic to many other procedures done in the chemistry laboratory. The method to be discussed in this section involves the use of the photometer as the device for accurate quantitative measurement and the use of an enzyme reaction procedure (see under Methods for Quantitative Determination).

Nitrogen (N) exists in the body in many forms, most of them being as components of complex substances. Nitrogen-containing substances are classified in two main groups: protein nitrogen (nitrogen which is found in protein) and nonprotein nitrogen (nitrogen-containing substances which are not protein). The nonprotein nitrogen, or NPN, is the nitrogen of whole blood that is not precipitated by the usual protein-precipitating reagents.

In the human being, nonprotein nitrogen is found in urea, uric acid, creatinine, creatine, amino acid, and other substances. For analysis of these or for nonprotein nitrogen as a whole, all protein must first be removed from the sample.

Normally, urea comprises about 45 percent of the total nonprotein nitrogen. The concentration of nonprotein nitrogen is, therefore, determined predominantly by the concentration of urea. In a healthy individual, amino acids comprise about 20 percent and uric acid about 20 percent of the total nonprotein nitrogen.

Since urea is the chief component of the nonprotein nitrogenous material in the blood, it is also quantitatively the most important. Urea is the chief end product of protein metabolism. It is distributed throughout the total body water and is of equal concentration in the intracellular and extracellular fluid. Gross alterations in the nonprotein nitrogen usually reflects a change in the concentration of urea. Because the concentration of urea is directly related to protein metabolism, the protein content of the diet will affect the amount of urea in the blood. The ability of the kidneys to remove the urea from the blood will also affect the urea content. However, the urea concentration is primarily influenced by the protein intake. In the normal kidney, the urea is removed from the blood and excreted in the urine. If kidney function is impaired, the urea will not be removed from the blood, and the result will be a high urea concentration in the blood.

The liver is the sole site of urea formation. It is the only organ which contains all the necessary enzymes needed for the formation of urea.

SPECIMENS

Specimens of whole blood, serum, or plasma may be used for this determination. They will all give much the same value. However, by convention, whole blood is usually tested. The use of whole blood requires an anticoagulant. The choice of anticoagulants is very important, as certain of the available anticoagulants will produce interfering reactions. One anticoagulant which is used frequently and with good results is potassium oxalate. Sodium fluoride anticoagulants must not be used for urea nitrogen procedures employing an enzyme reaction. Many of the more common methods of urea nitrogen determination use the enzyme urease in their reactions, and any enzyme present will be destroyed by fluoride, with falsely low results. Another anticoagulant which should not be used is "double oxalate," or potassium and ammonium oxalate. The ammonium slats present in this anticoagulant will also be measured in the determination (most determinations ultimately measure ammonium present), and falsely high urea nitrogen values will be seen.

After being properly collected and preserved, the blood may be safely kept in a refrigerator for at least 72 hours without measurable change in the urea nitrogen concentration.

METHODS FOR QUANTITATIVE DETERMINATION

A wide variety of methods have been devised for the determination of urea nitrogen. Some of these methods may be performed directly on whole blood, serum, or plasma, while others require a protein-free filtrate. The variety of methods available would indicate that the ideal method has not yet been found.

The group of manual methods used most frequently to determine urea nitrogen concentration, and the most reliable, are those requiring the addition of the enzyme urease to whole blood. During incubation, urea is converted to ammonium carbonate by urease. The ammonia in the ammonium carbonate is analyzed in one of three ways: (1) a protein-free filtrate is prepared, a portion is treated with Nessler's reagent to develop a color, and the color formed is measured using a photometer; (2) the blood is transferred to the Van Slyke apparatus for gas analysis; or (3) the blood is alkalinized, the ammonia aerated into an acid solution, and a titration performed. Whenever a protein-free filtrate is required, one may be prepared by using either the tungstic acid or the barium hydroxide–zinc sulfate methods.

The method involving Nessler's reagent is used most commonly. Nessler's reagent splits the ammonium carbonate to form ammonia and carbon dioxide. The reagent then reacts with the ammonia to produce a yellow color. This color is measured in a photometer and compared with standard solutions which also have been treated with Nessler's reagent.

The enzyme urease is obtained from jack beans, sword beans, or soybeans. It can be purchased in tablet form or in powder form. Urease is capable of hydrolyzing the urea to ammonium carbonate according to the reaction

$$CO(NH_2)_2 + 2H_2O \xrightarrow{\text{urease}} (NH_4)_2CO_3$$

Urea   Ammonium carbonate

This reaction is complete and highly specific. Only at a certain pH and temperature will the urease convert urea into ammonium carbonate. The amount of urease recommended in the procedure to be used, along with the incubation times and temperature, is adequate to deal with any concentration of urea that may occur in human blood. Urease obeys the general laws of most enzymes. Enzymes are protein in nature; therefore, urease is a protein. Any of the urease which is not used in the hydrolyzing step is removed in the protein-precipitation step.

The substance on which an enzyme acts is called the *substrate*. The new substance formed as a result of enzyme reaction is called the *end product*. In the urea nitrogen procedure, the substrate is the urea, and the end product is the ammonium carbonate.

There are many factors which affect the action of the enzyme. The concentration of the substrate is one factor which can affect enzyme action, although only in certain instances does this affect it to any degree. The concentration of the enzyme is very important. The speed of the reaction is proportional to the concentration of the enzyme. Therefore, in a clinical laboratory procedure employing enzyme reactions, the concentration of the enzyme must be constant.

The pH is also an important factor to consider. Every enzyme has an optimum pH at which it is most efficient. The optimal pH for urease activity is approximately 7. A buffer is present in the urease solution used in most urea nitrogen procedures to ensure that the pH is kept constant.

The temperature used for the enzyme reaction is another important factor. There is a definite relationship between temperature and activity of the enzyme. The speed of such reactions is increased two to three times for each 10°C rise in temperature. This rate of increase is known as the Q^{10}. Each enzyme has its own particular Q^{10}. The Q^{10} is usually around 2 for most enzymes. If the Q^{10} is 2, this means that for each 10°C rise in temperature, the activity of the enzyme is doubled. If the Q^{10} is 3, for each 10°C rise in temperature the activity of the enzyme is tripled. Each enzyme also has its optimal temperature. The optimal temperature is that temperature at which the greatest amount of substrate is changed per unit time. In other words, the highest temperature at which the enzyme will react without danger of being inactivated is its optimal temperature. The optimal temperature for urease is 48 to 50°C. Above 55°C, the urease begins to be destroyed because of its protein nature.

There is a definite relationship between time and enzyme activity. A given amount of enzyme will decompose a given amount of substrate (urea, in the case of this discussion) per minute. Therefore, the enzyme reaction must be stopped at a definite time.

The presence of enzyme poisons or inhibitors must be avoided in using any procedure employing enzyme reactions. If such an inhibitor is present, the reaction will not take place satisfactorily. One enzyme inhibitor already discussed is the fluoride present in the anticoagulant sodium fluoride used in the glucose procedure. For this reason, sodium fluoride must not be used as an anticoagulant for specimens in any urea nitrogen procedure employing the enzyme urease. Other enzyme inhibitors are mercury, gold, silver, and ultraviolet light. Any substance that precipitates protein would stop the enzyme action also.

UREA NITROGEN METHOD EMPLOYING COLOR DEVELOPMENT WITH NESSLER'S REAGENT

Since color development with Nessler's reagent[10] is the most commonly used method for determination of urea nitrogen, this method is described in detail in the paragraphs that follow.

Principle

Whole blood (preserved with potassium oxalate) is incubated with urease, which breaks down urea to form ammonium carbonate. From this incubated blood, a modified Folin-Wu filtrate is prepared. Nessler's reagent is added to the protein-free filtrate. In the alkaline pH of Nessler's reagent, the ammonium carbonate forms ammonium ions and carbon dioxide. The ammonium ions combine with the mercury–potassium iodide complex in Nessler's reagent to form a yellow-colored compound. The intensity of the yellow color developed is compared with that formed in a series of standard tubes containing ammonium sulfate which has been nesslerized.

The reactions taking place in this procedure are given below:

1. $$CO(NH_2)_2 + 2H_2O \xrightarrow{\text{urease}} (NH_4)_2CO_3$$
   Urea (in whole blood) $\qquad$ Ammonium carbonate

2. Protein-free filtrate is prepared using modified Folin-Wu method.

3. $$(NH_4)_2CO_3 + \text{Nessler's reagent} \xrightarrow[\text{pH}]{\text{alkaline}} NH_4^+ + CO_2$$

4. NH_4^+ + mercury–potassium iodide complex $\rightarrow$ yellow compound
   (in Nessler's Reagent)

Reagents

All reagents must be prepared using ammonia-free water.

For incubation of blood with the enzyme urease:

1. Stock urease solution. Two percent jack bean urease prepared from powder (available from Sigma Chemical Company, St. Louis, Missouri).

2. Phosphate buffer (pH 7.0). Prepare $M/15$ primary phosphate by weighing 9.0 g of KH_2PO_4 per liter. Prepare $M/15$ secondary phosphate by weighing 9.47 g of anhydrous Na_2HPO_4 per liter. To make 1 liter of buffer (pH 7.0), mix 389 ml of $M/15$ KH_2PO_4 and 611 ml of $M/15$ Na_2HPO_4; check the pH of the resulting solution on a pH meter. The acceptable range is pH 6.95 to 7.05.

3. Working urease solution. This solution must be prepared fresh each day. Mix 1 part of stock urease solution, 2 parts of phosphate buffer (pH 7.0), and 2 parts of ammonia-free water.

4. Stock urea solution (1 ml = 10 mg of nitrogen). Dissolve 2.143 g of urea in ammonia-free water, and dilute to 100 ml.

5. Urea working solution (1 ml = 1 mg of nitrogen). Dilute 10 ml of the stock urea solution to 100 ml with ammonia-free water.

For preparation of the protein-free filtrate:

1. 0.095 N H_2SO_4.

2. Ten percent sodium tungstate. Weigh 10 g of sodium tungstate, and dilute to 100 ml with ammonia-free water.

For color development:

1. Stock ammonium sulfate standard (1 ml = 1 mg of nitrogen). Dis-

solve 4.7165 g of $(NH_4)_2SO_4$ (dessicated overnight) in ammonia-free water, and dilute to 1 liter.

2. Working ammonium sulfate standard (1 ml of 0.01 mg of nitrogen). Dilute 1 ml of the stock standard solution to 100 ml with ammonia-free water.

3. Stock Nessler's reagent. Buy commercially available Nessler's reagent powder, and prepare it by following directions on the bottle.

4. One percent potassium gluconate. Dissolve 2 g of potassium gluconate in ammonia-free water, and dilute to 200 ml. Store in refrigerator. Make a fresh solution weekly.

5. 2.5% potassium persulfate. Dissolve 5 g of potassium persulfate in ammonia-free water, and dilute to 200 ml. Make a fresh solution weekly. Store in refrigerator. During warm weather, remove the solution only long enough to measure the amount required, because decomposition is rapid at high temperatures.

6. Working Nessler's reagent. Mix 1 part of 1% potassium gluconate and 1 part of 2.5% potassium persulfate. Pour this mixture into an equal volume of stock Nessler's solution (1 part gluconate, 1 part persulfate, and 2 parts Nessler's). This mixture must be used within 15 minutes after it is prepared.

Stock urease may be made from soybean meal instead of jack bean meal. It may also be made from urease tablets. The tablets are ground finely and mixed with a specific amount of water. The ammonia-free (double-distilled) water is very important in this procedure and must be used wherever water is needed.

The addition of the persulfate and gluconate solution to Nessler's reagent helps to stabilize the final color reaction. The normality of the sulfuric acid used in the protein-precipitating step (0.095 N) is more concentrated than the usual acid used in the modified Folin-Wu filtrate (0.083 N). It must be more concentrated to correct for the water present in the urease solution.

Procedure for Direct Nesslerization Method

This procedure requires the use of a recovery solution, along with a control sample, to ensure that the results will be reliable. The measured sample of recovery solution is added to a control sample or to a known normal blood sample. Theoretically, the amount of nitrogen in the recovery solution added to the control should be recovered at the end of the procedure. That is, none should be lost or gained along the way. The use of a recovery solution checks the accuracy of the method. The recovery solution added is the same substance as is being measured in the sample of unknown concentration. For this procedure, the recovery is a solution of urea which has been accurately prepared and measured.

Incubation with Urease

1. Pipet 1 ml of well-mixed whole blood into labeled test tubes. Treat undetermined specimens and control sample alike. Pipet a duplicate sample of one undetermined specimen and the control.

2. To one of the control tubes (labeled "R") pipet 0.2 ml of working urea solution (the recovery solution). This must be done very carefully, as the accuracy of the whole batch depends on it. Mix well.

3. To each of the tubes add 1 ml of working urease solution (this solution must be prepared fresh each day). Mix by shaking. Do not invert.

4. Immediately place tubes in a water incubator having a temperature of 48 to 50°C.

5. Incubate the tubes for 15 minutes. Shake the tubes every 5 minutes. Do not invert. At the end of the 15 minutes, remove the tubes, and immediately go on with the next step.

Preparation of Protein-free Filtrates

1. Immediately after removing the tubes from the incubator, add 7 ml of 0.095 N H_2SO_4. Cork and mix well by inversion.

2. Add 1 ml of 10% Na_2WO_4. Cork the tubes and shake vigorously.

3. Pour mixture into filter paper previously placed in funnels, and filter into labeled test tubes. The filtrate should be clear and colorless.

Preparation of Reagents

These are to be made fresh daily.
1. Working urease.
2. Working Nessler's reagent. This is stable for 15 minutes only.

Color Development

1. Into labeled photometer cuvettes, pipet:

Tubes	Ammonia-free Water, ml	Standard $(NH_4)_2SO_4$, ml	Filtrate, ml
Blank.............	5		
Standard 1........	4	1	
Standard 3........	2	3	
Standard 5........	....	5	
Control...........	4	....	1
Recovery..........	4	....	1
Unknown..........	4	....	1

2. Cover the tubes with parafilm, hold them firmly, and invert the mixture several times.

3. Prepare working Nessler's reagent.

4. To each photometer cuvette, add 1 ml of working Nessler's reagent. Mix immediately after each addition. Set the timer for 15 minutes after addition of Nessler's reagent.

5. The color formed is stable for at least 1 hour and may be stable for up to 3 hours. Read the photometer cuvettes at the end of the 15-minute waiting period, using a wavelength setting of 505 mμ.

Reading Tubes in the Photometer

1. Polish the tubes.
2. Read them in the photometer using a wavelength setting of 505 mμ.
3. Enter galvanometer readings for standards, control, recovery solution, and undetermined specimens on a work sheet. Prepare a standard graph and calculate the milligrams of urea nitrogen per 100 ml of blood.

Calculations

Urea nitrogen results are reported in units of milligrams percent, or milligrams of urea nitrogen per 100 ml of blood. Several factors must be taken into consideration before the final results can be calculated. The calculation of final results is accomplished by reviewing the various steps taken in the procedure:

1. *To determine how much of the specimen was actually present in the protein-free filtrate:*

In this procedure, 1 ml of whole blood is incubated with 1 ml of working urease solution. After incubation, 7 ml of 0.095 N H$_2$SO$_4$ and 1 ml of 10% Na$_2$WO$_4$ are added. This is a total of 10 ml in the tube. Of this 10 ml, 1 ml of filtrate is pipetted into the photometer curvette. Using the following formula, the amount of blood actually being treated in the photometer cuvette and the amount which the percent transmission reading represents are found:

$$\frac{10 \text{ ml filtrate}}{1 \text{ ml blood}} = \frac{1 \text{ ml filtrate}}{x \text{ ml blood}}$$
$$x = 0.1 \text{ ml blood/ml filtrate}$$

The result read from the graph therefore represents the milligrams of urea nitrogen in 0.1 ml of blood.

2. *To determine how many milligrams of urea nitrogen is present in 100 ml of blood:*

As stated above, the result as read from the graph is the milligrams of urea nitrogen present in 0.1 ml of blood. The following formulas may be used to find the result in milligrams percent:

$$\frac{\text{Graph reading, mg N}}{0.1 \text{ ml blood}} = \frac{x \text{ mg N}}{100 \text{ ml blood}}$$

or

Graph reading, mg N $\times$ (100/0.1) = x mg N per 100 ml blood (mg%)

If any other dilutions have been made during the procedure, this must be accounted for in the calculations.

3. *To calculate the recovery concentration:*

In the beginning of the procedure, 0.2 ml of working urea recovery solution was added to one of the control tubes and labeled "R." The concentration of the working urea solution is 1 mg nitrogen/ml. Therefore, in the 0.2 ml of recovery solution that was added, there is 0.2 mg nitrogen. 0.2 mg of urea nitrogen was added to the R tube and should be measured (or recovered) at the end of the procedure. This tube was diluted through the incubation and preparation of protein-free filtrate steps, as the other tubes were. The resulting total amount in the R tube is, however, 10.2 ml, not 10 ml as it was in the rest of the tubes (the other tubes do not have the addition of the 0.2 ml of working urea solution). To calculate the amount of urea in the 1 ml of filtrate pipetted into the photometer cuvette for the R tube, use the following formula:

$$\frac{10.2 \text{ ml filtrate}}{0.2 \text{ mg N in urea}} = \frac{1 \text{ ml filtrate}}{x \text{ mg N in urea}}$$
$$x = 0.0196 \text{ mg N added to recovery tube}$$

Taking this into consideration, the values obtained for the R tube should be 0.0196 mg nitrogen *more* than for the control tube (the same specimen as used for the R tube, but no recovery solution added). The control value as read from the graph is subtracted from the R tube value as also read from the graph. One hundred percent recovery is 0.0196 mg of nitrogen. Calculate the percent recovery using 0.0196 mg of nitrogen as 100 percent, using the following formula:

$$\frac{0.0196 \text{ mg N}}{100\%} = \frac{\text{mg N actually recovered in determination}}{x\% \text{ recovery}}$$

The acceptable recovery range is from 90 to 110 percent. If the percent recovery is outside these limits, the procedure must be repeated and the results not given out until the recovery is within the limits established. The use of a recovery solution tells us just how good the method really is.

Technical Factors and Sources of Error

The blood specimens must contain no fluoride or ammonium salts. Both will interfere with the final results (the presence of fluoride will give low results and the ammonium salts high results). The glassware used must be free from contamination by substances such as mercury, fluoride, and ammonia compounds. Ammonia-free water must be used to prepare all reagents and for any step in the procedure requiring the use of water. Ammonia-free water can be prepared from tap water by the process of double distillation.

The protein-free filtrates must be clear and colorless. If the urea content is high, the filtrate will be colored with hemoglobin, because the ammonium carbonate formed by the action of the urease will neutralize part of the acid, leaving an insufficient amount for the precipitation of the protein. To a colored filtrate, 2 N H_2SO_4 is added in small drops until all the color has been precipitated.

Dilutions of the filtrates must be prepared in any instance where, in the routine procedure, any unknown filtrate gives a galvanometer reading lower than the most concentrated standard solution used (S_5, in most cases). Using ammonia-free water, 1:5 or 1:10 dilutions of the filtrate are prepared. The color is developed using 1 ml of this diluted filtrate, and a reading is taken with a new set of standards and a blank. This additional dilution factor must be taken into consideration in the final calculations.

Incubation time, temperature, and pH are critical factors in any enzyme reaction. These factors must be watched carefully to ensure good results.

Reporting Results and Recording Laboratory Data

The usual way of reporting urea nitrogen results is in milligrams percent. This result is reported to the nearest whole number. The laboratory retains the standard graph and the work sheet with the galvanometer readings obtained for a particular procedure for a time. The results for the various specimens are recorded permanently in some manner by the laboratory. Results are reported to the physician only when the control values check out and when the recovery is within the acceptable range, 90 to 110 percent for the urea nitrogen procedure.

Normal Values for Direct Nesslerization

The normal range for whole blood urea nitrogen concentration is from 8 to 22 mg%.

CLINICAL SIGNIFICANCE

The concentration of urea in the blood serves as an index of the ability of the kidney to remove waste materials from the blood. An increase in the blood urea nitrogen concentration often indicates kidney damage or disease. The urea itself is not toxic, but its presence is associated with other waste products which are toxic. The term for the condition in which urea is found in the blood in increased amounts is *uremia*. Considerable deterioration of kidney function is usually present before the urea nitrogen level rises above the normal range.

Normally, the urea nitrogen of whole blood varies between 8 and 22 mg%. In early nephritis, the urea nitrogen level may rise to 30 or 40 mg%, but in terminal stages of chronic nephritis and in some cases of acute nephritis marked urea retention may occur. High values may also be found in other conditions associated with damaged renal function. Conditions such as intestinal obstruction, lead poisoning, certain infections, or cardiac failure can cause a rise in the urea nitrogen level in the blood.

A low urea nitrogen level is not usually clinically significant unless a case of liver damage is suspected. The liver is the site of urea formation, and a damaged liver can result in inability to form urea at all.

In summary, the measurement of urea nitrogen, and of nonprotein nitrogen as a whole, is used to determine the function or impairment of the kidney. In the normal kidney, the urea is removed from the blood and excreted in the urine. If the kidney is impaired and not functioning properly, the urea is not removed from the blood, and it accumulates. Thus the urea nitrogen level rises in the blood (uremia occurs). The main purpose of any test for renal function is to determine the nature and extent of the impairment.

TO THE STUDENT LABORATORY TECHNICIAN

It is inevitable that the medical laboratory technician will be called upon to perform other chemistry tests than the ones described in this textbook. For example, the tests for bilirubin and cholesterol are routinely performed, even in physicians' offices. The laboratory technician should be able to apply the basic knowledge learned from this textbook to new laboratory tests. These new tests employ many of the basic principles and techniques which have been covered and which by now should be familiar to the student.

Each new procedure should be approached with a definite pattern in mind. The laboratory technician should be aware of the type of specimen the test requires and should make certain that the specimen is collected, prepared, and preserved properly. Any reagents necessary for the procedure must be prepared by following the directions carefully. The laboratory technician should review the procedure beforehand, and extra research in laboratory medicine textbooks is suggested in regard to clinical implications and background material for the determination. The principle of the test, why the reagents are used and what they do in the reactions that occur, the actual stepwise method to be followed, the technical factors and sources of error for the particular method, the calculations, the reporting of results to the physician, and something about the normal values for the substance to be measured are all essential pieces of information that must be understood by the person performing the test. The three procedures discussed in this chapter (chloride, glucose, and urea nitrogen) were all approached by means of this pattern. By reviewing these three procedures and how they were discussed, the student will be better able to approach a new procedure and, most likely, will do an accurate job in the laboratory analysis too.

A procedure should never become a "cookbook" method. Specific directions are necessary in performing any laboratory determination, but there is so much to know about even the simplest procedure that the directions alone are not enough. It is the job of the well-trained laboratory technician to do some additional research if necessary to gain as much knowledge as possible about every laboratory test that is performed.

REFERENCES

1. Testing of Glass Volumetric Apparatus, *Nat. Bur. Std. Circ.* 602, 1959.
2. Joseph S. Annino, "Clinical Chemistry: Principles and Procedures," 3d. ed., pp. 34–36, Little, Brown and Company, Boston, 1964.
3. O. Folin and H. Wu, A System of Blood Analysis, *J. Biol. Chem.*, 38:81, 1919.
4. Annino, *op. cit.*, p. 86.
5. O. Schales and S. S. Schales, Simple and Accurate Method for Determination of Chloride in Biological Fluids, *J. Biol. Chem.*, 140:879, 1949.
6. Annino, *op. cit.*, p. 134.
7. Norton Nelson, A Photometric Adaptation of the Somogyi Method for the Determination of Glucose, *J. Biol. Chem.*, 153:375, 1944.
8. Michael Somogyi, Determination of Blood Sugars, *J. Biol. Chem.*, 160:169, 1945.
9. *Ibid.*, 195:19, 1952.
10. C. J. Gentzkow, An Accurate Method for the Determination of Blood Urea Nitrogen by Direct Nesslerization, *J. Biol. Chem.*, 143:531, 1942.

BIBLIOGRAPHY

Davidsohn, Israel, and Benjamin B. Wells: "Clinical Diagnosis by Laboratory Methods (Todd-Sanford)," 13th ed, W. B. Saunders Company, Philadelphia, 1962.

Freier, E. F., and V. L. Rausch: Quality Control in Clinical Chemistry, *Am. J. Med. Technol.* vol. 24, 1958.

Hoffman, W. S.: "The Biochemistry of Clinical Medicine," 2d ed., The Year Book Medical Publishers, Inc., Chicago, 1959.

MacFate, Robert P.: "Introduction to the Clinical Laboratory," The Year Book Medical Publishers, Inc., Chicago, 1961.

Oser, Bernard L. (ed.): "Hawk's Physiological Chemistry," 14th ed., McGraw-Hill Book Company, New York, 1967.

Page, Lot B., and Perry J. Culver: "A Syllabus of Laboratory Examinations in Clinical Diagnosis," rev. ed., Harvard University Press, Cambridge, Mass., 1960.

Peters, J. P., and D. D. Van Slyke: "Quantitative Clinical Chemistry," vol. II, "Methods," The Williams & Wilkins Company, Baltimore, 1932.

Reiner, Miriam (ed.): "Standard Methods of Clinical Chemistry," vol. I, Academic Press Inc., New York, 1953.

Simons, J. S., and C. J. Gentzkow: "Medical and Public Health Laboratory Methods," 5th ed., Lea & Febiger, Philadelphia, 1955.

3

Hematology

The word "hematology" comes from the Greek *haima,* meaning "blood," and *-logia,* or *logos,* meaning "discourse" and, hence, "the science of," or "the study of." Hematology is therefore the science, or study, of blood. In a hematology course, the laboratory worker is concerned with the main constituents of the blood. Blood is composed of plasma (55 percent) and cells (45 percent); the plasma is the fluid portion of the blood. The blood cells, or formed elements, to be discussed in this chapter are the red blood cells (called *erythrocytes*), the white blood cells (called *leukocytes*), and the platelets (called *thrombocytes*). The laboratory tests performed by a medical laboratory technician in the area of hematology center around the cells and some of their constituents, such as hemoglobin found in the red blood cell.

Blood functions as a part of the circulatory system of the body. It nourishes the cells of the body. An average adult contains 5 to 6 qt, or 10 to 12 pints, of blood.

Several hematologic tests are required as part of every patient's initial hospital admission report and are also a part of physical examinations done by a physician in his office. For this reason, many hematologic tests are considered "routine" and are definitely the type of test which a laboratory technician with a limited training can very adequately perform. That these tests are done frequently does not mean that they are unimportant. Quite to the contrary, the physician can obtain valuable information about a patient's physical condition from accurately performed routine hematologic determinations.

In this chapter, the student should gain enough basic knowledge concerning the formed elements of the blood, their enumeration, and their characteristics so that routine tests can be performed accurately and conscientiously in the clinical laboratory. This knowledge should include the necessary basic theory of the determinations, use and care of the equipment used to perform the tests, the proper preparation of the reagents used, ability to recognize problems when encountered, proper collection and handling of the specimens, calculation of the results, and an appreciation of the need for accuracy and care in performing any and all hematologic determinations.

Performing accurate hematologic determinations requires repeated practice before any degree of accuracy is attained. The clinical laboratory student should not become discouraged if the first practice periods in the hematology laboratory result in little advancement. Many of the techniques required in performing accurate hematologic determinations are gained only through practice, employing good manual dexterity, and experience in the manipulation of the necessary laboratory equipment.

Clinical application of the various hematologic tests discussed will be found throughout the chapter. Again, it is important that the student remember the reason for the laboratory determination's being ordered in the first place. The *patient* is the ultimate concern of the laboratory and of the physician who uses the information provided by the laboratory.

Procedures performed in the hematology laboratory require microscopic observation, macroscopic observation, and, in some instances, a combination of both. In certain of the routine procedures photometry is used. The discussion of the various hematologic procedures will be grouped according to these broad categories. Since samples for hematologic study are so often obtained by means of a finger prick, a thorough section concerning the collection of specimens and the approach to the patient in general is included in this chapter.

APPROACHING THE PATIENT

Anyone who plans to assume a duty or occupation where contact with patients is required must consider several factors: The medical laboratory technician is providing a service to the patient. The adequate performance of this service involves not only technical knowledge but sincere and concerned interest in human beings. This is a quality which, unfortunately, cannot be taught readily. It is a quality which each one must learn for himself as a part of reaching maturity. Those in the medical laboratory field must not only be academically capable but must also be psychologically adjusted.

When approaching a patient for the first time, there are certain procedures to remember.

First make certain that the patient on whom the test is being done is actually the right patient. Checking the hospital number of the patient is essential. Mix-ups in labeling tubes or in the initial drawing of blood from the wrong patient can be disastrous. Always label tubes of blood at the bedside of the patient, as well as any slides, hemoglobin pipets, white blood cell pipets, or other materials from tests taken. Proper and immediate labeling is essential.

When working with a pediatric patient, you must first gain his confidence. Get acquainted with the child by using a book or a toy, for example. Keep your equipment tray as inconspicuous as possible. Be frank with the child. Sometimes you may be able to tell a story about what you are doing. It is important in working with a pediatric patient to bolster his morale as much as possible. If the child is very small or uncooperative, ask for help in restraining him. Before leaving the room, double-check to make certain that the rails of the bed are up as you found them.

Older children may be more responsive when permitted to "help" by holding the gauze, for example. If your technique is efficient and you talk to the patient convincingly, you will be able to "take a picture from his finger" before he realizes what has happened. Handling a child often involves handling the parents also. This is best accomplished by allowing the parents to know, by your attitude, that you are kind but very definitely in charge of the situation. This attitude so basic for laboratory personnel can be developed only with practice.

In the nursery, each hospital will have its own rules, but a few general precautions apply: After working with an infant in a crib, be sure to put up the crib sides. If an infant is in an Isolette, keep the portholes closed. When an oxygen tent is in use, do not forget to close the openings when you have finished with the baby. Never leave laboratory equipment, especially blades or needles, in the bed or room.

The adult patient must be told briefly what is expected of him and what the test involves. With adults and especially when dealing with children, complete honesty is most important. It is unwise to say that a finger puncture will not hurt, when it really will. However, if it is possible, avoid saying that the puncture will hurt.

When entering the patient's room, greet him in a friendly and tactful manner. Do not become overly familiar; carry on any conversation in a pleasant and calm manner. Tell the patient why you are there and what you are going to do. Speak quietly at all times. Discuss personal information the patient relates to you softly; this is being told to you in confidence. Respect the religious beliefs of the patient. Keep all laboratory reports confidential, and also keep any personal information about the patient confidential. Firmly refuse information about other patients or physicians. If you continue to see the same patient frequently, become familiar with his interests, hobbies, or family and use these as topics of conversation. Many patients in the hospital are lonely and need a friend. Occasionally you will find, especially with extremely ill patients, that the patient does not wish to talk at all; in this case, respect his wishes. Do not irritate the patient. It is important to be honest, but boost his morale as much as possible. Smile, be cordial, and leave the room in a friendly fashion.

Even if the patient is disagreeable (and many are), remain pleasant. It is important to repeat at this point that it is most helpful if you enter the patient's room wearing a pleasant expression; a smile will often work miracles. Be firm when the patient is unpleasant, remain cheerful, and express confidence in the work to be done. Young children who do not understand words seem pacified by the sound of a confident voice. Talking pleasantly to any patient is essential.

Always check before leaving the patient's room to see that you have returned everything to your laboratory tray. Keep the tray holding your supplies and equipment out of reach of the patient. This is especially important when working with children, but it applies to all patients.

Always follow the orders of the hospital or patient station regarding the procedure for isolation patients. Generally there are two types of isolation patients: One called protective isolation is used to protect the patient from outsiders. For example, a burn patient is greatly susceptible to infection, so that anyone entering the room of this type of patient must use isolation procedure. The other type of isolation is used to prevent spread of a communicable disease from a patient. Whether protective or strict isolation is observed, a nurse on the ward will provide instructions about procedure. Follow all instructions of this type explicitly.

COLLECTION OF SAMPLES

There are two general sources of blood for laboratory tests: peripheral, or capillary, blood and venous blood. This statement applies to all areas of the clinical laboratory, not just to the hematology department. Since, however, so many hematologic tests are done on blood obtained by means of a finger prick (capillary blood), proper collection of blood samples in general is discussed in this chapter. Many hematologic determinations require venous blood, which necessitates discussion of the venipuncture technique. Collection of capillary blood (by finger prick) and venous blood (by venipuncture) will be discussed in the following paragraphs.

PERIPHERAL, OR CAPILLARY, BLOOD

For the small quantities of blood required for most hematologic procedures, an adequate sample may be obtained from the capillary bed by puncture of the skin. In adults and older children, the tip of the finger is pricked (Fig. 3-1); in infants, the plantar surface of the heel is pricked. Blood obtained from the puncture of the ear lobe has been found to contain a higher concentration of hemoglobin than fingertip or venous blood and also is not reliable for white blood cell counts.[1] The ear lobe is the desirable source of blood needed for the preparation of blood films used

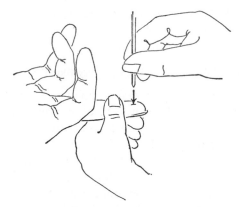

Fig. 3-1. Finger puncture technique.

to study leukocyte abnormalities, since larger cells are frequently trapped in the capillary bed because of the slowed circulation in the ear lobe.

There are various types of lancets or blades used for skin puncture. The best type of blade to use is one which is disposable. Generally, the nondisposable blades are hard to clean and are painful to the patient. Some blades require the operator to gauge the depth of the puncture, while others have a safety gauge on them. It is important that all used blades be destroyed and that none remain in the laboratory. Infectious hepatitis can be transmitted if blades are reused or improperly disposed of.

Procedure for Puncture

1. The area to be punctured must be free from cyanosis or edema. *blueishness* *swelling* The skin is cleansed thoroughly with 70% *isopropl* medicated alcohol. All the necessary pipets, diluents, slides, and other equipment must be ready.

2. The finger or heel is grasped firmly, and a quick, firm puncture *done with a rolling motion* is made approximately 2 mm deep with a sterile, disposable blade. If blood does not flow immediately, the puncture is repeated quickly in the same place. The puncture should be made across the grain of lines in the finger and near the top of the finger, that is, not too far down or too close to the fingernail.

3. The first drop of blood is always removed with gauze or tissue. It is contaminated with the alcohol used to cleanse the finger. The succeeding drops are used for the various tests to be done. *also tissue fluid*

4. A good puncture is freely flowing. If blood does not flow freely, the flow can be coaxed by gentle pressure and release. Excessive squeezing will cause contamination of the blood with tissue fluid. *will make it clot faster + will dilute the sample*

5. With the necessary equipment ready, the blood is pipetted. Rapid pipetting is necessary to prevent coagulation, especially when several tests are to be done using blood from the same puncture. *How do you do rapid pipetting if the blood isn't flowing freely?*

6. When the taking of the sample has been completed, the patient is given a piece of gauze to hold on his finger. The technician remains with the patient until the bleeding ceases.

Precautions to Be Noted When Obtaining Capillary Blood

If the patient's fingers are cold, slight rubbing may help to warm them. The finger or heel must not be squeezed excessively, because tissue fluid may dilute the blood sample or cause the blood to clot faster than it normally would. The first drop of blood is always removed, because it contains tissue fluid, alcohol, or perspiration which will dilute the blood. Immediately after an operation patients with low blood pressure and in surgical shock may require more than one puncture. Only one sterile blade is used at a time. The tip of the blade should not touch anything until it punctures the skin of the patient. Contaminated blades are thrown away and new ones used. After the puncture is made, the blade is disposed of. The laboratory technician must always have clean hands when working with patients.

When blood is taken for blood cell counts and the hemoglobin determination (these tests involve the use of special diluting pipets), the tip of the pipet is placed in the drop of blood. The pipet is not touched to the skin. Usually the hemoglobin test is taken first. The blood measured in the hemoglobin pipet must be put into the diluent immediately and mixed well. It can be read in the photometer later. Hemoglobin pipets require more blood than the red or white cell diluting pipets; that is, a larger drop of blood is required.

White and red cell counts are done next. Blood measured in the red and white cell diluting pipets must be diluted immediately with the proper diluting fluid. After dilution, the pipets must be immediately shaken for 15 seconds. If blood and diluent are not shaken immediately after dilution, proper mixing will not occur, and clots may form. The pipets can then be placed in the equipment tray until there is time to shake them for 5 minutes in the laboratory prior to doing the cell counts.

After the red and white cell counts, any other tests, such as reticulocyte counts, are done. Platelet counts are always done first. The blood films are prepared last, following the directions given under Cell Morphology.

VENOUS BLOOD

There is no significant difference between cell counts from venous blood and capillary blood if freely flowing samples are obtained. When several hematologic procedures are to be carried out, it is often more efficient to collect blood from a vein rather than from the finger. Blood collected in this manner requires an anticoagulant. The choice of anticoagulant is dictated by the test or tests which are to be performed. Two anticoagulants suitable for most hematologic procedures are balanced oxalate (a mixture of ammonium and potassium oxalate) or Sequestrene (or EDTA, disodium ethylenediaminetetracetate). Both these anticoagulants prevent coagulation by binding the calcium. The balanced, or double, oxalate consists of a mixture of 3 parts ammonium oxalate to 2 parts potassium oxalate and has the advantage of preserving the volume of the red blood cells. Two milligrams of the dry mixture is used per milliliter of blood. Oxalated blood may be used for hemoglobin, hematocrit, cell counts, and the erythrocyte sedimentation rate tests but cannot be used for blood films or for platelet counts. Sequestrene has the advantage over balanced oxalate of preserving the white blood cells and the platelets, in addition to the red blood cells. Sequestrene can be used most satisfactorily for blood films and platelet counts as well as for the other tests. One milligram of Sequestrene per milliliter of blood is used.

The veins which are generally used for venipuncture are those in the forearm, wrist, or ankle. The first choice for a venipuncture site are the veins in the forearm, because they are larger than those in the wrist or ankle regions. The wrist and ankle veins are used only if the forearm site is not available.

The venipuncture may be made by either the syringe method or the vacuum tube method. In the syringe method, a needle is attached to a syringe and inserted into the vein. The plunger of the syringe is drawn back, which creates suction drawing the blood into the syringe. In the vacuum tube methods, one end of a two-way needle is partially attached to the rubber stopper of a specially purchased vacuum tube. The other end of the two-way needle is inserted into the vein. The needle in the rubber stopper is pushed through the stopper to make a direct connection to the vacuum tube. The vacuum tube creates a suction which draws the blood into the tube.

When doing a venipuncture, the medical technician should remain in a standing position, which gives the greatest freedom of movement. The patient should assume a comfortable position. Bed patients should remain lying down, and ambulatory patients should be seated. The patient sitting down should put one of his arms on a table or other firm support and extent it for the technician.

The use of a tourniquet is desirable to enlarge the veins, so that they become more prominent. A piece of rubber tubing serves as a tourniquet. It is applied around the arm just above the bend in the elbow and should be just tight enough to stop the blood flow. The patient should also be instructed to clench his fist, to aid in building up the blood pressure in the area of the puncture. The proper way to apply a tourniquet is as follows:

1. Place the tourniquet under the patient's arm just above the bend in the elbow.

2. With each hand grasping the ends of the tourniquet, pull up so

that tension is applied to the tourniquet. This tension must be maintained throughout the procedure.

3. With the proper tension, tie a loop in the tourniquet. Do not tie a bow or a knot. The loop must be made in such a way that it can easily be released when the tourniquet is to be removed.

The most prominent vein is usually chosen for the venipuncture. If the veins are difficult to find, have the patient open and close his fist a few times; this will build up more pressure. The veins can be felt by touching or palpating with the index finger. They reveal themselves as elastic tubes under the surface of the skin. By pressing up and down on the vein gently several times, the path of the vein can be felt.

Once the site for the venipuncture has been chosen and the vein observed or palpated, the area is cleansed with an antiseptic solution. One suitable antiseptic is 70% medicated alcohol. The area of puncture is rubbed thoroughly with the antiseptic. After application of the antiseptic, the area must not be touched until after the actual puncture is made.

To insert the needle properly into the vein, the index finger is placed alongside the hub of the needle with the bevel of the needle facing up. The vein is fixed by grasping the patient's arm with the other hand and pulling the skin taut. This can be accomplished by using the thumb and by placing it about 1 or 2 in. below the puncture site (Fig. 3-2). The needle should be pointing in the same direction as the vein. The syringe or vacuum tube apparatus should be held so that it makes a

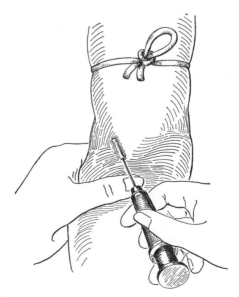

Fig. 3-2. Venipuncture technique.

15-degree angle with the patient's arm. The tip of the needle is then placed on the vein and pushed deliberately forward. When the vein has been punctured and the suitable amount of blood removed into the tube or syringe, the patient releases his clenched fist, the tourniquet is released, gauze moistened with the antiseptic solution or sterile, dry gauze is placed —*QUICKLY* over the puncture site, and the needle is withdrawn slowly. After removing the needle, pressure may be applied on the puncture site using gauze.

It is most important that the tourniquet be released *before* the needle is removed from the vein. If this is not done, excessive bleeding will occur. If the venipuncture is poorly done (if there is trauma to the tissues) a hematoma (collection of blood under the skin) may result. This should be avoided, if at all possible. *as clots form and can travel up the arm to the heart and cause heart attacks*

Procedure for Venipuncture

1. A suitable vein is chosen and the puncture area cleansed.

2. A tourniquet is applied so that it is easily released.

3. The patient's arm is firmly grasped, and the skin over the vein is drawn taut.

4. Using a sharp, dry, sterile needle attached to a dry, clean syringe or vacuum tube, the skin and then the vein are punctured.

5. The desired amount of blood is withdrawn, the tourniquet is released, and the needle is removed from the vein.

6. The flow of blood from the wound is stopped by using pressure with a sterile, dry gauze.

7. If the blood is to be transferred from a syringe into a tube, the needle is first removed and the blood then gently expelled into the tube. This action prevents hemolysis.

SPECIMENS FOR HEMATOLOGY AND THE USE OF ANTICOAGULANTS

After the blood specimen has been collected from the patient, it must be transported to the laboratory for analysis. Assuming that the specimen is properly labeled immediately after drawing and in good condition, it is examined in the laboratory as quickly as possible to prevent deterioration. Laboratory tests are always done on fresh specimens, whenever possible. Special handling of specimens for the various hematologic determinations will be discussed later in this chapter in connection with the specific tests covered.

If the sample has been drawn from the arm by using a syringe and needle or a special vacuum tube device, it must be preserved in some way in order that the required tests be done on unclotted blood. It is often best to do the test on fresh blood obtained from puncture of the patient's finger, but many times this is not feasible, and venipuncture blood must be used. However, only if it is properly preserved can it be used for hematologic studies. Clotted blood cannot be used for tests in hematology; therefore, special anticoagulants must be employed. The anticoagulant used removes, by chemical action, the calcium of the blood so that the clotting mechanism cannot take place.

Only certain anticoagulants are acceptable for hematologic tests. In addition to keeping the blood in a liquid form (preventing clotting), the anticoagulant must maintain the natural appearance of the red blood cells, white blood cells, and platelets. Sequestrene is the only anticoagulant in general use which can do all these things. Another anticoagulant which is used in some laboratories is balanced, or double, oxalate, as mentioned under Collection of Samples. This anticoagulant is a composite of ammonium and potassium oxalate balanced in such a way that the size and shape of the red blood cells are preserved. Balanced oxalate does not preserve the morphologic features of the white blood cells or the platelets and for this reason cannot be used for all the hematologic tests. Sequestrene is the anticoagulant of choice for most routine hematologic tests.

After the blood has been properly drawn and placed in the tube containing the anticoagulant, it should be gently mixed by repeated inversions immediately. This mixing is necessary to ensure thorough contact with the anticoagulant. Clotted specimens are absolutely unacceptable for most tests done in the hematology laboratory, especially cell counts. If there is even a tiny clot in a specimen, the cell count will be grossly inaccurate.

Immediately before a test is performed on a blood specimen, the blood sample must be mixed by repeated inversion for 5 minutes. This can be accomplished by hand or with a mechanical tube inverter. If the blood sample has stood for a few minutes, it should be mixed again for at least 1 minute.

When a preserved blood specimen is allowed to stand for a period of time, the components will settle into three distinct layers: (1) the plasma, or the top layer, (2) the buffy coat, a grayish-white cellular layer composed of the nucleated cells and platelets, and (3) the red blood cells, comprising the bottom layer. There are some hematologic procedures which are based on the ability of the blood specimen to settle into layers when it has been preserved by use of an anticoagulant.

When the blood specimen has been properly drawn and placed in preservative in the prescribed manner, the plasma will have its natural color, a very light yellow or straw hue. There are occasions when the plasma may have an altered color due to a disease process, but there are also changes which can result from improper handling of the specimen by the laboratory worker. The color change most often seen is a red appearance in the plasma due to hemoglobin released into the solution by the breakup of some of the red blood cells. This breakup, or rupturing, of the red cells is called *hemolysis*. Hemolysis is one of the changes due to alterations in the osmotic pressure in the solution surrounding the red cells. Hemolysis can also occur when the membrane surrounding the red cells has been mechanically ruptured.

The principle of osmotic pressure and osmosis is very important whenever a solution or diluent is used as part of a procedure. In many hematologic procedures, diluents are used. In simple terms, osmosis is the passage of a solvent through a membrane from a dilute solution into a more concentrated solution. The difference in concentration of the solutions on each side of the membrane causes the phenomenon called *osmotic pressure.* If the concentrations of the solutions on each side of the membrane are the same, there will not be any pressure. When the concentration is the same in the diluent solution as it is inside the red blood cell, the solution, or diluent, is called an *isotonic* solution. If the diluent solution is less concentrated than the inside of the red blood cell, the solution is called a *hypotonic* one. From the definition of osmosis it can be seen that in the case of a hypotonic solution (dilute), the passage of diluent will be from outside the red cell into the red cell, causing the cell to swell and eventually to rupture, or hemolyze. If the solution on the outside of the red blood cell is more concentrated than that inside the red cell, the outside solution is called *hypertonic.* In the case of a hypertonic solution, the osmosis of the solvent is from the inside of the red cell to the surrounding solution. When this happens, the red cell will shrink from loss of liquid, and it will become crenated.

When red cells are in plasma, they are in an isotonic solution. For this reason, any diluent used to dilute blood in doing the various hematology tests must have the same concentration as plasma. When a solution has the same concentration as, or is isotonic with, plasma, it is called a *physiologic solution.* One very common physiologic solution used in hospitals is isotonic saline solution, a 0.85% solution of sodium chloride. If red blood cells are placed in an isotonic saline solution, their size is preserved. If red cells are placed in a hypotonic solution, that is, one less concentrated than the concentration inside the red cell, the cell will swell until it bursts; that is, hemolysis will take place. Crenation, or shrinking, of the red cell takes place when the cell is placed in a hypertonic solution. Either situation is unsatisfactory for doing accurate hematologic studies.

As previously indicated, in general there are two types of blood samples which are unsuitable for hematology tests: the clotted sample and the hemolyzed sample. Clotted specimens are not suitable for cell counts because the cells are trapped in the clot and therefore not counted. The result of a cell count on a clotted sample will be falsely low. A red appearance of the plasma indicates that hemolysis has taken place. The red cells have burst and are no longer present intact. Red cell counts done on hemolyzed samples will also result in falsely low cell counts.

FORMATION OF THE BLOOD CELLS AND THEIR APPEARANCE

During early fetal life, blood cells are formed in many of the body tissues. During this period, the liver and the spleen are the most active sites of blood cell production, or hematopoiesis. At about the fifth month of fetal life, the bone marrow begins functioning as a blood cell producer. Shortly after birth, under normal conditions, the marrow is the only tissue which continues to produce red cells, granular leukocytes (granulocytes), and platelets. Until the age of five, the marrow in all the bones is red and cellular, and actively produces cells. Between the ages of five and seven years, the long bones become inactive, and fat cells appear to replace the active marrow. Red marrow is gradually displaced by fat cells in the other bones through the maturing years. In other words, red marrow is transformed to yellow marrow. After the ages of eighteen to twenty years, red marrow remains only in the following bones: the vertebrae, the ribs, the sternum, the skull, and partially in the femur and the humerus. Bone marrow aspirations are often taken to detect any abnormal changes in the newly formed cells or in their quantity. Beginning blood disease may be detected by examination of the bone marrow.

The bone marrow produces only the red cells, granulocytes, and platelets. Lymphocytes are produced by the lymphoid tissue (the lymph nodes and nodules, and the spleen). The origin of the monocytes is uncertain.

The red blood cells, or erythrocytes, are biconcave disks which carry hemoglobin, an iron compound which combines chemically with oxygen and carbon dioxide. The red blood cells carry the hemoglobin to and from all parts of the body. The total life span of the red blood cells is about 120 days, making it necessary for the body to release some new red cells into the circulating system every day. There is a never-ending, constant process within the body—formation of new red cells and tearing down the old, worn-out ones, storing the cell components which are reusable, and eliminating the "waste" products resulting from the breakdown of the red cell. The components of the red cell which are reusable and are stored by the body include iron and protein. Other components of the breakdown process are waste products and must be removed from the body. These waste products are called the *bile pigments*. The bile pigments are composed of urobilins and urobilinogens which can be excreted in the urine or the feces (see Chapter 4). A schematic representation of the blood formation and destruction process is seen in Fig. 3-3.

When one of the steps in the blood formation and destruction process is not functioning properly or is occurring too rapidly, a blood disorder will result causing alterations in the other steps as well, since they are all closely related. When tests are performed in the hematology laboratory,

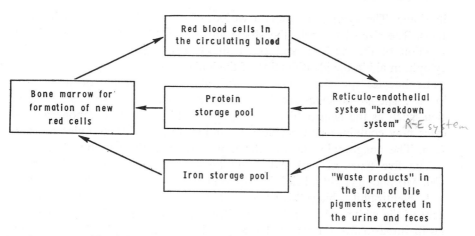

Fig. 3-3. Blood formation and destruction process.

changes in the appearance of the red cell or changes in the manner in which whole blood reacts under certain test conditions are noted in order to determine whether alterations in function have occurred.

Dead red cells are broken down through the reticuloendothelial (R-E) system of the body. The R-E system is composed of many connective tissue cells that carry on phagocytosis, a process by which a cell engulfs, or eats, foreign material. The R-E cells are important in the body's defense mechanism. These cells are located in many sites in the body: in the blood sinusoids (tiny blood vessels), liver, spleen, bone marrow, and lining of the lymph channels in the lymph nodes.

The red blood cell is only one of the three formed elements of the blood. The second formed element to be discussed is the white blood cell, or leukocyte. The leukocytes are nucleated and are a part of the defense mechanism of the body. They are able to engulf and carry away harmful particles, such as bacteria, which may attempt to invade the body. As mentioned previously, this engulfing process is called phagocytosis. Under normal conditions, there are five types of leukocytes found in the blood: lymphocytes, neutrophils, monocytes, eosinophils, and basophils.

When a stained blood film is examined with the microscope, the majority of the cells seen will be the red blood cells. They appear as small, rounded, reddish orange bodies. By far, they are the most numerous of the blood cells seen. Scattered among the red-staining cells are the less numerous leukocytes (white blood cells). These are larger and more complex in appearance than the red blood cells. They consist of the nucleus surrounded by the cytoplasm. Usually the nucleus is in the center of the cell and is a prominent purple-staining body. The nucleus can be round or oval (as in the lymphocyte) or lobulated (as in the neutrophil and eosinophil). The cytoplasm, which surrounds the nucleus gives the cell its shape. The cytoplasm stains a variety of colors, depending on its contents. The size of the cell, the shape and size of the nucleus, the staining reaction of the nucleus, and the contents and staining reactions of the cytoplasm aid in the identification of the leukocytes.

Leukocytes are sometimes categorized as granulocytes or nongranulocytes. The granulocytes are the leukocytes which contain specific granulation, such as the neutrophils, eosinophils, and basophils. The nongranulocytes may contain a nonspecific granulation, but specific granules are not seen. The nongranulocytes are the monocytes and the lymphocytes.

The five types of leukocytes will be studied more thoroughly under Cell Morphology, but a brief description of each of the five cells follows:

1. Neutrophil. This cell is normally the most numerous and most prominent of the white cells seen in an adult blood film. The nucleus is lobulated (with three to five lobes), and the cytoplasm stains pinkish lavender and contains numerous fine dark granules.

2. Lymphocyte. This cell is second to the neutrophil in number in adult blood samples (usually about three neutrophils are seen to every one lymphocyte). The nucleus is round or oval, and the cytoplasm stains blue and is usually free from any granules.

3. Monocyte. This cell is the largest of the white cells and is often confused with lymphocytes. It has a horseshoe-shaped or kidney-shaped nucleus that stains lavender. The cytoplasm stains a muddy blue and can be vacuolated.

4. Eosinophil. This cell is easily recognized because of large red beadlike granules seen in the cytoplasm. There usually are not many eosinophils present (only about 4 per 100 total white cells counted are normally eosinophils).

5. Basophil. This cell is the one least likely to be seen (only 1 basophil per 100 total white cells counted). It is easily distinguished, however, because of purple-blue beadlike granules seen in the cytoplasm.

The third formed element of the blood is the platelet, or thrombocyte. Thrombocytes are small, colorless bodies (usually spherical, oval, or rod-shaped). Like the red cell, they do not have nuclei. Platelets are produced in the bone marrow by a cell called a *megakaryocyte*. They function as a part of the blood clotting system and act in two general ways in this function: (1) as "plugs" around the opening of a wound and (2) to contain certain factors necessary for the formation of a blood clot.

The formed elements—the red blood cells, white blood cells, and platelets—are suspended in the fluid called plasma. Plasma is the protein fraction of the blood, and it contains many substances in solution for maintenance of the body. Calcium and fibrinogen are two substances present in the plasma, both of which are necessary in the clotting system of the blood, along with the platelets.

COUNTING THE FORMED ELEMENTS OF THE BLOOD

The procedures used for enumeration of the formed elements of the blood employ microscopic observation. These procedures include those for counting red cells, white cells, and platelets. Since the numbers of formed elements (red cells, white cells, and platelets) are relatively great per unit volume of blood, it is necessary to dilute the blood to an appropriate volume before attempting to count them. Methods for performing reliable counts of formed elements of the blood are designed to obtain the number of cells in 1 mm³ of whole blood. Whether an electronic cell counter or one of the manual methods is used, the various steps in the procedure will include a way to dilute the blood sample quantitatively by using special pipets and diluents, to determine a reliable estimate of cells in the diluted sample, and to convert, by calculation, the number of cells in the diluted sample to the final result—the number of cells in 1 mm³ of whole blood.

Any blood cell count is done on a minute sample of an already small sample of the total volume of blood in an individual's body. For this reason, inherent errors exist in the most adequately designed methods, and the steps in a given procedure must be performed as carefully as possible in order to reduce the variation of the final result from the "actual count."

In most student practice laboratories, a widely used manual method will be employed to provide the experience necessary for counting formed elements of the blood. Most of the practice will be done on preserved blood samples. Before using any blood sample, the technician or student must always make certain that the sample has been preserved with the proper anticoagulant and has been properly labeled, and that the appearance indicates that a good collection technique was used. Each sample should be checked for hemolysis and small clots (known as fibrin clots) as soon as it is received.

COUNTING ERYTHROCYTES AND LEUKOCYTES

The leukocyte count is routinely included in every initial study of a new patient. It is a basic hematology laboratory procedure. The erythrocyte count is not considered a basic laboratory examination, and knowledge of the limits of significance of the erythrocyte count must be understood thoroughly. Both counts may be performed using either manual or electronic counting devices. For teaching purposes only manual methods will be discussed in detail in this chapter. The use of electronic devices may be taught where they are used. As in the case of any electronic apparatus, the manufacturer of the instrument supplies the purchaser with specific details on the use and care of the instrument in question. When a new instrument is used by student in a laboratory course, instructions must be followed explicitly.

The normal leukocyte count varies from 5,000 to 10,000 cells/mm³. An increase in the leukocytes counted above the normal upper limit is termed *leukocytosis*. A decrease, below the normal value is termed *leukopenia*. Leukopenia may occur following the use of x-ray therapy, after the administration of certain drugs, in infections with such agents as the typhoid group, certain viruses, and malaria, and pernicious anemia. Leukocytosis may occur in many acute infections, in severe malaria, hemorrhage, during pregnancy, postoperatively, in some forms of anemia, in some carcinomas, and in leukemia. Leukemia is a condition of unknown cause, of usually fatal termination, and characterized by proliferation of the leukocytes and their precursors in the tissues of the body. It is associated with many changes in the circulating cells of the blood. Blood films prepared from leukemia patients should be examined only by qualified persons, a pathologist or experienced medical technologist. There are two main classifications of leukemia, myelogenous and lymphatic, according to the predominant type of leukocyte seen. Leukemias are further divided into subclassifications, acute and chronic. In the acute condition, the disease progresses rapidly, and morphologic changes are marked. In the chronic condition, these changes are not as rapid, nor are they as marked.

Anemia is a term generally applied to a decrease in the number of erythrocytes. There are many types of anemias. Anemia can be caused by excessive blood loss or blood destruction (called *hemolytic anemia*). Anemia can also be due to decreased blood cell or hemoglobin formation. Examples of these include pernicious anemia, bone marrow failure anemia, or iron deficiency anemia. Polycythemia is a condition whereby the number of erythrocytes is increased.

Diluents

As stated previously, because the blood cells are so numerous, they cannot be counted accurately without dilution. When red blood cells are counted, it is obvious from the principles involved in osmosis that the most important characteristic of the diluent is isotonicity. Two other necessary properties of a diluent for red cell counts are prevention of clumping, or clotting, of the cells and provision of the proper specific gravity, so that all the cells will settle as evenly as possible. The most commonly used diluent for hand cell-counting methods for the enumeration of red cells is Hayem's solution. Hayem's solution meets all three of the necessary requirements. It contains mercuric chloride to prevent clumping of the red cells, and sodium sulfate and sodium chloride to provide the proper specific gravity and isotonicity. Other diluents for red cell counts include

0.85% saline solution, Gower's solution, Toison's solution, and Rees-Ecker solution.

In the methods for leukocyte counts, the diluting fluid must fulfill one very different requirement. Specifically, the white cell diluting fluid must destroy the red cells so that the white cells may be counted more readily. It is necessary to eliminate the red cells when counting white cells, because red cells are much more numerous than white cells. (The white cells are not eliminated, however, when counting red cells.) The principles of osmotic pressure are again employed, but in a different way from that necessary for counting the red cells. The diluent used most commonly for white cell counts is 2% acetic acid, which functions in two ways: (1) it darkens the nuclei of the white cells, so that they are easier to see, and (2) it hemolyzes the red cells. When the acetic acid hemolyzes the red cells, it converts the hemoglobin released from the red cells into acid hematin, which gives the resulting solution a brown color. The intensity of the brown color is directly related to how much hemoglobin is present in the red cells. Another diluting fluid which is used for white cell counts is 0.1 N hydrochloric acid (HCl). The principle is the same with either 2% acetic acid or 0.1 N HCl.

Any diluent used must be filtered immediately before use to ensure elimination of foreign particles which might be confused with the cells to be counted.

Directions for Preparation of Diluents

1. Hayem's solution for red cell counts. Dissolve 15 g sodium chloride, 33 g anhydrous sodium sulfate, and 7.5 g mercuric chloride, and dilute to 3,000 ml with deionized water.

2. Two percent acetic acid for white cell counts. Dilute 60 ml of glacial acetic acid to 3,000 ml with deionized water.

Pipets for Red and White Blood Cell Counts

To ensure proper dilution of the sample to be used for counting red and white blood cells, the correct diluent is used with pipets manufactured for this purpose. Laboratories employ various brands of diluting pipets, all of which are generally of the same structure. The important differences are determined by the grade of glass used in the manufacture of the pipet and in the calibration of the pipet. Precalibration by the manufacturer and calibration checking in the hematology laboratory may appear complex. The procedure is more easily understood if it is compared to a matching process. The pipets can be matched with U.S. Bureau of Standards pipets either by comparing the weight of some substance, such as mercuy, contained in the "unknown" pipet and the weight of the same substance contained in the "standard" pipet or by actually counting blood cells on equivalent cell samples. The mark (if any) on the pipet to indicate that it has been checked will vary from laboratory to laboratory. It is therefore necessary to identify the calibration check mark and use only those pipets which have been properly calibrated. Using matched pipets reduces one source of error in blood cell counts by increasing consistency in the dilution.

Several companies manufacture a type of pipet for white blood cell and red blood cell counts known as the *Thoma pipet*. It is important to distinguish between brand names and pipet types. The Thoma pipet is not a brand name but rather is a type of pipet used for blood cell dilution. Most hematology laboratories use a pipet of the Thoma type. This pipet, like all cell-counting pipets, does not measure blood or diluent in definite amounts such as milliliters or millimeters but rather provides the proper dilution in terms of a certain part of its volume to the total volume. The Thoma pipet consists of a graduated capillary tube divided into 10 parts and marked 0.5 at the fifth mark and 1.0 at the tenth, a mixing bulb above the capillary tube containing a glass bead (the glass bead facilitates mixing of the blood and diluent), and, above the bulb, another short capillary tube with an engraved graduation marked 11.0 on the white cell pipet and 101.0 on the red cell pipet (Fig. 3-4). The graduation marks on these pipets are relative. The 0.5 and 1.0 marks do not denote a measurement of milliliters or millimeters. Some of the brand names for Thoma diluting pipets include K-exax, Normax, Glasco, Yankee certified, Tri-Lyne, Sargent, and American Optical. It is most important to select only those brands of pipets which are reliable and accurate.

The marks on the Thoma white cell pipet indicate that there are a total of 11 units of volume contained in the pipet from the tip to the 11.0 mark above the bulb (Fig. 3-4). The 1.0 mark on the stem means

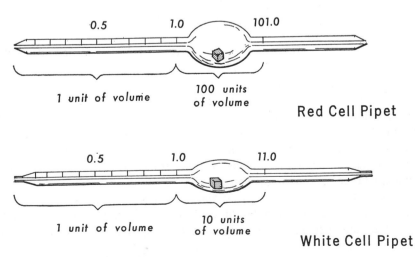

Fig. 3-4. Red cell and white cell diluting pipets.

that one of the units of volume for that pipet is contained in the stem from the tip of the pipet to the 1.0 mark. The 1 unit of volume in the stem is divided into 10 equal portions by measuring from the tip. The bulb is defined as extending from the 1.0 mark on the stem to the 11.0 mark on the short stem above the bulb. The volume contained in the bulb portion of the pipet is 10 units of volume.

Routinely, the dilution made for the white cell count is 1:20. This is accomplished by measuring whole blood from a well-mixed sample to the 0.5 mark and washing the sample into the bulb with the diluent to the 11.0 mark. The mixture in the bulb will contain 0.5 part of blood and 9.5 parts of diluent in the total of 10 units of volume in the bulb. The 1 unit in the stem contains diluent only and does not enter into the calculation of the dilution. The dilution factor is calculated by dividing 10 by 0.5. This is the same as determining what the total volume would have to be if 1 unit of blood were used and the same relationship of blood to diluent maintained.

The red blood cell count is measured in exactly the same way and the dilution factor determined by the same general method. The difference between the white cell pipet and the red cell pipet is that the red cell pipet allows a dilution which is ten times greater than the dilution in the white cell pipet. Rather than 11.0 total units of volume, the red cell pipet has 101.0 units of volume (Fig. 3-4). Therefore, when 0.5 unit of blood is measured and diluted to the 101.0 mark, the dilution is 1:200. There are 0.5 unit of blood and 99.5 units of diluent in the mixture contained in the bulb, which contains a total of 100 units. The 1 unit in the stem of the red cell pipet contains only diluent, as in the white cell pipet stem.

Procedure for Diluting Red and White Cell Counts

1. Filter the appropriate diluting fluid from the stock bottle into a small diluting bottle.

2. Using a properly mixed whole blood sample and the diluting pipet with tubing and mouthpiece attached, draw blood into the capillary bore of the pipet to slightly above the 0.5 mark.

3. Wipe off the *outside* of the pipet with gauze, and adjust the blood level to the 0.5 mark *exactly* by tapping the tip of the pipet with a finger or other nonabsorptive material. Do not use gauze for this adjustment, because the liquid portion of the sample inside the stem will be drawn into the gauze, leaving a higher concentration of cells inside the stem (thus giving an inaccurate result for the cell count).

4. Maintain the blood level at the 0.5 mark by placing the tongue over the plastic mouthpiece on the tubing or by holding the breath. Place the tip of the pipet into the diluting fluid well below the surface of the liquid.

5. Using constant mouth suction, draw the diluent into the pipet while

at the same time lightly twirling the pipet between the fingers. Draw the mixture to the top mark above the bulb. During the time the bulb is being filled, tap the pipet with the finger to knock the bead down below the surface of the solution in the bulb. This will help to prevent bubbles from forming.

6. While removing the pipet from the diluent bottle, maintain the level of the mixture exactly on, or slightly above (never more than 1 mm), the top mark by closing the pipet tip with the index finger and holding the breath or covering the sucker mouthpiece with the tongue. Holding the pipet in a horizontal position is also important. Remove the rubber sucker tubing carefully by continuing to hold the index finger over the pipet tip.

7. As soon as the rubber tubing is removed, hold the pipet horizontally with the thumb and third finger at either end. Shake the pipet vigorously at right angles to the long axis of the pipet for a few seconds. The glass bead in the pipet should be moved from one side to the other during the mixing. After shaking, the pipet may be put aside in a horizontal position, preventing any leakage until the actual cell count is done.

General Precautions for Pipetting Red and White Cell Counts

There are several precautions which can be taken to avoid errors when doing a red or white blood cell count in the hematology laboratory. Pipets must be clean, dry, and without chipped or broken tips. Technique must be practiced until completed pipets are free from bubbles, packing, or clumping of cells. Contaminated diluting fluid must not be used. Periodic checking of the fluid on the diluting bottle is a useful indicator of how carefully the pipet is being placed into the fluid and the blood level maintained at the 0.5 mark. No blood should be allowed to go into the diluent, because this will affect subsequent cell counts using the same diluent.

The upper dilution mark on the pipets may be exceeded by no more than 1 mm, and the mixture must not be corrected back to the top mark if overdilution has occurred. Adjusting the upper dilution back to the mark forces cells from the bulb into the lower stem of the pipet. The fluid in the stem of the pipet must be free from cells when dilution has been completed. Absorptive material such as gauze must not be used to adjust the upper blood level to the 0.5 mark. The sample in the stem can be falsely concentrated if gauze or other absorptive materials are used to adjust the blood level.

Preserved blood samples must not be hemolyzed or contain fibrin clots.

The Counting Chamber for Red and White Blood Cell Counts

The first steps in the production of a valid cell count, proper handling of the blood sample and careful dilution to obtain a less concentrated solution of known quantity, are followed by counting the number of cells in a known volume of the diluted sample. The counting chamber is often called a *hemacytometer*. Technically, however, a hemacytometer consists of a counting chamber, a coverglass for the counting chamber, and the blood cell diluting pipets. In this section the counting chamber and the hemacytometer will be used in accordance with common usage as interchangeable terms. For a routine count employing a hand method, the counting chamber used most often is the Levy-Hausser hemacytometer with Neubauer ruling.

To understand how the counting chamber allows the result to be reported in terms of volume when it has a flat surface, it is easier to start with a cube and work backward. Picture a cube 1 mm on each side. The counting chamber allows the cube to be divided into equal units which are $\frac{1}{10}$ mm in depth. When the counting chamber is viewed from the side, one can see that when the coverglass is placed on the chamber, it rests on supports (Fig. 3-5). When the coverglass is used, the space between the bottom of the coverglass and the surface of the counting chamber is $\frac{1}{10}$ mm. Essentially, the chamber provides a series of "slices" of the cube which are 1 mm² in area and $\frac{1}{10}$ mm in depth. The only way to be sure that the depth is $\frac{1}{10}$ mm is to use the plane ground coverglasses which have a constant weight and even surface. The method used to arrange the $\frac{1}{10}$-mm slices so that one may count the cells in one of the slices or count the cells in only certain portions of one slice is to vary the areas of the ruled surface of the chamber. Each counting chamber has two precision-ruled counting areas which are composed of 9 mm² (Fig. 3-6).

When the ruled area of the counting chamber is viewed for the first time under the microscope, it may be difficult to see the nine basic 1-mm squares, because each one has been ruled into smaller areas. The 1-mm² sections in the four corners are ruled into 16 equal portions (Fig. 3-7). The square in the center of the ruled area is divided into 25 equal portions

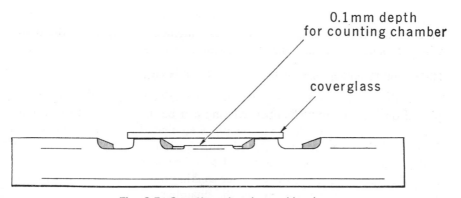

0.1mm depth
for counting chamber

coverglass

Fig. 3-5. Counting chamber—side view.

(9 square millimeters)

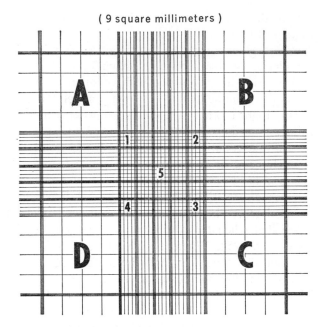

White blood cells are counted in areas A, B, C, and D (4 sq. mm.)
Red blood cells are counted in areas 1, 2, 3, 4, and 5
(80/400 sq. mm.)

Fig. 3-6. Improved Neubauer ruling for one counting chamber area.

(Fig. 3-7). In turn, each of the $\frac{1}{25}$-mm squares is divided into 16 parts providing an area of $\frac{1}{400}$ mm (Fig. 3-7). With the ruled surface of the counting chamber constructed in this manner, it is possible to measure aliquots of the diluted blood sample which are contained in 1-mm, $\frac{1}{16}$-mm, $\frac{1}{25}$-mm, $\frac{1}{80}$-mm, and $\frac{1}{400}$-mm squares, all of which are $\frac{1}{10}$-mm in depth. The area to be counted will depend on the type of count to be done and the situation.

There are other types of counting chambers which can also be used in counting blood cells. Some of these include the Spencer Brightline with Neubauer ruling and the Levy chamber with Fuchs-Rosenthal ruling.

Mixing and Mounting Samples in the Counting Chamber

The diluted blood in the pipet must be mixed before the mixture is placed on the counting chamber. Mixing can be done by hand for a minimum of 5 minutes by holding the pipet so that the mixing bead moves freely and the cells are not pushed into the stem. Usually, a mechanical shaker will be available for use, and the time will vary according to the type of shaker used. Immediately after shaking the pipet and before placing a small portion of the mixture on the chamber, three drops are expelled from the white cell pipet and five drops from the red cell pipet, and

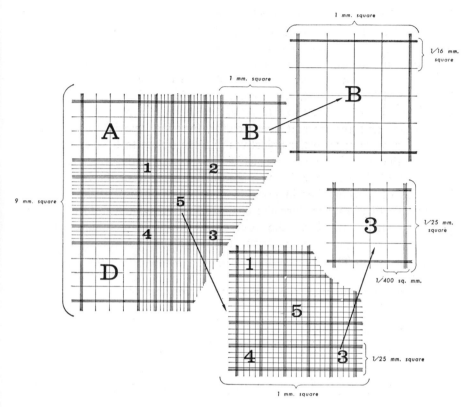

Fig. 3-7. Counting areas of the hemacytometer.

the tip is wiped. The cell-free diluent contained in the capillary bore is discarded in this manner, and the cells are counted in the next drop, which is a representative drop of the well-mixed cell suspension. Pipets may vary in size so that discarding three to five drops may not be adequate. In that case, approximately one-third of the mixture in the bulb should be expelled before mounting.

While the pipet is held at an angle of about 40 degrees, the chamber between the rule area and the coverglass is filled with a single drop which should be drawn rapidly into the chamber by capillarity. If the fluid spills into the dividing moats or is otherwise filled unevenly, mounting must be repeated. Only one drop can be used to fill the chamber. It should not be filled partially with a small drop and filled completely with a second drop; this would result in an uneven distribution of cells.

Shaking the pipet and proper filling of the counting chamber are important factors in obtaining good cell distribution in the counting areas and, finally, in obtaining accurate cell counts. The counting chamber is filled in the same manner for both red cell and white cell counts. Both sides of the hemacytometer must be filled to use the chamber properly. The drops following the three to five expelled drops are the most representative. For practice in mounting, however, more of the fluid remaining in the pipet can be used.

Before any counting is done, the microscope must be properly adjusted. To do this, the essentials concerning the use of the microscope should be reviewed. Important things to keep in mind include knowing which side of the mirror to use, how to adjust the necessary parts for proper illumination, and the correct method for focusing (paying attention to prevention of damage to the objectives and the object to be viewed).

Place the counting chamber, which has been filled properly, on the stage of the microscope and fasten securely. Place one of the ruled counting areas of the chamber in position over the condenser. With the low-power objective in place, turn the coarse-adjustment knob until the objective is about $\frac{1}{4}$ in. above the coverglass. Move the condenser all the way up with the diaphragm open. Look through the microscope, and move the mirror and light until the light is reflected up the body tube to the eye and the field looks evenly lighted. Turn the coarse-adjustment knob slowly upward until the ruled area comes into focus. Use the fine-adjustment knob to bring the area into perfect focus. Use the iris diaphragm to adjust the light. If this technique is used, there is little danger of damaging the coverglass with the objective. If the objective touches the coverglass, cell distribution is altered, necessitating a new mounting. After the ruled area is in focus, scan it quickly to identify the various ruled portions. Approximately 1 mm² can be seen in each field using the low-power (10×) objective.

When the counting chamber is properly in place on the microscope and the various ruled areas identified and understood, counting of cells can begin.

Counting and Calculating White Blood Cells Using a Manual Method

White blood cells are counted under low magnification (10× objective) in the four corner square millimeters of the ruled area of the counting chamber. Each square measures 1 mm² and is divided into 16 equal divisions. Cells touching the lines on the left side or on the top of the squares are included in the count. Cells touching the lines on the right side or on the bottom of the squares are *not* counted (Fig. 3-8). In this way, every cell is assigned to a square, and cells are not counted twice or omitted from the count.

The count obtained in each of the 1-mm² sections in the four corners is tabulated separately in the practice laboratories. The cells in each of the four squares should not vary by more than 10. Tallying the squares separately provides a check of the distribution of the cells and indicates whether mixing and mounting was adequate. When the numbers of cells counted per square do not agree within 10, another pipet must be used,

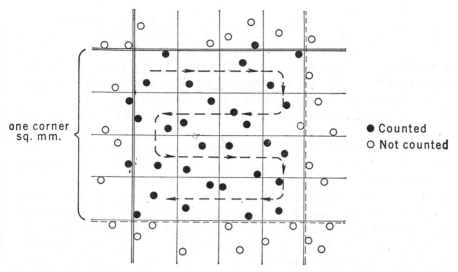

one corner
sq. mm.

● Counted
○ Not counted

Fig. 3-8. Example of which blood cells are counted in a representative area.

because remounts from the previously used pipet usually result in progressively higher counts.

In calculating the total count per cubic millimeter of blood four important facts must be considered: (1) the total number of cells counted in the four 1-mm squares, (2) the dilution of the blood sample, (3) the square area counted, and (4) the depth of the counting chamber. The square area and the depth can be considered together as volume. Using the four factors in calculating the count, the following general formula holds true:

No. cells counted in 1-mm² areas × dilution of blood
$$\times \text{ square area counted} \times \text{ depth of chamber}$$
$$= \text{no. white cells/mm}^3 \text{ whole blood}$$

To illustrate this calculation: The sum of the cells counted in the four 1-mm² corner areas is 32 plus 38 plus 39 plus 31, giving a total of 140. In this case, the calculation would be

$$\frac{140}{1} \times \frac{20}{1} \times \frac{1}{4} \times \frac{1}{0.1} = 7,000$$ white blood cells per mm³. If the square areas and the depth are considered as volume, the general formula is:

$$\frac{\text{No. cells counted in 4 squares} \times \text{dilution of blood}}{\text{Volume (area} \times \text{depth)}} = \text{white cells/mm}^3$$

A count with a total of 140 cells counted in the four squares would be calculated as

$$\frac{140 \times 20}{4 \times 0.1} = 7,000 \text{ white cells/mm}^3$$

For each white cell count completed in the routine manner, the dilution of the blood and the volume of diluted blood used for counting is the same. Therefore, a constant factor may be used for multiplying the total cells counted to find the final result. If the number of cells in the illustrations were omitted, the result of 20 divided by 0.4 would be 50. Any total number of cells can be converted to the number of white cells per cubic millimeter of blood by multiplying by 50. Fifty is the constant factor for counting white cells in the routine manner using the manual method presented.

White cells should be counted in duplicate until accuracy is established, after which duplicate determinations may be done at will (for low counts or counts of grave clinical importance).

The allowable difference[2,3] between duplicate pipets for the same blood sample is 500 cells/mm³ for counts within the normal range and 10 percent of the lowest count when the total count is less than 5,000 or over 10,000 cells/mm³. Five to ten thousand white cells per cubic millimeter is considered to be the normal range. The white cell count result is always rounded off to the nearest 50 cells, since the constant in the equation is 50. For example, a white cell count calculated to be 8,044 would be reported as 8,050, and a count calculated to be 8,022 would be reported as 8,000. The general rule for rounding off numbers to the next significant figure is used.

Counting and Calculating Red Blood Cells Using a Manual Method

Red blood cells are counted under high-dry magnification ($43\times$ objective). The central square millimeter area on the counting chamber is used. It is best to find this area with the low-power objective and then change to the high-dry objective. The cells in 80 of the squares measuring $\frac{1}{400}$ mm are counted. This is equivalent to counting the cells in $\frac{1}{5}$ of 1 mm² ($\frac{80}{400}$). The volume is determined by multiplying the depth (0.1 mm) by $\frac{1}{5}$, which is equal to 0.02 mm.³

The preferred method for counting the cells in $\frac{1}{5}$ mm² is to count the cells in five of the $\frac{1}{25}$ squares (Fig. 3-9). Since each $\frac{1}{25}$-mm square contains sixteen smaller squares, eighty $\frac{1}{400}$ mm squares will have been counted. Distribution is checked by duplicate mounts.

The calculation of the red cell count is based upon the same principles as those used for the white cell count. The usual blood dilution is 1:200, the area counted is $\frac{1}{5}$ mm², and the depth is 0.1 mm. An example of calculations for a red cell count with a total of 475 cells counted in the proper area is

$$475\tfrac{/}{1} \times 200\tfrac{/}{1} \times 400\tfrac{/}{80} \times 10\tfrac{/}{1} = 4{,}750{,}000 \text{ red cells/mm}^3$$

If the area and depth are converted to volume first, the general equation would be

$$\frac{\text{No. cells counted in } \frac{1}{5} \text{ mm} \times \text{dilution}}{0.2 \text{ area} \times 0.1 \text{ depth}} = \text{no. red cells/mm}^3$$

(Center Square Millimeter)

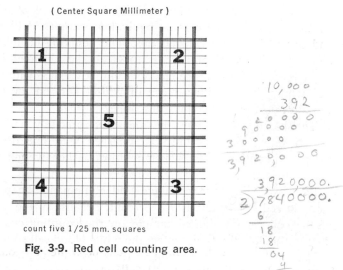

count five 1/25 mm. squares

Fig. 3-9. Red cell counting area.

The constant factor for the red blood cell count is 10,000, since 200/0.02 represents the general equation in a shortened form.

The red blood cell count is one of the least accurate procedures done in the hematology laboratory. For this reason, every sample is pipetted in duplicate, and each pipet is mounted on two sides of the counting chamber, giving four possible counting areas. If the counts on the two pipets do not check within 10 percent, the count is repeated.* A generally accepted normal range for red cell counts is 4.00 to 5.00 million cells/mm³ for women and 4.50 to 5.50 million cells/mm³ for men.

The rules for counting the cells touching the top and left lines of any given area are the same for red cell counts as those described for the white cell count.

Precautions to be Noted When Counting Red and White Blood Cells

Errors in counting white and red blood cells may be categorized as errors related to the extremely small size of the sample, the nature of the sample, faulty laboratory equipment, faulty technique, and the inherent error of cell distribution in the counting chamber which is subject to the laws of chance.[2]

The minute size of the blood sample is illustrated by the fact that a variation of even 1 cell in the red cell count changes the count by 10,000 cells in the final result.

Venous blood must be free of clots and mixed well immediately before it is used for dilution purposes. Peripheral blood or capillary blood must be obtained from a freely flowing puncture and must be diluted rapidly to prevent coagulation.

* Allowable error used by the hematology laboratory of the University of Minnesota Hospitals.

Pipets must be checked against U.S. Bureau of Standards pipets with an agreement of 7 percent on equivalent samples.[2,3] Pipets must be clean and dry and without chipped tips. The counting chamber must be clean and dry. The usual practice is to clean the chamber immediately prior to each use by flooding the chamber and coverglass with medicated alcohol and wiping it dry with a piece of gauze. Dirt on the counting chamber can alter the eventual count being done.

The blood sample must be measured precisely and diluted properly. The counting chamber must be charged with one drop of the diluted sample without an excess, which could raise the coverglass and thus change the depth factor.

Even with excellent technique and equipment, the probable minimum error in red cell counts is 7.8 percent, because of the chance distribution of the cells in the diluted sample on the counting chamber.[3] This same distribution factor can also affect the white blood cell count.

Use of electronic cell counters does not relieve the laboratory worker of the responsibility for being constantly alert for sources of error. Unless equipment is properly calibrated and unless fundamental aspects such as the quality of the sample are considered carefully, electronic counters become merely tools for producing inadequate results at a faster rate.

COUNTING PLATELETS

Platelets, or thrombocytes, function in the coagulation of the blood and are therefore associated with the bleeding and clotting, or hemostatic, mechanism of the body. The platelets are formed in the bone marrow from megakaryocytes. Platelets are rather difficult to count accurately for several reasons: They are small and difficult to discern. They have an adhesive character and become attached readily to glassware or to particles of debris in the diluting fluid. They clump easily and are probably not evenly distributed in the blood in the first place. With good technique and experience, however, platelets can be counted accurately.

The normal number of platelets, depending in part on the method employed for their enumeration, ranges from 170,000 to 400,000 cells/mm³ of whole blood.[4] A decrease in the number of platelets from normal may be associated with a generalized bleeding tendency and a prolonged bleeding time. An increase in platelets may be associated with a tendency toward thrombosis.

There are several diseases in which a change in the platelet count, either higher or lower than normal, can result. Thrombocytopenia, or a decrease in platelets, is found in thrombocytopenia purpura, in some infectious diseases, in some leukemias, in some anemias, and when the patient is undergoing x-ray treatment. Thrombocytosis, or an increase in platelets, can be found in rheumatic fever, asphyxiation, following surgical treatment, following splenectomy, with acute blood loss, and with some types of drug therapy used in relation to leukemia treatment.

There are several manual methods for counting platelets. In general, the best results are obtained by using some variation of the direct methods. Some hospitals have discontinued platelet counts altogether, because a well-prepared blood smear can be used for an estimation of the platelets and the error in platelet counts can be very great. Electronic counting devices may also be used for platelet counts.

When using any of the direct methods, the blood source used either must be preserved with Sequestrene or must be fresh finger-prick blood. Balanced oxalate does not preserve the white blood cells or the platelets.

Diluents

The diluent used for counting platelets must meet certain requirements. It must serve the following purposes: (1) fixation to reduce the adhesiveness of the platelets, (2) prevention of coagulation, (3) prevention of hemolysis (unless the method chosen eliminates the red blood cells), and (4) provision of a low specific gravity, so that the platelets will settle in one plane. One diluent which meets all these requirements is Rees-Ecker solution. All diluents used, including Rees-Ecker, must be stored in the refrigerator and filtered before each use. Rees-Ecker solution contains sodium citrate, which prevents coagulation, preserves the red blood cells, and provides the necessary low specific gravity; it also contains Formalin, which is a fixative, and brilliant cresyl blue, a dye used for identification of the diluent. This dye does not stain the platelets; it merely acts to identify the diluent from other similar solutions. It is not essential for the counting procedure.

Directions for Preparation of Rees-Ecker Diluting Fluid

In a volumetric flask, 3.8 g of sodium citrate and 0.2 ml of Formalin are diluted to 100 ml, using deionized water. A small amount of brilliant cresyl blue is added to color the solution a light blue.

Equipment for the Platelet Count

The pipets used for platelet dilution must be scrupulously clean, preferably acid-cleaned, although hot-detergent cleaning appears to give good results. Anything in the pipet to which the platelets could adhere must be removed.

The Spencer Brightline counting chamber appears to have definite advantages over other types of counting chambers for counting platelets. The platelets seem to be easier to see against the metallic-coated surface of the Spencer Brightline chamber. The cell distribution also seems to be better, since the chamber's surface is smoother. However, other types of counting chambers can be used. In the Spencer Brightline chamber the lines appear white against a dark background. This type of chamber is more difficult to mount correctly, however, so care must be taken in this regard.

Procedure Using a Manual Method

1. The capillary bore of a red cell diluting pipet is rinsed with Rees-Ecker diluting fluid. Any excess fluid is thoroughly expelled from the pipet.

2. Blood from a freely flowing finger puncture or venous blood preserved with Sequestrene is drawn rapidly into the pipet to the 0.5 mark.

3. The blood is diluted rapidly with Rees-Ecker fluid to the 101 mark on the pipet. Two pipets are always diluted for each platelet count, and each pipet is mounted on both sides of the counting chamber. Blood smears are also made at this time in order to check the platelet count.

4. The pipet is shaken immediately after dilution for a minimum of 1 minute.

5. After thorough mixing (for at least 5 minutes), six to eight drops are expelled from the pipet and discarded before mounting. Mount one drop from the pipet on both sides of the chamber. Repeat with the duplicate pipet.

6. The platelets are allowed to settle in the chambers for 10 minutes. The chambers are covered to prevent evaporation. One such cover is a Petri plate containing moistened gauze.

7. The platelets, which appear as small, round, refractile bodies, are counted in the center square millimeter of each of the four counting areas using the high-power objective (4 mm). The counts on the four center squares must agree within 20,000 cells for duplicate mounts and 40,000 cells for duplicate pipets.

Calculations

Next, the number of platelets per cubic millimeter of whole blood must be calculated. Several factors are important: (1) the average number of platelets counted in 1 mm^2, (2) the dilution of the blood (usually 1:200), and (3) the volume of the diluted blood counted, which is equal to the depth of the chamber (0.1 mm) times the area in which the cells are counted (1 mm^2); this volume is equal to 0.1 mm^3. Therefore, the following general formula applies:

$$\text{Number of platelets counted (average of four squares)} \times \frac{1 \text{ mm}^3 \times 200}{0.1 \text{ mm}^3}$$
$$= \text{platelets/mm}^3$$

In this case, a calculation factor of 2,000 can be used. The normal range for the platelet count is 170,000 to 400,000 platelets/mm^3, using Rees-Ecker diluent.

Precautions

Many of the same precautions as described for counting erythrocytes and leukocytes also apply to platelet counts. In platelet counts, however, it is imperative that peripheral blood must be freely flowing when obtained from a finger prick. Pipets and counting chambers must be clean and free from lint, since platelets may be confused with dirt and debris. Rapid dilution of the blood is essential, or the platelets may form clumps and the blood may clot. The pipet must be rinsed with the diluent immediately prior to the dilution procedure to prevent the platelets from sticking to the walls of the pipet.

Since the erythrocytes and leukocytes are not destroyed by the Rees-Ecker solution, constant focusing of the microscope is necessary to identify the platelets among these larger, more numerous cells. A blood film is made, stained, and viewed microscopically to check each platelet count.

If a platelet count is requested in combination with other counts to be collected from the same patient and one wishes to utilize the same finger puncture, it is necessary to take the blood for the platelet count first and then the remaining counts. The finger must not be squeezed excessively when drawing the necessary blood into the pipet.

COUNTING EOSINOPHILS

Occasionally it will be necessary to count specific types of leukocytes. One such test is the eosinophil count. It has been shown that the administration of a single 25-mg dose of ACTH intramuscularly to subjects with normal adrenocortical function results in a reduction of the total number of circulating eosinophils.[5,6] This finding has been used as a test of adrenocortical function, but it is not specific, and the value of the test is limited.[7] An inverse relation exists between adrenocortical activity and the number of circulating eosinophils. A modification of the Randolph method is used for random eosinophil counts before and after the administration of ACTH.[8,9] The eosinophil count is not a routine hematologic test.

An increase in the number of eosinophils (termed *eosinophilia*) may be seen in cases of trichinosis, widespread metastatic carcinoma, allergies (particularly asthma), skin disease (eczema), and infectious diseases (scarlet fever, for one).

Normal % = 4/100
Mainly parasites and allergies cause increase in eosinophils

Diluent

The diluent used is a combination of phloxine B and methylene blue in propylene glycol. Another diluent which can be used is a hypotonic solution of eosin. *Pilot Solution*

Directions for Preparation

Solution A. Dissolve 0.5 g of phloxine B in 1,000 ml of 50% propylene glycol in deionized water.

Solution B. Dissolve 0.5 g of methylene blue and 1,000 ml of 50% propylene glycol in deionized water.

Mix 1 part solution B in 9 parts solution A immediately before use.

Equipment for Eosinophil Count

The blood for the eosinophil count is diluted in a white blood cell diluting pipet. A special counting chamber is used for this procedure—the Levy chamber with Fuchs-Rosenthal ruling. This chamber usually has a depth of 0.2 mm and has two ruled areas of 16 mm² each.

Procedure

1. Blood is drawn to the 1.0 mark in a leukocyte pipet (a 1:10 dilution is usually needed for this procedure) and the pipet diluted to the 11.0 mark with the propylene glycol dye diluent. Duplicate pipets should be made.

2. The pipets are shaken for 20 minutes, and each of the duplicate pipets is mounted on two sides of a counting chamber.

3. The cells are allowed to settle for 20 minutes. The chambers are covered to prevent evaporation during this waiting period.

4. Eosinophils are counted under low power in each of the four ruled areas (the total area counted is 64 mm²). The eosinophils are identified in the counting chamber by their brightly red-stained granules. The remainder of the leukocytes do not stain, and the erythrocytes are destroyed by the diluent.

Calculations

In calculating the total eosinophil count, the following factors are taken into consideration: (1) the total number of eosinophils counted, (2) the dilution of the blood (usually 1:10), and (3) the volume of the diluted blood, which is equal to the depth of the chamber (0.2 mm) times the area in which the cells are counted (64 mm²); this volume is equal to 12.8 mm³. Therefore, the eosinophils per cubic millimeter of blood is equal to the following equation:

$$\text{No. eosinophils counted (in 64 mm}^2) \times \frac{1 \text{ mm}^3 \times 10}{12.8 \text{ mm}^3}$$

Using this formula, a calculation factor of 0.78 is found. The normal value for the eosinophil count is from 100 to 300 cells/mm³.

Precautions

Venous blood or capillary blood may be used for this test. The type of blood sample used should be noted, as simultaneous counts using venous and capillary blood have resulted in values 25 percent higher for the capillary blood as opposed to the venous blood.[9]

The two solutions used for the diluting fluid, solution A and solution B, are stable separately, but the final mixture of the two dyes must be used within 4 to 8 hours. After 8 hours, the dyes will precipitate.[9]

Technical errors should be minimized. The same technical factors apply as those described for the other cell counts. To avoid undue rupture of the eosinophil membrane, gentle shaking of the pipets is suggested.

COUNTING RETICULOCYTES

Reticulocytes are nonnucleated immature red cells. The number of reticulocytes evaluates regeneration or production of red blood cells. Reticulocytes are young red cells which have matured enough to have lost their nuclei but not their cytoplasmic ribonucleic acid (RNA). They do have the full amount of hemoglobin. As seen in a blood film stained with Wright's stain, reticulocytes appear as polychromatic red blood cells because of the young cytoplasm. Their polychromatic nature is due to the basophilic cytoplasmic remnant of the immature red cell, RNA. Basophilic stippling are inclusions seen in pathologic abnormal conditions in which the RNA precipitates in the red cells as small pinpoint particles due to a toxic condition such as lead or heavy metal poisoning. Basophilic stippling may also be due to iron. It also is visible with Wright's staining of the blood film. Howell-Jolly bodies are seen in pathologic conditions where one or more larger spherical bodies which consist of nuclear material are found in the red cell.

The circulating blood usually contains 0.8 to 1.5 percent of the red cells as the younger form known as reticulocytes. When the reticulocyte count increases above this level (reticulocytosis), it is clinically significant, indicating that the body is attempting to compensate for an increased need for red cells. In order to meet this need, more immature reticulocytes are being released from the bone marrow to the circulating blood. Such an increase in reticulocytes is noted when red cells are being hemolyzed within the body. The bone marrow sends out red cells at an increased rate until only the younger cells are available to be released, although increased red cell production is probably taking place at the same time. The demand may be so great in some instances that nucleated red cells will be sent from the bone marrow.

The reticulocyte count is used to follow therapeutic measures for some anemias. In these anemias, the patient is deficient in, or lacking, one of the essential substances for manufacturing red cells. When the deficiency has been diagnosed, therapy is begun which consists of supplying the missing essential substances to the body and waiting for the body to react by increasing red cell production. New red cells will be released rapidly into the circulating blood, many before they are fully matured, in response to therapy. The corresponding increase in the reticulocyte count indicates favorable response to therapy. Iron deficiency anemia (treatment is with iron) and pernicious anemia (treatment is with vitamin B_{12}) are two forms of anemia which are followed by reticulocyte counts. As the total red cell count and the hemoglobin concentration reach normal levels, the increased red cell regeneration slows to the normal level, allowing more time for maturation of the red cells in the bone marrow. This is indicated by the presence of fewer young red cells (reticulocytes) in the circulating blood.

The methods for preparing reticulocyte films all require supravital staining of the red cells, whether the end result is a dry film or not. Supravital staining requires the mixture of living blood cells with the stain as opposed to making a film and staining it. Some methods consist of spreading the stain on the slide and drying it; the blood is then added to the dried stain and mixed, and the usual blood smear is prepared. Another method uses the same slide preparation, but the stain is mixed with a drop of blood and, cover-slipped, and the mixture is sealed on the slide and viewed in the liquid form under the microscope. A third method is to mix blood and stain in a small test tube, allow time for the staining reaction to occur, and then prepare a blood film from the mixture. The prepared blood film is then viewed microscopically. The first two methods described employ an alcoholic solution of the dye, and the third method uses a saline solution of the dye.

The blood sample used for reticulocyte counts may be obtained from a finger puncture or venipuncture. The anticoagulant Sequestrene is recommended if preservation is necessary, because balanced oxalate can interfere with the action of the dye. Two dyes are available, both of which seem to give comparable results.

Dyes Used to Stain Reticulocytes

Brilliant cresyl blue or new methylene blue is used for the staining of reticulocytes. Some workers claim that when the new methylene blue dye is used, the reticulum of the reticulocyte is easier to see. In addition to the dye used, the stain should contain an ingredient to preserve the red cells (provide an isotonic condition), if the third method is used, and prevent coagulation. Ingredients for the brilliant cresyl blue stain are sodium citrate (which prevents coagulation) and sodium chloride (which provides isotonicity). Ingredients for the new methylene blue are sodium oxalate (which prevents coagulation) and sodium chloride. These supravital dyes precipitate the basophilic material (RNA) in the reticulocytes, coloring it blue.

Directions for Preparation

1. Brilliant cresyl blue. Dilute 1.0 g of brilliant cresyl blue and 0.4 g of sodium citrate to 100 ml with 0.85% sodium chloride. Filter before using.

2. New methylene blue. Dilute 0.50 g of new methylene blue N, 0.70 g of sodium chloride (C.P. grade), and 0.13 g of sodium oxalate (C.P. grade) to 100 ml with deionized water. Filter before using.

Procedure*

1. Two drops of blood (capillary or venous) are added to three drops of reticulocyte dye in a small test tube. If the patient is very anemic, more blood should be used to ensure proper staining and good smears.

2. The blood and dye are mixed for 30 seconds and allowed to stand for 15 minutes.

3. The cells are resuspended by mixing for 1 minute, and at least three thin films are made on slides using small drops of the blood-stain mixture. The films are dried rapidly.

4. When dry, the reticulocytes are counted. Two thousand erythrocytes (one thousand on each of two slides) are counted using the oil-immersion objective. The reticulocytes seen in the count are included and recorded separately. If the two slides counted do not agree within five to seven reticulocytes, the third slide is used. The count should be made in an area of the smear considered to be medium-thin (about 70 erythrocytes per oil-immersion field). The reticulocytes appear as greenish blue cells with the reticulum showing as a dark purple network, or precipitate, in the cells. Precipitated stain must not be confused with reticulocytes.

Calculations

The reticulocyte count is reported as the percentage of reticulocytes seen in the total number of red cells counted. The following general formula can be used:

$$\frac{\text{No. reticulocytes counted}}{\text{No. erythrocytes counted}} \times 100 = \text{percentage reticulocytes}$$

The normal range for reticulocytes is from ~~0.8 to 1.5~~ percent.

1.5 to 3.0 %

Precautions to be Noted

Careful focusing of the microscope is essential when counting reticulocytes. Platelet granules and leukocyte granules will stain with the dye and must not be mistaken for reticulocytes. Precipitated stain might also be mistaken for reticulum within the erythrocytes. To minimize this possibility, the dye must be filtered immediately before use. Immediate drying of the smear will prevent the formation of the crystalline-like artifacts which sometimes appear in the red cells.

The proportion of dye to blood must be altered if the patient is anemic. More blood must be used. If the procedure is followed carefully, the distribution of reticulocytes on the blood films will be good. The allowable

* Procedure used by the hematology laboratory of the University of Minnesota Hospitals.

difference between the number of reticulocytes on the films per 1,000 erythrocytes should be within 5 to 7 cells.*

CELL MORPHOLOGY: THE PREPARATION, STAINING, AND EXAMINATION OF BLOOD FILMS

The preparation of a blood film is part of the routine hematologic tests done on most new hospital patients. The blood film is part of the complete blood count (CBC) in most hospitals or physicians' offices. The CBC can consist of different tests depending on the laboratory, but generally tests for hemoglobin, the white blood cell count, microhematocrit, and examination of a blood film are included in the CBC.

The blood film is the only permanent record of hematologic work done on a patient which can be retained in the laboratory. Occasionally, it may be necessary to examine a blood film again to check for errors or evaluate changes in the clinical status of the patient. The blood film has many uses. It is used to study the morphologic features of both the red cells and the white cells. (Morphology is the study of the form and structure of an organism.) The various types of white blood cells are classified and recorded as percentages. The blood film can also be used to verify the hemoglobin value and the red cell count. It is used to check or estimate the white cell count, reticulocyte count, red cell indices, and platelet count. Because the blood film is used for so many purposes, a well-made smear is essential. Generally, two good films are prepared with each blood count (white cell count, platelet count, red cell count, etc.). One of these films is stained, and the other is kept in reserve.

The source of blood used for the smear is an important consideration. Fresh blood from a finger prick is the best source of blood for morphologic examination of the white blood cells and the red blood cells. The finger must not be squeezed excessively to obtain the drop of blood, and the finger must not be touched with the glass slide. If the slide touches the finger, oils or moisture from the finger will lead to a poorly prepared film. The ear lobe is used for making blood smears if the finger site is unavailable or if special morphologic studies are to be made. When the ear lobe is used, it must be wiped thoroughly with alcohol and dried well, as the ear lobe is waxy and wax may lead to bubbles in the smear. If the blood must be preserved in some way, Sequestrene is the anticoagulant of choice. It is the best preservative for hematologic work and preserves the morphologic features of the white cells as well as the shape and size of the red cells. Balanced, or double, oxalate is not an acceptable anticoagulant for morphologic studies, because it distorts the shape and

* Allowable error used by the hematology laboratory of the University of Minnesota Hospitals.

characteristics of some of the white cells. However, balanced oxalate maintains the shape and size of the red cell.

PREPARATION OF THE BLOOD FILM

The equipment used for making blood films must be meticulously clean. Precleaned glass slides or slides cleaned with alcohol and wiped dry are to be used for the best results. Use of a spreading device is recommended. One example of this device is a margin-free spreader slide with ground-glass edges used for spreading the film of blood on the clean, lint-free slide. The edges of this spreader slide must be clean and free from chips in order to obtain a well-made blood film. Coverslips can also be used as spreading devices. The spreading devices must be cleaned thoroughly with alcohol and dried between each film and must be discarded when chipped or broken.

Procedure for Making a Blood Film

1. A drop of capillary or venous blood preserved with Sequestrene is placed on one end of the slide, about one-fourth of the slide from the edge. The drop should measure about 2 mm in diameter (about the size of a match head).

2. Immediately after the drop of blood has been placed on the slide, the spreader slide is drawn backward into the drop of blood at an angle of approximately 45 degrees with respect to the first slide. The blood is allowed to flow evenly across the spreader slide.

3. When the blood has spread evenly across the edge of the spreader slide, the spreader slide is moved quickly along the surface of the first slide. The spreader slide should be balanced on one or two fingers (for a freer, smoother movement) rather than held between the thumb and forefinger. As the spreader slide is moved, a thin film of blood is deposited behind it. The blood film should be at least 1 in. in length.

4. The blood film is dried immediately by waving the slide through the air or by placing it in front of an electric fan.

5. The film should be labeled by writing the name of the patient in the blood at the thick end using a lead pencil. Proper labeling is essential.

There are many criteria of a good blood smear. The body of the smear should be smooth and not interrupted (the smear should not have thick areas and thin areas). The smear should have a good feather edge (thin end of the smear); that is, the film should fade away without a defined border on the end. Chipped or dirty spreader slides will cause abrupt endings or tails with blood streaks out beyond the feather edge. When the feather edge is defined, there is an indication that the majority of the white cells have been piled up on the feather edge. When this occurs, the heavier neutrophils accumulate in the feather edge in a greater amount than the other types of white cells, leaving incorrect percentages of the types of white cells in the body of the smear. Platelets also tend to accumulate on the feather edge of the smear, decreasing the number in the smear proper. When the smear is too thick, accurate counting of the cells is difficult because of piling up. A very thin smear is satisfactory for morphologic studies, but it may be tedious to examine. Smears which have vacuoles or bubbles result from dirty slides or fatty samples. When microscopic observations are made from a blood smear, only a small part of the smear is used. This area must be one where the cells are well distributed and about one cell thick.

STAINING THE BLOOD FILM

After preparing a smear, the next step is the staining procedure. The stain most often used is Wright's stain, which is one of a group of the polychrome Romanowsky stains. The method employs fixation of the dead cells as opposed to the supravital stain in which living cells are stained. The Romanowsky stains contain eosin, methylene blue, and azure dyes. Another stain used for blood films is Giemsa stain. A combination of Wright's stain and Giemsa stain can also be used. The dyes can be purchased as a powder, which is diluted in C.P. absolute methyl alcohol. The blood cells are fixed by the methyl alcohol, and the staining takes place when the dye is diluted with an aqueous solution. Fixation is the process by which the blood is made to adhere to the slide and cellular proteins coagulate. Heat can also be used for fixation but is not necessary when the stain contains methyl alcohol. The aqueous solution used in the staining procedure consists of a phosphate buffer with a pH of 6.4.

Directions for Preparation of Wright-Giemsa Stain and Buffer

1. Wright-Giemsa stain. Dissolve 2.0 g of Wright's dye and 0.1 g of Giemsa dye in 800 ml of C.P. absolute methyl alcohol. Shake the mixture vigorously at intervals for several days. Filter it before use.

2. Phosphate buffer (pH 6.4). Dilute 6.63 g of monobasic potassium phosphate and 2.56 g of anhydrous dibasic sodium phosphate to 1,000 ml with deionized water. Distilled water may be substituted for the buffer, if the pH is approximately 6.4. Check the pH of the prepared phosphate buffer with a pH meter before use.

Procedure for Staining

1. Fix the film by flooding the slide with the stain. Allow the stain to remain on the slide for 3 to 5 minutes. Determine the exact timing for each batch of stain used.

2. Add phosphate buffer using about 1 to $1\frac{1}{4}$ times as much buffer as the stain on the slide. Add the buffer dropwise, and blow on the surface to mix the stain and buffer. A metallic film should form. Allow the stain and buffer mixture to remain on the slide for 10 to 15 minutes. At this

time the staining takes place as a result of the combination of dye and buffer at the correct pH.

3. Wash the slide with deionized water, and pour off the staining solution at the same time. Remove all precipitated stain during this process.

4. Wipe the dye from the back of the slide, and place the slide in a vertical position to dry. Do not blot the slide. Place the heaviest part of the smear downward to allow precipitated stain to flow away from the thin edge, which will be used for counting. When dry, the slide is ready for microscopic examination.

It is important that the stain and buffer be made correctly. The stain should stand for 1 week before being used, and the pH of the buffer must be correct. For every new batch of stain and buffer used, the fixing and staining times should be checked by staining a few slides. If staining of the cells is satisfactory, the times used for fixing and staining should be noted and used for that particular batch of reagents. If the pH is too acid or too alkaline, the stain will give false color and appearance to the cells.

The red blood cells should appear red-orange in color through the microscope. The white blood cells should appear as described under Examination of the Blood Film. The following situations will indicate staining errors: Faded or washed out cells are caused by overwashing, understaining, or improperly made stain. When the red cells are all blue-red, the slide has been underwashed or overstained, or the stain too alkaline. When the white cells appear indistinct and the nuclei blue instead of purple, the stain was too acid or the film overwashed or understained. When white cells appear darker and more granular, the stain was too alkaline or overstained and underwashed. Bright red red cells result from an acid stain. Large amounts of precipitated stain on the smear result from either the improper washing (not enough washing to remove the metallic scum) or using an old stain which has started to precipitate.

Precautions to Be Noted When Preparing and Staining Blood Films

All equipment used in the initial preparation of the blood smear must be meticulously clean and in good condition. The thickness of the film on the slide is determined by the size of the drop of blood used, the speed of the stroke used to move the spreader slide, and the angle at which the spreader slide is moved. A thick film results when the drop of blood is large, the angle used is greater than 45 degrees, and the speed of the spreading motion is fast. A thin film results when the drop of blood is small, the angle used is less than 35 degrees, and the speed of motion is slow.

The feather edge of the smear must be free from accumulation of white cells. When white cells are numerous on the feather edge, the distribution of the different types of white cells in the counting area will not be representative of the blood sample. Using a dirty spreader slide or too slow a stroke in the preparation of the film can result in this error. Rapid drying of the blood film is essential. When blood films are not dried rapidly, the red cells become crenated, the white cells shrink, and there is an increase in rouleaux of the red cells.

Adequate fixing time must be allowed. A minimum of 3 minutes is recommended for the initial staining time. Since inadequate fixation allows dissolution of the nuclear chromatin, overfixation is preferable. To achieve the proper staining reactions in the cells, the stain and buffer must be prepared correctly, and the correct technique must be used for the staining procedure. Accumulation of the metallic scum on the film may be avoided by washing and tipping the slides simultaneously. The fixing time and staining time varies with each batch of dye used. For this reason, new batches must be checked in order to determine the correct staining times.

EXAMINATION OF THE BLOOD FILM

Since the proper use of the microscope is important in the accurate examination of a blood film, a general review of the procedure to be used is presented for the student viewing a blood film for the first time. When looking at a blood film, first the smear should be viewed with the low-power objective, various areas of the smear being examined by moving the slide with the mechanical stage. The difference in appearance of the various areas is due to the technique used in preparing the smear. In spreading the blood on the slide, the smear is relatively thick at its beginning and gradually thins out to a very thin feather edge. The majority of the cells seen under the low-power objective are red blood cells, appearing as small, round, reddish-orange bodies.

Scattered among the red-staining cells are the less numerous white blood cells. These cells are larger and more complex in appearance than the red blood cells. The white cells consist of nuclei surrounded by cytoplasms. The nuclei are purple-staining bodies, and the cytoplasms stain various colors, depending upon contents. The size of the cell, the shape and size of the nucleus, and the contents and staining reaction of the cytoplasm are used in identification of white blood cells.

Procedure

With the low-power objective, an area of the smear is found where the red cells are just touching each other and are not piled on top of one another. This area will be found near the feather edge of the smear. When this area has been found, the oil-immersion objective should be used instead of the low-power objective. It is pertinent to point out now that the high-dry objective ($45\times$) is not suitable for examination of blood films. When the high-dry objective is used, a blurred image is seen.

A drop of immersion oil is placed on the selected site (where the red blood cells are just touching each other). The coarse-adjustment knob should be turned until the lens is well into the drop of oil. The oil must be in direct contact with the lens for effective use of the oil-immersion objective. While the technician is looking through the eyepiece, the objective is slowly raised using the fine-adjustment knob, since the oil-immersion lens does not have to be raised very far.

When red blood cells are viewed with the oil-immersion objective, they appear as round structureless bodies and contain no nuclei, granules, or discrete material. The red color is darker at the edge of the cell than in the center. This variation is due to the biconcave shape of the red blood cell. The thinner center of the red cell contains a lesser quantity of pigment. The pigment, or red color, of the cell is due to the hemoglobin present. Normally, there is little variation in the size of the red cells. With oil immersion, most of the red cells in a normal blood smear are about the same size. The average diameter of the red cell is about 7.2 μ. The shape of the normal red cell is uniformly round on a dry film, although variation in shape can be produced with a poor spreading technique in the preparation of the blood film.

When experience has been gained in using the microscope properly in the viewing of blood smears, a more specific technique is used to observe the morphologic features of the blood cells. Every examination of a blood film should include the following steps:

1. Evaluation of the quality of the blood film using the low-power objective. The film should be thin enough so that the red cells and the white cells are clearly separated. There should be no precipitated dye. The red cells and the white cells should be properly stained, and there should not be a large accumulation of white cells at the feather edge of the blood film. If the blood film does not meet these criteria, it should not be examined further, and a new film must be made.

2. Estimate of the white cell count and general scanning for abnormal cells using the low-power objective. A blood film should be used to check every white cell count. The number of white cells is estimated in the counting area of the film (that area where the red cells are lying side by side with no overlapping) with the low-power objective. Using the low-power objective ($10\times$) and the usual eyepiece ($10\times$), with a total magnification of $100\times$, approximately 20 to 30 white cells per field are equivalent to a white cell count of approximately 5,000 cells/mm^3. Using this same magnification, 40 to 60 white cells per field are equivalent to a white cell count of approximately 10,000 cells/mm^3. The bulk of the film should be scanned for the presence of any abnormal cells.

3. Oil-immersion examination of the red cells for alterations and variations in morphologic features. The red cells must be examined for morphologic alterations. The normal red cell is a nonnucleated biconcave

disk containing hemoglobin, and its function is to transport oxygen to the various cells of the body. The majority of red cells measure between 7.0 and 7.4 μ, the average diameter being 7.2 μ. The minimum thickness of the red cell is 0.8 μ, and the maximum is 1.3 μ. The mean volume for red cells is 87 μ^3. In estimating the diameters of white blood cells, it is often advantageous to use the red cell as a 7-μ measuring stick.

There are various terms used to describe changes in the red cell shape, size, and staining reaction observed. Alterations in the size of the red cell are described by the following terms: *anisocytosis*—excessive variation in cell size; *macrocytosis*—predominance of large red cells, with an MCD greater than 7.5 μ; and *microcytosis*—predominance of small red cells, with an MCD less than 6.9 μ. Alterations in the shape of the red blood cell include such descriptive terms as *poikilocytes*—red cells which show marked irregularity in shape; *sickle cells*—red cells which are sickle-shaped or long and clublike in appearance; *spherocytes*—small, spherical red cells which appear round and completely filled with hemoglobin; and *ovalocytes*—red cells which are oval. Variations in the staining reaction of the red cell are described by terms such as *hypochromasia* (or hypochromatic)—pale-staining red cells with very pale central areas; *anochromasia* (or anochromatic)—extremely pale-staining red cells which exhibit only a narrow, peripheral rim of pale-staining hemoglobin; *orthochromasia* (or orthochromatic) or *normochromasia* (or normochromatic)—red cells which contain the normal amount of hemoglobin and stain accordingly; and *polychromasia* (or polychromatic)—mixed staining reaction due to the presence of RNA and hemoglobin. These polychromatic "red" cells vary in color from a muddy blue to a gray red-orange and appear as reticulocytes when stained supravitally. The degree of the observed red cell alterations is noted as slight, moderate, or marked.

Several inclusions are also seen, under certain conditions, in the red cells. These inclusions must be readily identified. *Basophilic stippling* is seen as pinpoint to granular, blue-green– to blue-black–staining particles in red cells. These particles consist of precipitated RNA. Some red cells which contain basophilic stippling, upon observation of the smear stained with Wright's stain, will prove to be siderocytes. *Siderocytes* are red cells which contain particulate iron, which stains a bright blue-green color after treatment with acid–potassium ferrocyanide (Prussian blue). *Jolly bodies* are spherical, purple- to black-staining bodies (1 to 2 μ in diameter) present in red cells. These particles are also nuclear remnants. One or more of these bodies may be present within the same red blood cell.

When nucleated red cells (normoblasts) are seen, the number of these cells per 100 white cells is counted and reported. It is necessary to correct the total white cell count when normoblasts are present, since they are not destroyed by the 2% acetic acid used for the white cell count (normoblasts would be counted along with the white cells). The total white cell count can be corrected in the following way:

$$\text{Corrected white cell count} = \frac{\text{uncorrected white cell count/mm}^3}{100 + \text{no. nucleated red cells}}$$

The presence of rouleau formation of the red cells is also to be noted. Rouleau is the term used for piling up of the red cells as in a roll of coins. This formation is seen in certain diseased conditions but more often is caused by poor technique used in the slide preparation. When the blood film is not dried immediately after the film has been spread on the slide, rouleau can result.

4. Evaluation of platelet count and morphologic changes using the oil-immersion objective. The blood film is examined with the oil-immersion objective to estimate the number of platelets and to detect morphologic alterations. The platelet count is estimated as low, normal, or increased. If the blood film is well made without aggregates at the feather edge of the smear and platelets can be found only with great difficulty, the platelet count is most likely reduced. However, if there are a few platelets in almost every oil-immersion field, the platelet count is probably within the normal range. When the platelets are sufficiently abundant to attract the attention of the observer almost automatically, it is reasonable that the platelet count is increased. Examination of the stained film provides an invaluable check on platelet counts, and a check of the smear is automatically done with each platelet count made in the laboratory.

Platelets generally vary from 2 to 4 μ in diameter. They are ovoid structures having a colorless to pale blue background substance containing centrally located, reddish to violet granules. They are often increased in size when there is active regeneration of the blood. Bizarre forms are also noted under these circumstances.

5. Differential count of the white cells and examination of the white cells for morphologic alterations, using the oil-immersion objective. The differential count consists of identification and counting of a minimum of 100 white cells. After red cells and platelets have been examined, white cells are classified and counted. The slide should be moved in a way which will allow continuous counting and classification of white cells from margin to margin of the smear. When a margin is reached, the slide should be moved to the left or to the right (a distance of a few microscopic fields) and the white cells counted and classified from margin to margin again. When exactly 100 white cells are counted, the number of different white cells recorded is an estimate of the approximate percentages of the respective types of white cells comprising the total white cell count. For example, when 3 of the 100 cells counted are eosinophils, then 3 percent of the circulating white cells are eosinophils. If the relative

numbers of specific types of white cells differ markedly from the accepted normal values, it is advisable (except in cases of leukopenia) to count 200 cells or even more before recording percentages. The percentages of a specific cell type must then be calculated.

One hundred successive white cells must be counted to obtain an accurate differential percentage. A white cell cannot be skipped or not tabulated because it cannot be identified. Experience is necessary in morphologic studies of white cells, especially when any immature or abnormal cell is seen. Individuals with limited training in the field of hematology should not attempt to identify abnormal white cells. This identification should be made by a more qualified person, such as the pathologist. Persons with limited training should, however, be able to identify and classify the normal white cells but should be encouraged to seek assistance when a questionable cell is seen.

Types of White Cells

In addition to the five types of white cells to be described in the paragraphs that follow,* there is another cell, the plasma cell (or plasmacyte), which can occur in certain blood specimens. The plasma cell is thought to be a derivative of the lymphocyte or primitive connective tissue cell. Plasma cells can be found in cases of measles, chickenpox, scarlet fever, multiple myeloma, and plasmacytic leukemia.

Neutrophils   60 to 70% in adults
18 to 40% in infants

The most numerous of the granulocytes is the polymorphonuclear neutrophil leukocyte (PMN). Neutrophils comprise from 60 to 70 percent of the total number of leukocytes in adults and from 18 to 40 percent in infants. Neutrophils vary in diameter from about 9 to 12 μ, and the nucleus forms a relatively small part of the cell. The nucleus can assume various shapes, but its usual configuration is lobular. That is, the elongated nucleus is usually constricted in one to four places, forming a series of bulges or lobes connected by narrow strands of chromatin; it may exhibit two to five lobes. The chromatin is irregularly arranged in fairly compact masses, and it takes a deep reddish purple stain. The chromatin masses are distinct and clearly distinguishable from the lighter-staining (generally pink-staining) parachromatin (karyoplasm). The nuclear membrane is distinct, and no nucleoli are visible. The cytoplasm has a faint pink color and contains a large number of very small, often indiscrete, granules distributed throughout it in a rather irregular fashion. These granules are usually light pink or very light violet. A few darker granules may be present.

Generally, *leukocytosis* is due to an increase in the absolute number of neutrophils and is then designated as *neutrophilia*. Neutrophilia is found

* From the University of Minnesota Hospitals hematology laboratory procedure manual.

in acute infections and metabolic, chemical, and drug intoxications; acute hemorrhage; postoperative states; certain noninflammatory conditions such as coronary thrombosis; malignant neoplasms; and following acute hemolytic episodes. Neutrophilia is usually accompanied by a "shift to the left," or an increase in the number of immature cells, and cytoplasmic toxic changes. In normal blood, 3 to 5 percent band forms (nonsegmented neutrophils) can be seen. An increase in the number of band forms, which may be accompanied by the presence of immature neutrophils, is significant, and these cells should be reported in percent when present. Toxic changes in the neutrophils are indicated by the presence of deeply stained basophilic granules, pale blue Döhle bodies, or vacuolization of cytoplasm.

Eosinophils 2 to 4 %

The eosinophilic granular leukocytes, or eosinophils, make up 2 to 4 percent of the total number of leukocytes. They are slightly larger than neutrophils, and their nuclei occupy a relatively small part of the cell. The nucleus is also polymorphic, but it usually has fewer lobes than that of a neutrophil. Commonly only two lobes are present; occasionally three may be seen. The nuclear structure is much like that of the neutrophil, but the lobes are plumper, and the chromatin often stains a lighter purple. The nuclear membrane is distinct, and no nucleoli are visible. The cytoplasm is usually colorless, but it may be faintly basophilic; it is crowded with spherical acidophilic granules which stain a red-orange with eosin and are larger and more distinct than neutrophilic granules. The eosinophilic granules are hard, firm bodies which are not easily damaged. The granules remain intact when pressed into the nucleus or even when the whole cell is damaged and the cell membrane broken. Eosinophilic granules are also highly refractile, a feature which often proves a valuable distinguishing characteristic.

Basophils 0 to 1 %

The basophilic granular leukocytes, or basophils, comprise zero to 1 percent of the total leukocytes. They are about the same size as neutrophils, but their nuclei usually occupy a relatively greater portion of the cell. The nucleus is often extremely irregular in shape, varying from a lobular form to a form showing indentations which are not deep enough to divide it into definite lobes. The nuclear pattern is indistinct. There appears to be a mixture of the chromatin and parachromatin, and this mixture stains purple or blue and shows little structure. One is often able to recognize a basophil by this lack of nuclear structure. The nuclear membrane is fairly distinct, and there are no nucleoli visible. The cytoplasm is usually colorless; it contains a variable number of deeply stained, coarse, round or angular basophilic granules. The granules (meta-chromatic) stain deep purple or black; occasionally a few smaller, brown-ish granules may be present. Since the granules are soluble in water, occasionally a few or even most of the granules can be dissolved during the staining procedure. When this occurs, the cell will contain vacuoles in place of granules, and the cytoplasm may appear grayish or brownish in their vicinity. The cytoplasm of a *mature* basophil is colorless. An immature basophil has a pale blue cytoplasm and is seen only in myelogenous leukemia.

Lymphocytes   22 to 30% in adults
                40 to 70% in infants & children

Lymphocytes constitute 22 to 30 percent of the leukocytes of the normal adult and 40 to 70 percent of the leukocytes in infants and young children. Lymphocytes assume three classically cited sizes: small (6 to 8 μ), medium (9 to 11 μ), and large (12 to 15 μ). There are numerous gradations of size and form from one type to the other; some lymphocytes can be as large as monocytes.

The *small lymphocyte* is composed chiefly of nucleus. The nucleus is round or slightly notched, and the nuclear chromatin is in the form of coarse, dense, deeply staining blocks. There is relatively little parachromatin, and that visible is not very distinct. Almost the entire nucleus stains a deep purple. The nuclear membrane is heavy and distinct, and nucleoli are not usually seen. The cytoplasm appears in the form of a narrow, relatively dark-blue-staining band, usually free from azure granules.

The *medium-sized lymphocyte* has a larger nucleus but relatively more cytoplasm than nucleus. The nucleus is round, oval, or slightly notched, and the nuclear chromatin stains a dark purple. The chromatin, as in the small lymphocyte, is in the form of heavy blocks, or clumps. Some lighter staining parachromatin is present, but for the most part it blends with the chromatin and is not distinct. The nuclear membrane is heavy and distinct, and nucleoli usually are not seen. The cytoplasm can appear smooth and homogenous or somewhat spongy. It may be almost colorless or may vary from a pale blue-green to a deeper but somewhat powdery blue. If azure granules are present in the cytoplasm, they are usually spherical and light pink; they vary in size, from slightly larger than neutrophil granules to the size of eosinophil granules.

The *large lymphocyte* shows a further increase in the size of the nucleus and an increase in the relative amount of cytoplasm. The nucleus contains more parachromatin, and so it stains more lightly than do the nuclei of the smaller forms. However, the chromatin is still present in the form of heavy blocks, or clumps, without distinct marginal outlines because of the blending of chromatin and parachromatin. The nuclear membrane is distinct, and nucleoli usually are not seen. The cytoplasm in this form can be abundant and is most frequently smooth and hyaline in appearance;

it may, however, be spongy. It stains as does the cytoplasm of medium-sized lymphocytes, and azure granules are frequently seen. Nucleoli are rarely seen in lymphocytes of normal blood, but they may be seen in cells which have been crushed in the spreading of the film. It is possible that blood lymphocytes contain nucleoli which are normally obscured by the coarse nuclear chromatin.

It is sometimes difficult to distinguish between the nucleated red cells (normoblasts) and small lymphocytes. The staining reaction of the parachromatin of the two cells is an important diagnostic criterion; the parachromatin of the lymphocyte is a pale blue or violet, and that of the normoblasts in red or pink.

Monocytes 4 to 8 %

The monocytes constitute 4 to 8 percent of the leukocytes in the blood of normal adults. They are the largest of the normal leukocytes, measuring from 12 to 20 μ in diameter. The nucleus is fairly large; it may be oval, lobulated, notched, or polymorphic but most frequently assumes a kidney shape. The nucleus stains faintly, and the nuclear pattern is usually very characteristic. There is sharp segregation of chromatin and parachromatin, and the chromatin is distributed in a linear arrangement of delicate strands which gives the nucleus a "stringy" appearance. (Occasionally the nuclear pattern resembles that of a lymphocyte, and the cytoplasmic differences must be relied upon for distinction.) The nuclear membrane is delicate but distinct, and nucleoli usually are not seen. The cytoplasm is abundant, slightly basophilic, and often vacuolated, and has a slate-gray or muddy blue color. Extremely fine and abundant azurophilic granules are present; this dustlike azure granulation is called "azure dust" and is seen only in monocytes. The granules vary in color from a light pink to a bright purplish red.

Blood Cell Changes

Morphologic changes in the red and white blood cells as seen on the stained blood film aid in determining the nature of many blood diseases. Certain diseases give fairly characteristic alterations in red blood cells, white blood cells, and platelets, in addition to other clinical signs. The physician uses the information obtained from the laboratory in regard to the morphologic appearance of the blood cells to assist him in the diagnosis of and treatment for many diseases.

It is most important that the laboratory technician be well informed as to the appearance of normal blood cells, so that when blood films with abnormal cells or immature cells in them are seen, the technician will recognize these immediately. Any abnormal or immature cells should be identified by someone experienced in cell morphology. The technician should screen the films and give questionable ones to the pathologist or experienced medical technologist for final evaluation.

Most abnormalities found in white blood cells relate to the age of the cell. All white blood cells in the circulating blood should be mature, and the presence of young, or immature, white cells in the blood is considered abnormal. Some general observations for differentiating immature white cells from mature ones are morphologic changes in the cell size, the appearance of the intracellular structure (presence of granules, changes in the nucleoli, chromatin, or nucleus, for example), the staining properties, and the cell function. There is a progressive decrease in the cell size with maturity; the nucleus of the cell gets smaller, resulting in an increased cytoplasmic ratio with the increasing age of the cell. In the granulocyte, granules appear with maturity. In young, immature white cells the nucleus is round; with cell maturity the nucleus becomes lobed or indented. Chromatin, the background substance in the nucleus, is fine and lacy in the young cell and eventually becomes coarse and clumped. Nucleoli may be present in young cells and absent in the mature ones. In young granulocytes, the cytoplasm stains basophilic (blue) and eventually turns pink with maturity. The young nucleus stains reddish violet and turns intensely basophilic with maturity. The granules in the cytoplasm assume specific staining qualities with increasing maturity.

Certain evidence of cell function is observed which is characteristic of specific developmental stages of the white cells. Examples are the presence of nucleoli, which would indicate a young cell; mitotic figures, which indicate a young cell; cytoplasmic inclusions, which are characteristic of a mature cell; phagocytosis, which is seen in mature cells; and appearance of hemoglobin, which is seen in mature red cells.

It has already been stressed that a person with a limited training in the field of hematology should not identify abnormal cells on a blood film. It must also be stressed, however, that this person should be able to differentiate a young, or immature, cell from a normal one. There are many stages of young cells, and it is not necessary for the technician to be able to differentiate between these stages; the trained medical technologist or pathologist makes this evaluation. It is interesting, however, for the medical laboratory technician to be at least aware of the various developmental stages of the blood cells, and for this reason, a brief resumé of the blood cell developmental series follows:

1. Erythrocyte series. Pronormoblast, basophilic normoblast, polychromatic normoblast, orthochromatic normoblast, reticulocyte, and erythrocyte.

2. Granulocyte series. R-E cell, myeloblast, leukoblast, promyelocyte, myelocyte, metamyelocyte, and mature granulocyte.

3. Lymphocyte series. Lymphocytes are formed by the lymphoid tissues throughout the body (spleen and lymph nodes). The evidence of maturity is indistinct, and the developmental stages are poorly defined. One listing of developmental stages for the lymphocyte is R-E cell, reticular lympho-

cyte, immature lymphocyte, and mature lymphocyte. Normally three sizes of mature lymphocytes are found in the blood: small, medium, and large. An immature lymphocyte, called a *lymphoblast,* is found in pathologic conditions.

4. Monocyte series. The origin of the monocyte has not been definitely established, but it is thought to arise from phagocytic reticular cells of the connective tissue (the R-E system is involved). One monocytic series is R-E cell, myeloblast, monoblast, and mature monocyte.

5. Thrombocyte series. Megakaryoblast, megakaryocyte, and thrombocyte (platelet).

THE HEMATOCRIT DETERMINATION

for size of red cell and hemoglobin content - evaluation & classification of anemia

The hematocrit is a macroscopic observation by which the percentage volume of the packed red blood cells is measured. This test is relatively simple and reliable. It gives useful information concerning the size of the red blood cell which may be correlated with the information obtained concerning the number of red cells (red cell count) and hemoglobin content of the cells. The hematocrit is a useful test in the evaluation and classification of the various types of anemia. There are two widely used methods for determination of the hematocrit: one test is the Wintrobe method, and the other is the microhematocrit method. Most laboratory technicians obtain agreement with both methods. In some instances, however, when the hematocrit measurement is being used to calculate the red cell indices, the Wintrobe method is the better one to use. The microhematocrit method offers advantages to the technician such as its utilizing less time, labor, and amount of blood sample when compared with the Wintrobe method.

The hematocrit, or percentage volume of packed red blood cells, is one of the most important and precise measurements that can be made on a blood sample for the evaluation of anemia and polycythemia.[10] It is more accurate and less time-consuming than running a red cell count. The normal range of values for both the Wintrobe method and the microhematocrit method is from 40 to 50 percent for males and 37 to 45 percent for females.

The Wintrobe hematocrit method is a macro method which requires the use of venous blood preserved with either balanced oxalate or Sequestrene.[11] The microhematocrit method requires a small amount of blood, using blood from a free-flowing puncture.

Equipment

For the Wintrobe method, a special hematocrit tube called the *Wintrobe tube* is used. This tube is a thick-walled glass tube with a uniform inner diameter and is graduated from zero to 10.5 cm. The tube is filled with blood using a special type of pipet called a *Pasteur pipet.* This pipet is a long-stemmed capillary pipet. A standard laboratory centrifuge capable of generating a relative centrifugal force of 2,260 g (in this instance "g" designates the acceleration due to gravity) is necessary to pack the red cells suitably in the Wintrobe tube.[11]

For the microhematocrit method, special ungraduated glass capillary tubes are used. These tubes are 1 mm in diameter and 7 cm in length and are lined with dried heparin, which prevents coagulation. Microhematocrit tubes are purchased specifically for this procedure, and a special microchematocrit centrifuge is also used. This centrifuge is capable of a speed of 10,000 rpm and holds the hematocrit tubes in a disk-type apparatus. A reading device must be used, since the capillary tubes are not graduated. The length of the whole column of blood and the length of the column of packed red cells may be measured with a millimeter ruler and a magnifying glass or with one of several commercially available devices.

Procedure for Wintrobe Hematocrit Determination[11]

1. The Pasteur pipet is used to transfer well-mixed venous blood to the clean, dry Wintrobe hematocrit tube. This is properly done by first placing the pipet in the bottom of the tube and gradually withdrawing the pipet while expelling blood until the tube is filled to the 10-cm mark. Bubbles in the tube must be avoided.

2. The tube is sealed with a cap and centrifuged at full speed in a suitable centrifuge for 30 minutes. During centrifugation, the red cells, which have the highest specific gravity of the blood elements, settle to the bottom. The Wintrobe tube is calibrated from 0 to 10.5 cm, and the height of the various layers may be easily read.

3. After centrifugation, three layers are apparent in the tube. These layers are, reading from the bottom of the tube, (1) red cells, (2) buffy coat, containing platelets, leukocytes, and other nucleated cells when present, and (3) plasma.

4. The level of the red cell column and the total height of the column of blood are noted. If the tube has been filled to exactly the 10-cm mark, the hematocrit in volumes percent is equal to the direct reading at the top of the layer of packed red blood cells times 10. When the height of the column of cells and plasma is not exactly 10 cm, a simple calculation to correct for this can be made. The following general formula applies:

$$\text{Hematocrit } \% = \frac{\text{height of column of packed RBC}}{\text{height of column of cells and plasma}} \times 100$$

This is exactly the same as setting up a proportion, as illustrated below:

$$\frac{\text{Reading of packed RBC}}{\text{Reading of plasma level}} = \frac{x}{10}$$

$$x \times 10 = \text{hematocrit } \%$$

Procedure for Microhematocrit Determination[12]

1. A freely flowing puncture is made in a finger (or in the heel of an infant).

2. Two microhematocrit capillary tubes are filled to within 2 cm of the end (one-half to two-thirds full).

3. The vacant end of the tube is sealed with Plasticene, a specially manufactured plastic seal for these tubes. The tubes can also be heat-sealed.

4. The sealed tubes are centrifuged in a microhematocrit centrifuge for 4 to 5 minutes at 10,000 rpm.

5. The microhematocrit result is read from a graphic reading device or with some other accurate measuring device. The hematocrit is read as the percentage of the volume of packed red cells per volume of blood used. The graphic reading devices enable direct reading in percentage.

Precautions

The blood sample must be properly collected and preserved. If the Wintrobe method is used, Sequestrene or balanced oxalate are the anticoagulants of choice. The blood cannot be clotted or hemolyzed. If clotted blood is used, there will be a false packing of the red cells, and the true packing in the tube will not be noted (a falsely increased result will be observed). In using a hemolyzed specimen, some of the red cells have been destroyed, so again the packing of the red cells will not be true (a falsely decreased result will be observed). Centrifugation must be sufficient to yield maximum packing of the red cells. Preferably the centrifugation should be done with the hematocrit tube in an upright position, because it is sometimes difficult to read the level of the packed cells when this level is on a sl⁻nt.

The hematocrit value is frequently accompanied by a hemoglobin determination. There should be a correlation between the two results: the hematocrit result should be approximately three times the hemoglobin result.

For the microhematocrit method, the capillary blood must be collected from a freely flowing puncture. The capillary tubes must be properly sealed, so that no leakage occurs. Since the capillary tubes used for this determination are not calibrated, it is essential that the level of packed red cells and the total volume of the cells and plasma be accurately measured by some convenient reading device.

THE ERYTHROCYTE SEDIMENTATION RATE

The erythrocyte sedimentation test is another hematologic determination that employs macroscopic observation. If blood is prevented from clotting (by using a suitable anticoagulant) and allowed to settle, sedimentation

of the erythrocytes will occur. The rate of sedimentation of the erythrocytes depends on three main factors: (1) the number of erythrocyte particles, (2) the size of the erythrocyte particles, and (3) certain technical
factors. The speed or rate of sedimentation also appears to be dependent
on the amount of fibrinogen or globulin present. The size of the erythrocyte
particle is altered in many pathologic conditions because the phenomenon
of erythrocyte aggregation which is caused by an alteration of the erythrocyte surface charge by plasma proteins. The protein that is most often
involved is fibrinogen, although increases in gamma globulins or abnormal
proteins will also produce this effect. These factors determine the size
of the aggregates of erythrocytes. With increased concentration of large
molecules in the plasma, there is a greater tendency for erythrocytes to
pile up in rouleau formation.

The sedimentation of the erythrocytes in any given sample of blood
may be plotted as a curve using graph paper with the millimeters of
fall as the ordinate and the minutes of time as the abscissa. In such
a curve it will be noted that there is at first a variable period of gradual
fall during which time the aggregates of erythrocytes are forming (rouleau
formation is taking place). Next, a very rapid and marked drop
or fall of the aggregates occurs, constituting the main portion of the sedimentation of the erythrocytes. The last part of the curve represents a
more gradual, but relatively slight, falling off of the sedimentation rate
during which time the erythrocyte aggregates are being packed at the
bottom of the sedimentation tube. If the patient is anemic, this packing
will be more marked than in an individual with the normal number of
erythrocytes. In any event, the effect of anemia on the sedimentation
rate will be relatively slight. By far the most important factor in determining the rate of sedimentation is the size of the erythrocyte aggregates,
or rouleau.

In the vast majority of infections there is at least some increase in
the sedimentation rate of the erythrocytes; chorea and undulant fever
are two exceptions. There is also an increased sedimentation rate in most
cases of carcinoma. In leukemia and in diseases of bone marrow the
sedimentation rate is generally very rapid. As patients recover from infectious diseases, the sedimentation rate slowly returns to normal. The sedimentation rate may still be increased long after other clinical manifesta-
tions have disappeared. It is still one of the best evidences that the defense
mechanisms of the body are still more active than normal. Increased numbers of erythrocytes, such as are seen in cases of polycythemia and failure
of the right side of the heart, tend to cause a marked slowing of the
sedimentation rate. When the hematocrit value is greater than 48 to 50
percent, the sedimentation rate is markedly slowed, regardless of any other
factors present which might otherwise accelerate it. A decrease in the
erythrocyte sedimentation rate will result when the plasma fibrinogen level

is decreased, as in cases of severe liver diseases (acute yellow atrophy, for one).

There are two methods for determination of the sedimentation rate: one is the Westergren method, and the other is the Wintrobe method. Normal values for the two methods agree well. The normal values for the sedimentation rate are 5 to 20 mm in 1 hour for women and 5 to 15 mm in 1 hour for men.

Equipment for Westergren Method *antiquated method, but be familiar with the procedure.*

A special Westergren "tube," which is really an open-ended pipet, is used. It is 300 millimeters long with an inner diameter of 2.5 millimeters and is graduated in millimeters from 0 at the top of the tube to 200 at the bottom. The graduated volume of the tube, or pipet, is 1.0 ml. A special rack to hold the Westergren pipets in a vertical position is also necessary for this test. This rack is known as a *Westergren sedimentation rack,* and it is constructed so that rubber stoppers attached to springs close the open ends of the pipet when this pipet is placed properly in the rack. In order to assure proper sedimentation of the red cells, the pipet must be held exactly in a vertical position, and use of the special rack will ensure this.

Procedure for Westergren Method[13]

1. Five milliliters of venous blood is drawn and placed in a tube containing either Sequestrene or double oxalate. Either of these anticoagulants is suitable for this test.

2. Before performing the test, the blood is mixed by repeated inversions for 3 to 5 minutes.

3. A Westergren pipet is filled to the zero mark and vertically placed in the Westergren rack.

4. The upper level to which the red cells fall is read in millimeters from the graduation marks on the pipet at intervals of 20, 40, and 60 minutes. Each of these readings is recorded.

Precautions

An anticoagulant which not only prevents clotting but preserves the shape and volume of the red cells must be used. Certain anticoagulants prevent erythrocyte sedimentation and are, therefore, unsuitable for this test. Since erythrocyte numbers influence the rate of fall, there must be no hemolysis of the specimen. The pipet used for the test must be placed in a vertical position in the rack; an angle different from this position can alter the rate of fall significantly. As the blood specimen stands after the venipuncture, the suspension stability of the erythrocytes increases. The test must be set up in a clean Westergren pipet within 2 hours after the blood has been drawn, to ensure a reliable sedimentation rate. Preferably the test should be set up within 1 hour after the specimen is collected from the patient. Temperature and vibrations can also affect the sedimentation rate, and these factors should be taken into consideration.

COAGULATION STUDIES

The blood coagulation mechanism is highly complicated and involves many factors. Knowing which factor is not performing its proper function is of critical importance to the physician. This knowledge is gained through the use of several different laboratory tests. The proper formation of a blood clot after a scratch or cut has been inflicted depends on the healthy functioning of all the numerous factors involved. In an individual having a weakness or deficiency in one or several of the numerous factors, severe trauma from a serious injury or from surgical treatment can result in collapse of the clotting mechanism. This in turn will result in a most drastic manifestation—severe hemorrhage. This has been dramatically demonstrated in those persons whose clotting mechanism is adequate for everyday living but who, during such common surgical procedures as dental extractions or tonsillectomies, erupt into severe bleeding. It is of the utmost importance, therefore, that the laboratory tests done in this area be done well. Most of these tests employ macroscopic observations of one sort or another. A great amount of responsibility rests upon the laboratory for producing valid results for these tests.

With the damage of a blood vessel wall, a variety of factors normally combine to stop the flow of blood. The term *hemostasis* refers to the stopping of the blood flow. When a blood vessel is damaged, the surrounding tissues exert pressure on it which slows the blood flow. Sometimes this pressure is sufficient to stop the flow of blood. Another of these factors is the positive reaction of the injured vessel. When injured, the muscle of the blood vessel walls contracts and retracts. Contraction and retraction of the injured vessels serve as the first line of defense against bleeding. When a capillary is injured, it appears that the tissue pressure factors play an important role in arresting the blood flow. The platelets also contribute to hemostasis and act as a second line of defense against hemorrhage. They are of fundamental importance in at least four ways: (1) platelets alone or with fibrin form the hemostatic plug, (2) platelets are very important in the blood coagulation mechanism, (3) platelets may be essential to prevent the passage of red cells through the capillary walls, and (4) platelets carry a local vasoconstrictor identified as serotonin.

The actual coagulation of blood occurs because fibrinogen is converted to fibrin. Coagulation is the third line of defense against hemorrhage. The first two lines of defense (the retraction and contraction of the blood vessel and the platelet plug) stop or slow the flow of blood so that the clotting mechanism can occur. The general topic of blood coagulation is highly controversial, and much research is still in progress in this field. It is generally agreed that all the elements necessary for clot formation are normally present in the circulating blood. The fluidity of the blood, therefore, depends on a balance between the coagulant and anticoagulant factors.

The mechanism of coagulation takes place in three major steps: (1) the formation of thromboplastin, (2) the formation of thrombin, and (3) the formation of fibrin. Various clotting factors, or constituents, are involved in this mechanism. The following is a list of several of these factors and their abbreviations and synonyms:[14]

Factor V—proaccelerin
Factor VII—proconvertin
Factor VIII—antihemophilic factor (AHF), antihemophilic globulin (AHG), or thromboplastinogen
Factor IX—plasma thromboplastin component (PTC)
Factor X—Stuart-Prower factor
Factor XI—plasma thromboplastin antecedent (PTA)

Abnormal formation of a clot results from a deficiency of any of these factors or the presence of an inhibitor or anticoagulant. The following schematic presentation details the interactions of the various clotting factors according to the three stages discussed previously:

Stage 1:
$$\left. \begin{array}{l} \text{Platelets} \\ \text{VIII (AHF)} \\ \text{IX (PTC)} \\ \text{XI (PTA)} \end{array} \right\} \xrightarrow[X]{V} \text{plasma thromboplastin}$$

Stage 2:
$$\left. \begin{array}{l} \text{Prothrombin} \\ \text{Plasma thromboplastin} \\ \text{Calcium} \\ \text{V} \\ \text{X} \end{array} \right\} \rightarrow \text{thrombin}$$

Stage 3:
$$\left. \begin{array}{l} \text{Thrombin} \\ \text{Fibrinogen} \end{array} \right\} \rightarrow \text{fibrin (clot)}$$

The presence of an anticoagulant prevents coagulation. The anticoagulants Sequestrene, oxalate, and citrate remove calcium to prevent clotting in vitro. Heparin and Dicumarol prevent conversion of prothrombin to thrombin, also preventing the clotting mechanism from functioning in vivo.

Besides having a system for clot formation, the body also has a means by which the fibrin clot may be removed. The mechanism for clot, or fibrin, removal is not completely understood. It can be briefly described as a two-stage reaction. In stage 1, profibrinolysin (normally present in the blood) and the enzyme fibrinokinase (released under a variety of conditions such as trauma, surgical treatment, or transfusion reaction) form fibrinolysin. In stage 2, fibrinolysin reacts with the fibrin to break it down, forming fibrin derivatives. Fibrinolysin also destroys fibrinogen and prothrombin, in addition to destroying the fibrin.

Tests involved in the study of hemostasis may be divided into three main categories according to the three lines of defense against hemorrhage which were discussed earlier in this section: (1) tests for the vascular factor, (2) tests for the platelets, and (3) tests for the plasma factors involved in coagulation. Tests for the vascular factor include the cuff test (also known as the tourniquet test or capillary resistance test) and tests for bleeding time. Tests for the platelet factor include the platelet count, the bleeding time, and the clot retraction test. There are numerous tests for the plasma factors involved in coagulation. Some of these include the venous clotting time and the prothrombin time tests.

CUFF TEST

In the cuff test, a blood pressure cuff is placed above the patient's elbow and inflated to a pressure of 100 mm Hg. The arm is examined before the pressure is applied to see if any petechiae are present. Petechiae are collections of red blood cells around minute vessels; when these are present, small reddish spots will be seen on the skin. Any petechiae are noted by marking a circle around them with ink. The pressure is maintained for 10 minutes, the cuff is removed, and the number of petechiae are counted which have appeared in a circle 5 cm in diameter drawn below the bend of the elbow. A normal value is 0 to 10 petechiae, and a positive reaction is indicated by more than 10 petechiae. A positive test result indicates capillary weakness, thrombocytopenia, or both.

Bleeding time tests measure the time required for cessation of bleeding following a stab wound of a capillary bed. The time required will depend upon capillary integrity, the number of platelets, and the platelet function.

BLEEDING TIME TESTS   How long one bleeds before clotting

There are two commonly used bleeding time tests, the Ivy bleeding time test and the Duke bleeding time test.[15,16] The chief difficulty in performing bleeding time tests is in the production of an adequate and standardized skin puncture. An adequate test depends greatly on the skin wound and, therefore, upon the skill of the technician. Capillary bleeding is tested; wounds greater than 3 mm in depth are likely to involve vessels of greater than capillary size. On the other hand, wounds that are shallow are not likely to test adequately the capillaries and the other hemostatic factors involved.

Bleeding is believed to be controlled in the conditions of the test by capillary retraction and the formation of a platelet plug in the wounds. Tissue factors are also thought to play a role; the most important of these is tissue tonus. Defects in the clotting mechanism have little effect on the bleeding time. The bleeding time is prolonged in conditions where there is a combination of poor capillary retraction and platelet deficiency.

The bleeding test is positive in thrombocytopenic purpura and in constitutional capillary inferiority. Normal bleeding times are found in hemophilia and other defects of the clotting mechanism. It is important to realize that the value ascribed to bleeding and capillary clotting tests has undergone a change. With the availability of more specific and sensitive methods, bleeding and clotting tests (especially capillary clotting tests) have very little to offer as diagnostic aids. Bleeding and clotting tests may give the physician a false sense of security about the bleeding tendencies of his patient. Some hospitals have discontinued the use of capillary clotting tests in the battery of hematologic tests done.

Procedure for Duke Bleeding Time Test

1. An ear lobe (or heel, in an infant) is cleansed carefully with 70% medicated alcohol. Use of an ear lobe on which the patient has been lying is avoided.

2. A stab wound 3 mm deep is made in the margin of the ear lobe (or heel of an infant).

3. Timing is begun as soon as bleeding begins.

4. Drops of blood are removed with blotting paper every 10 to 20 seconds without touching the wound. The patient must remain quiet throughout the test.

5. The time at which bleeding ceases is reported to the nearest 30 seconds.

6. Normal values are 1 to 6 minutes.

Procedure for Ivy Bleeding Time Test

1. A blood pressure cuff is placed on the upper arm, and the forearm is cleaned with 70% medicated alcohol below the antecubital fossa area and allowed to dry. The area used should be relatively vein-free.

2. The cuff is inflated to 40 mm Hg, and this pressure is maintained throughout the test.

3. Three skin punctures 3 mm deep are made in the cleansed area. The punctures should be made in rapid succession using a new number 11 surgical blade.

4. Timing is begun as soon as bleeding begins.

5. Blood is removed every 10 to 20 seconds as it accumulates over the wounds by blotting lightly with the flat side of a piece of blotting paper or other absorbent paper. Care should be taken not to apply any pressure or disturb the lips of the wounds.

6. The time at which bleeding ceases is reported to the nearest 30 seconds.

7. Normal values are from 1 to 6 minutes.

Precautions to Be Noted in Bleeding Time Tests

It is important to note again at this point that the bleeding time tests are not always significant, because normal bleeding times are found in patients where there are defects in the actual clotting mechanism. The bleeding time is prolonged in conditions where there is a combination of poor muscle retraction is the blood vessels and a platelet deficiency. The performance of an adequate bleeding time depends greatly on the depth of the skin puncture; a standard depth of 3 mm must be used. When the Duke bleeding time test is performed, the ear must not be congested, and the patient must be instructed not to move his head. In the Ivy bleeding time test, the blood pressure cuff must be maintained at 40 mm Hg throughout the test.

Prolonged bleeding times (over 6 minutes) and shortened bleeding times (under 1 minute) must be repeated on the other arm or ear. The Duke bleeding time test is not used to check the Ivy method.

Tests for the platelet factor involved in hemostatis include the platelet count (previously described); the bleeding time test, in which prolonged bleeding time indicates that platelets are reduced below the minimum normal level; the clot retraction test; and the prothrombin consumption (or serum prothrombin time) test.

CLOT RETRACTION TESTS How long it takes to clot

Normal blood will clot completely and begin to retract within 1 hour. At the end of 18 hours, the clot should have retracted completely, and serum is expressed. The clot should be tough and elastic and not easily broken with an applicator stick. The retraction is primarily dependent on normal platelet function. The extent of the retraction is influenced by the amount of fibrin formed, the presence of intact platelets within the fibrin network, and physical interference from trapped red blood cells. When the platelet count is less than 100,000 cells/mm^3, poor clot retractibility is usually seen.

There are several ways by which the coagulation mechanism can be altered; if any one of the many factors is deficient, the coagulation of blood will not take place normally. Tests for venous clotting time and prothrombin time, described in this section, are coagulation tests done routinely in the laboratory. More specific tests such as the partial thromboplastin time, prothrombin consumption test, thromboplastin generation test, and determination of increased fibrinolysin will not be discussed, since these are tests which are not done in the routine of the hematology or coagulation laboratory but are specific assays performed by specially trained technologists.

VENOUS CLOTTING TIME TESTS

The Lee-White method for determining venous blood coagulation time is in general use.[17] Capillary blood clotting tests are unreliable, because the sample is contaminated with a variable amount of thromboplastin obtained with the tissue juice. The Lee-White test provides a measurement of the time required for freely flowing blood to clot after it has been removed from the body. The results are influenced by the nature of the surface of the test tube used and by the diameter of the tube. Temperature and agitation of the sample of blood also influence the test results; vigorous agitation of the tubes will shorten the clotting time. Only when these factors are carefully controlled and there is no mixture of tissue fluid with the blood sample can the venous clotting time be regarded as representing the "intrinsic coagulative power" of the blood. Contamination with tissue thromboplastin (in tissue juices) because of a poor venipuncture will shorten the clotting time. This test in no way differentiates between the deficiencies in the clotting factors and the presence of anticoagulants, both of which can prolong the clotting time.

Procedure for Lee-White Venous Clotting Time Test

1. A clean venipuncture is made. In making the venipuncture, it is important that the vein be penetrated without excessive probing. A stopwatch is started as soon as the blood enters the syringe, and 5 ml of blood is drawn.

2. One milliliter of blood is carefully placed into each of three small serologic tubes having an internal diameter of 8 mm.

3. The tubes are allowed to stand undisturbed at room temperature for 10 minutes.

4. After the 10-minute waiting period, the first tube is tipped gently at 1-minute intervals until the blood is completely clotted.

5. After the blood in the first tube has clotted, the second tube is tipped in a similar fashion at 1-minute intervals until clotting is observed.

6. After the blood in the second tube has clotted, the third tube is tipped every 30 seconds until clotting is observed.

7. The clotting time of the third tube is reported to the nearest 30 seconds. The normal range is from 15 to 25 minutes.

Precautions to be Noted in Venous Clotting Time Tests

In doing the venipuncture to obtain the blood specimen, the vein should be penetrated cleanly with as little probing as possible. Any excessive probing could introduce tissue juices into the specimen which would contaminate it with thromboplastin and thus shorten the clotting time.

If the tubes containing the blood are clotted at the end of the initial 10-minute waiting period, the test is unsatisfactory and must be repeated. One cause for this early clotting could be contamination with tissue thromboplastin.

Vigorous agitation of the tubes can also shorten the clotting time. Some methods for this test require that the three tubes used for the blood specimen be rinsed out with saline solution prior to their use. The surface of the tubes used as well as their inner diameter influence the clotting time.

PROTHROMBIN TIME TEST *results can be converted to longer time % activity. The longer time takes, the less activity.*

This test was devised on the assumption that when an optimal amount of calcium ion and an excess of thromboplastin are added to decalcified plasma, the rate of coagulation depends upon the concentration of prothrombin in the plasma. The prothrombin time, therefore, is the time required for the plasma to clot after an excess of thromboplastin and an optimal concentration of calcium have been added. The prothrombin time test is a test of stages 2 and 3 of the clotting mechanism.

Specimens for the prothrombin time test must be preserved by using sodium oxalate. The calcium is removed by the anticoagulant to prevent coagulation from taking place. Exactly 4.5 ml of venous blood is drawn into a tube containing 0.5 ml of 0.1 M sodium oxalate (the final oxalate concentration should be 0.01 M). The blood must be free from clots and examined carefully before the test to ascertain that there are no clots visible. The prothrombin time should be tested within 4 hours after the blood is drawn. If a longer time elapses, there will be progressive inactivation of some of the necessary factors.

The normal values for the prothrombin time range from 11.2 to 14.5 seconds. A normal prothrombin time shows that the elements of stages 2 and 3 of the coagulation mechanism are probably not disturbed. This finding coupled with a prolonged venous clotting time places the abnormality within stage 1. The value of the prothrombin time is seen both in following the progress of patients treated with Dicumarol (a therapeutic anticoagulant drug used to slow down the tendency for clotting, especially helpful in preventing postoperative thrombosis and pulmonary embolism) and in screening factor deficiencies in hemorrhagic diseases.

Certain reagents are necessary for the prothrombin time test. Primarily, the reagents are calcium chloride and thromboplastin. These reagents must be prepared in specific concentrations.

Directions for Preparation of Prothrombin Time Reagents

1. Stock thromboplastin. A commercial preparation employing dehydrated rabbit brain is used. One ampule (1 g) of the dried material is

mixed with 30 ml of isotonic saline solution and incubated at 45 to 48°C for 10 minutes. The suspension is poured into two conical centrifuge tubes and centrifuged. The supernatant fluid is decanted through gauze to remove the remaining particles. The thromboplastin may be used when cool. It should be stored at 4°C.

2. 0.1 M calcium chloride. 11.09 g of anhydrous calcium chloride is diluted to 1,000 ml with deionized water.

3. 0.015 M calcium chloride. 150 ml of the 0.1 M calcium chloride is diluted to 1,000 ml with deionized water.

4. Thromboplastin–calcium chloride. Equal parts of 0.015 M calcium chloride and stock thromboplastin are mixed prior to use.

5. Control solution. A commercial control is tested with each batch of prothrombins. Each prothrombin control must be prepared before use according to the manufacturer's directions. Control values and limits will vary with each brand of control used. Proper use of a control can detect deterioration of the thromboplastin, a calcium solution of the wrong concentration, or the wrong incubation temperature.

Procedure

1. Exactly 4.5 ml blood is drawn into a tube containing 0.5 ml of 0.1 M sodium oxalate. The ratio of 1 part sodium oxalate anticoagulant to 9 parts whole blood must be observed.

2. As soon as possible, the blood is centrifuged at 3,000 rpm for at least 10 minutes. The plasma is removed after centrifugation.

3. 0.2 ml of thromboplastin–calcium chloride mixture is pipetted into small test tubes (8- by 75-mm size is suitable).

4. The tubes containing the thromboplastin–calcium chloride and the tubes containing an aliquot of the plasma are incubated at 37°C. One minute is allowed for the thromboplastin and plasma to reach 37°C.

5. 0.1 ml of plasma is pipetted (using 0.1-ml pipets) into the tube containing the thromboplastin–calcium chloride mixture, and the stopwatch is started simultaneously.

6. The tube is shaken and left in the water bath (37°C) for a minimum of 7 to 8 seconds. It is then removed and tipped gently until a clot is formed.

7. The stopwatch is stopped immediately when a clot is observed, and the time is recorded. All plasma samples are tested at least in duplicate and usually in triplicate. Determinations must agree within certain limits: the allowable error for difference in agreement between duplicate or triplicate tests varies with the length of the prothrombin time; according to one study, for prothrombin times up to 30 seconds, agreement should be within 1 second for duplicates and 2 seconds for triplicates; for prothrombin times between 30 and 60 seconds, agreement should be within 2 seconds for duplicates and 3 seconds for triplicates; and for prothrombin

times over 60 seconds, the result is reported as "over 60 seconds."* The test must be repeated if the allowable error is exceeded.

Precautions

The sample of venous blood must be preserved properly using the anticoagulant sodium oxalate. The blood must be free from clots; if any clots are present, a new specimen must be drawn. The ratio of anticoagulant to blood specimen must be 1:10 (0.5 ml of anticoagulant and 4.5 ml of whole blood). The prothrombin time test must be run within 4 hours of the drawing of blood, because of progressive inactivation of certain factors present. Those samples giving results of over 1 minute should be repeated on a new sample. All plasma samples are tested at least in triplicate. Deterioration of the thromboplastin should be noted by running a control specimen, because the control will serve to detect deterioration or inaccurately prepared reagents. The control can also detect an incorrect incubation temperature, which could result in inaccurate test values.

THE HEMOGLOBIN DETERMINATION

The hemoglobin determination is one of the most frequently performed hematologic tests. It is included in the routine CBC done on patients in most hospitals or physicians' offices. As discussed previously, the other parts of the CBC usually include a white blood cell count, a microhematocrit, and the examination of the stained blood film. In the modern clinical laboratory photometry is used to determine hemoglobin concentration. A thorough knowledge of the photometer is essential to obtain accurate hemoglobin results.

Hemoglobin is the oxygen-carrying pigment in the red blood cell. The hemoglobin molecule is made up of two parts: (1) heme, an iron complex, and (2) globin, the protein fraction. The red blood cells carry oxygen from the lungs to the tissues of the body. Hemoglobin combines with oxygen to form a compound called *oxyhemoglobin;* it is in this form that oxygen is carried to the tissues. In disturbances of the body, hemoglobin may combine with various abnormal substances other than oxygen. Carboxyhemoglobin is due to the combination of hemoglobin with carbon monoxide. In this form, hemoglobin cannot transport oxygen. Another abnormal hemoglobin derivative is methemoglobin, resulting from chemicals or drugs. Still another example of abnormal hemoglobins is sulfhemoglobin, resulting from an overdose of sulfa drugs or their derivatives.

When the hemoglobin is below the normal level, the patient is said

---

* Allowable error used by the coagulation laboratory of the University of Minnesota Hospitals.

to be anemic. Anemia has previously been discussed in connection with conditions with low erythrocyte counts. It is a condition in which the circulating erythrocytes may be deficient in number, deficient in total hemoglobin content per unit of blood volume, or a combination of both. A decrease in hemoglobin can result from bleeding conditions in which the patient loses erythrocytes and therefore loses hemoglobin too. An increase in hemoglobin, usually as a result of an increase in the number of erythrocytes (erythrocytosis), is seen in polycythemia and newborn infants.

Hemoglobin is determined as grams of hemoglobin per 100 ml of blood, or grams percent (g%). This is the most satisfactory way of reporting hemoglobin values, since there is a wide range of normal values dependent on age, sex, and altitude of habitation for the various methods used for hemoglobin tests. Reporting hemoglobin as a percentage of a normal value is not satisfactory. Since there are so many different methods and each method has its own normal value, using a percentage value causes confusion. For example, 80 percent of normal for one method may be the same as 98 percent of normal for another method. Various hemoglobin testing methods with their values (in grams percent) for 100 percent hemoglobin are listed below:

Grams Percent

Sahli	17.3
Dare	16.0
Haden	15.6
Wintrobe	14.5
Haldane	13.8

Some of the many methods which can be used to determine the amount of hemoglobin present in a blood specimen are much more commonly used than others. Many years ago, before the use of the now popular photometer, most of the hemoglobin methods were of the visual type. These methods involved using the human eye to determine the various changes in color intensities due to hemoglobin concentration differences; these methods were not very accurate. Some of the visual methods are the Tallqvist, Dare, and Sahli. The Sahli method is now rarely used in the physician's office. In the Sahli method, the hemoglobin in the blood sample is converted to acid hematin by the addition of 0.1 N hydrochloric acid. The addition of acid to blood converts red hemoglobin to brown. Since brown is more easily matched by the human eye than red, the Sahli visual method for testing hemoglobin is one of the more acceptable visual methods. The error in a visual method is great, however, and these methods are certainly not recommended.

Gasometric analysis for hemoglobin with the Van Slyke apparatus is the most accurate method for determination of hemoglobin, but it is not used routinely in the clinical laboratory, because it is time-consuming and complicated. It is used as a reference method to obtain the hemoglobin concentration in blood samples used for standardization of hemoglobin procedures.

The two hemoglobin methods most widely used, the oxyhemoglobin method and the cyanmethemoglobin method, require the use of a photometer.[18,19] One photometer generally used is the Coleman Junior Spectrophotometer discussed under Photometry in Chapter 2. Other photometers can be used quite satisfactorily, however, and the hemoglobin method employed will depend on the type of machine used by the laboratory. Methods employing photometry in the analysis of hemoglobin content are rapid and are capable of giving results which have a high degree of accuracy. The degree of accuracy will also depend on basic technique, accuracy of the equipment, stability of the reagents, and cleanliness of the glassware.

Reagents

Proper preparation and storage of reagents for the hemoglobin determination is essential. For the oxyhemoglobin method, a solution of 0.04% ammonium hydroxide is needed. For the cyanmethemoglobin method, Drabkin's reagent is used. Except for the reagents used, the two methods differ very little. When the reagent 0.04% ammonium hydroxide is used and the red blood cells are hemolyzed, the hemoglobin present in the blood specimen is converted to oxyhemoglobin. This conversion is complete and immediate. The resulting color is stable.

Drabkin's reagent, used for the cyanmethemoglobin method, consists of three components: sodium bicarbonate, potassium cyanide, and potassium ferricyanide. When Drabkin's reagent is mixed with the specimen of blood, the stable pigment cyanmethemoglobin is formed. When a sample of whole blood is diluted with Drabkin's reagent, the potassium ferricyanide in the reagent oxidizes the hemoglobin to methemoglobin. The methemoglobin reacts with the potassium cyanide to form cyanmethemoglobin. All forms of hemoglobin except sulfhemoglobin are measured by this method.

Although Drabkin's reagent contains only a small amount of cyanide, it is still regarded as a poison. This reagent should be carefully handled to avoid any laboratory accidents. Salts and solutions of cyanide are poisonous; they should not be taken into the mouth or their fumes inhaled.

A control solution should be used for any hemoglobin determination. Daily controls should be run using either a commercially prepared control specimen or one prepared by the laboratory. The use of daily control values gives information regarding the state of the hemoglobin reagent (whether or not deterioration has taken place), accuracy of the hemoglobin pipets, variation and cleanliness of the calibrated photometer cuvettes, and variation in the photometer used to measure quantitatively the amount of hemoglobin present in the samples. Technical skill is also tested. When the control value is not within the acceptable limits, hemoglobin values of the blood specimens being measured should not be reported until the reason for the control value's being out of limits is found. Included in the reasons for "out of control values" are deteriorated reagents, faulty equipment (photometer), dirty glassware, inaccurate photometer standardization, deterioration of the control specimen, inaccurate or broken pipets, or poor individual technique.

Directions for Preparation of Reagents

1. 0.04% ammonium hydroxide. 0.4 ml of concentrated ammonium hydroxide is diluted to 100 ml with deionized water.

2. Drabkin's reagent. 1 g of ammonium bicarbonate, 0.050 g of potassium cyanide, and 0.200 g of potassium ferricyanide are diluted to 1,000 ml with deionized water. This reagent should be prepared fresh at least once a month and should be stored in a brown bottle to prevent deterioration: it is unstable in light.

Equipment for Hemoglobin Determination

A special pipet called a *Sahli* is used for hemoglobin determination. The Sahli pipet is calibrated to contain 20 mm^3 of blood. Since it is a to-contain pipet, it must be rinsed with the diluent to ensure proper measurement of the blood sample. The accuracy of hemoglobin pipets must be checked before the pipets can be used for hematologic determinations. This can be done simply by comparing the new pipet with U.S. Bureau of Standards pipets, which have been very carefully calibrated.

Since most determinations of hemoglobin employ photometry, a photometer of good quality and in good working order is essential. Most brands of photometers can be used to obtain good results if certain precautions are noted. Before a photometer can be used to determine hemoglobin concentration, it must be standardized. Since the Coleman Junior Spectrophotometer is in general use and since this machine has already been discussed in some detail under Photometry in Chapter 2, the procedure presented here for standardization of the photometer will deal specifically with this instrument. It must be stressed at this point, however, that the same general procedure can be followed for any type of photometer.

Standardization of the Coleman Junior Spectrophotometer

1. Stable standard cyanmethemoglobin solutions of concentrations representing 1:250 dilutions of whole blood containing 5, 10, and 15 g of hemoglobin/100 ml of blood are available commercially and are certified by the American College of Pathologists. For the oxyhemoglobin method or cyanmethemoglobin method these standards can be prepared by obtaining a sample of blood on which the hemoglobin has already

been determined by oxygen capacity or iron content. The oxygen capacity is the most frequently used reference method for hemoglobin standardization. It is based on the assumption that 1 g of hemoglobin will combine with 1.34 ml of oxygen. The following formula can be used to find the hemoglobin, in grams percent:

$$\text{Hemoglobin, g\%} = \frac{\text{vol\% oxygen capacity}}{1.34}$$

This blood sample is used for the stock standard solution. The sample is diluted in a volumetric flask with the hemoglobin reagent so that the hemoglobin concentration relative to the method used is approximately 25 to 30 g%. This standard should be stored in a refrigerator until ready for use. From the stock standard, a series of working standards are prepared, including duplicate sets for each of 10 dilutions having a total volume in each tube of 10 ml. The first tube should contain 10 ml of stock standard only, the second tube 9 ml of stock standard and 1 ml of hemoglobin reagent, the third tube 8 ml of stock standard and 2 ml of hemoglobin reagent, and so on, ending with the tenth tube containing 1 ml of stock standard and 9 ml of hemoglobin reagent. The percentage transmission of each standard is obtained with the photometer.

2. To span the light beam of the Coleman Junior Spectrophotometer, there must be at least 6 ml of solution in the commonly used cuvettes (19-mm size). The instrument can be modified to permit accurate readings with other volumes using the proper tubes and adapters. If no other tubes or adapters are available, a 5-mm slice cut from a number one stopper and dropped into the cuvette adapter so that it lies flat on the bottom will elevate the cuvette sufficiently so that a lesser volume of fluid (5 mm in the cyanmethemoglobin procedure, for example) will span the light beam.[20]

3. A blank tube containing 5 ml of Drabkin's reagent or 0.04% ammonium hydroxide is placed in the cuvette well, and the galvanometer beam is adjusted to read 100% T with the wavelength scale set at 540 mμ.

4. The percent transmission for each of the standards is obtained by reading the samples in the photometer. The blank tube must be reinserted and read between each sample. The percent transmission reading for each of the standards is recorded.

5. The readings are transcribed on semilogarithmic graph paper. The abscissa represents grams per 100 ml of hemoglobin, and the ordinate represents the percentage of light transmitted. A line is drawn through the plotted points, and a table is prepared from this graph to show what each reading of the percentage of light transmittance corresponds to in grams of hemoglobin per 100 ml of blood.

An alternate method is to calculate a constant factor (called the *K* factor) for the instrument. The formula for calculating the *K* factor is

$K = A/C$ where A equals the absorbance, or optical density and C equals the concentration of hemoglobin represented by the working standards. Using the average K value, hemoglobin concentrations corresponding to all potential galvanometer readings are calculated, and a standard chart is prepared.

For one specific photometer, the standard chart will designate the range of hemoglobin in grams percent which can accurately be determined using that photometer. Only hemoglobin values in grams percent obtained from the linear portion of the graph, plotting percent transmission against hemoglobin in grams percent, may be used to prepare the standard chart. This chart can be used to obtain hemoglobin values for any tests done using that specific machine but not for tests using any other instrument.

Another essential piece of equipment for hemoglobin determination is the cuvette for the photometer. New cuvettes must be carefully tested for their optical perfection before they are used for hemoglobin determinations. This is done by comparing them in the photometer with previously calibrated cuvettes (see under Photometry in Chapter 2 for more specific details). Once the cuvettes have been calibrated, they should be carefully washed and stored until used. Using scratched and dirty cuvettes will result in inaccurate hemoglobin values.

Procedure for Cyanmethemoglobin Determination for Hemoglobin

1. The wavelength scale must be set at 540 mμ.
2. The spectrophotometer (or photometer) must be allowed to warm up.
3. The blank tube containing 5 ml of Drabkin's reagent is placed in the cuvette well and the galvanometer beam adjusted to read 100% T.
4. Blood is drawn into a Sahli hemoglobin pipet to the 20-mm^3 mark. Blood may be pipetted from a finger prick, or preserved venous blood may be used (Sequestrene or balanced oxalate are satisfactory anticoagulants).
5. The outside of the pipet is wiped free of blood and the amount of blood adjusted exactly to the calibration mark; the blood is then discharged into a calibrated cuvette containing 5 ml of Drabkin's reagent. The pipet must be rinsed with the reagent at least five or six times by drawing the solution up into it and blowing it out again.
6. The contents of the tube are effectively mixed by inserting the pipet to the bottom of the tube and blowing vigorously through the pipet. It is most important that the amounts of blood and diluent be accurately measured and that these solutions be thoroughly mixed in the calibrated cuvette.
7. After a lapse of 10 minutes for color development, the tube containing the hemoglobin solution is placed in the cuvette well in the photometer, and the percentage of light transmitted is read from the galvanometer scale.

8. The result is converted into grams per 100 ml of blood from a calibration curve or table prepared for each photometer.

The technique for the oxyhemoglobin method is essentially the same as for the cyanmethemoglobin method. The chief difference lies in the use of 0.04% ammonium hydroxide as the diluting reagent.

Precautions in Hemoglobin Determination

Several precautions necessary while carrying out this determination have already been discussed. Photometric methods for the determination of hemoglobin are rapid and give results with a high degree of accuracy only when the equipment is in good working condition. The photometer must be working well, and the pipets and calibrated cuvettes must be clean and free from breaks or scratches. The Sahli pipets should be calibrated before they are used. Drabkin's reagent, if used, must be prepared fresh each month and must be stored in a brown bottle to prevent deterioration. Photometers must be standardized before being used for the hemoglobin determination. Periodically photometers should be restandardized and the calibrated hemoglobin tables redone when changes occur in the values. Each photometer must have its own calibration table.

TEST FOR OSMOTIC FRAGILITY OF THE RED BLOOD CELL

When red blood cells are introduced into a hypotonic solution of sodium chloride, they begin to swell until a critical volume is reached, and then hemolysis occurs. When the critical volume is reached, the cells are spherical. In this shape, the cell contains the maximum volume for the surface area of the cell, and any further increase in volume would require an increase in the area of the cell membrane.

In certain diseases, the osmotic fragility of the red cell is characteristically increased or decreased. The osmotic fragility test is a measure of the resistance of the red cells to increasingly hypotonic sodium chloride solutions. The resistance of the red cell membrane corresponds to the geometric configuration of the red cell. That is, red cell populations comprised of spherocytes demonstrate increased hemolysis, while those red cell populations comprised of flattened cells (such as sickle cells, target cells, or hypochromic cells) will demonstrate decreased hemolysis.[21] In hypochromic anemia, the osmotic fragility is decreased, or the red cells exhibit an increased resistance to hypotonic solutions. Hypochromic cells are very thin, contain very little hemoglobin, and therefore swell to a large extent before reaching their critical volume.

In cases where the red cells are already spheroidal, as in congenital hemolytic anemia, an increased osmotic fragility is noted. These red cells have a decreased resistance to hypotonic solutions, because they can swell only a little before their critical volume is reached.

The osmotic fragility test consists of diluting the blood sample in increasingly hypotonic solutions of sodium chloride. These solutions are generally prepared in the following concentrations: 0.80%, 0.66%, 0.56%, 0.52%, 0.48%, 0.44%, 0.40%, and 0.32%. The solutions should be kept at room temperature; they should be titrated against mercuric nitrate, and their pH should be between 5.5 and 7.0. The solutions must be chemically pure.

Procedure

1. Ten milliliters of each of the working sodium chloride solutions and 0.04% ammonium hydroxide are pipetted into two sets of conical centrifuge tubes.

2. Five milliliters of venous blood preserved either with Sequestrene or balanced oxalate is well mixed. Using a Sahli pipet, 0.02 ml of blood is pipetted into each tube of sodium chloride and mixed gently (1:500 dilutions). Gentle mixing is extremely important. One set of tubes is used for the patient's blood and the other set for a control sample of normal blood. The normal control is run with each batch.

3. The cell suspensions are incubated at room temperature for 1 hour.

4. The cell suspensions are centrifuged and the supernatant fluids decanted into calibrated cuvettes for the photometer.

5. The percent transmission for each of the supernatant fluids is obtained with the photometer, using the same wavelength setting as that used for the hemoglobin determination.

6. The hemoglobin concentration for each saline solution concentration is obtained and a hemoglobin chart prepared for the photometer used. The results are recorded, and the percent hemolysis is calculated for each of the saline solution concentrations.

7. A hemoglobin determination is made of the patient's blood and of the control samples. The results are recorded.

Calculation

The following general formula can be used to calculate the percent hemolysis:

$$\text{Hemolysis, } \% = \frac{\text{hemoglobin in supernatant}}{\text{hemoglobin, g\%}} \times 100$$

The percent hemolysis for each concentration of saline solution is reported. The increment of hemolysis (the increase in the degree of hemolysis) may also be calculated. For a given saline solution concentration, this is the difference in percent hemolysis from the next highest saline concentration. For example, if the 0.48% saline solution gave 25% hemolysis and the 0.44% saline solution gave 60% hemolysis, the hemolysis increment would be 60 minus 25, or 35%.

The percent hemolysis may be graphed on a special chart which indicates the normal range. Other saline concentrations can be included, when necessary.

THE RED BLOOD CELL INDICES

In classification of anemias, quantitative measurements of the average size, hemoglobin content, and hemoglobin concentration of the red blood cells are of substantial aid to the physician. These measurements are obtained by calculation when the values for the total number of red cells, the hemoglobin content per unit volume, and the percentage volume of packed red blood cells (the hematocrit) are known. The measurements calculated from these values are the mean corpuscular volume (MCV), the mean corpuscular hemoglobin content (MCH), and the mean corpuscular hemoglobin concentration (MCHC, or MCC). Another quantitative measurement of the red cells, the mean corpuscular diameter (MCD), is made directly.

Mean Corpuscular Volume (MCV)

This measurement is an expression of the average volume of the red blood cells in cubic microns. It is calculated by dividing the volume of red cells per liter by the number of red blood cells per liter. The volume is calculated by use of the formula

$$\text{MCV} = \frac{\text{hematocrit} \times 10 \text{ (vol packed cells/liter)}}{\text{RBC in millions/mm}^3}$$

An example of such a calculation follows: The hematocrit reading is 40%. The red cell count is 5 million cells/mm³.

$$\text{MCV} = \frac{40 \times 10}{5} = 80 \ \mu^3$$

The MCV in normal adults is between 80 and 94 μ^3. In some macrocytic anemias (such as are encountered in pernicious anemia) the MCV may be as high as 150 μ^3. In microcytic anemia with marked iron deficiency, the values may be between 60 and 70 μ^3.

The chief source of error in the MCV is errors in the red blood cell count, in which, as is well known, a considerable amount of error is inherent.

Mean Corpuscular Hemoglobin (MCH)

The MCH is the average hemoglobin content (weight) of the red blood cells in micromicrograms ($\mu\mu$g). It is obtained by dividing the hemoglobin content of 1 liter of blood expressed in micromicrograms by the number of red blood cells in millions per cubic millimeter. A micromicrogram is a millionth part of a microgram. A simple formula can be used to calculate this value:

$$MCH = \frac{\text{hemoglobin in g/liter (or in g\% } \times 10)}{\text{RBC in millions/mm}^3}$$

An example of this calculation follows: The hemoglobin is 15 g%. The red blood cell count is 5 million cells/mm³.

$$MCH = \frac{15 \times 10}{5} = 30 \ \mu\mu g$$

The normal range for the MCH is from 27 to 32 $\mu\mu$g. The value may be as high as 50 $\mu\mu$g in macrocytic anemias or as low as 20 $\mu\mu$g or less in the hypochromic anemias.

Again, the chief source of error is the red blood cell count, which must be done with accuracy if this calculation is to be of use to the physician.

Mean Corpuscular Hemoglobin Concentration (MCHC)

The MCHC is an expression of the average hemoglobin concentration per cell in percent. It may be calculated from the MCV and the MCH or from the hemoglobin and hematocrit values by using the following formula:

$$MCHC = \frac{MCH}{MCV} \times 100$$

or

$$MCHC = \frac{\text{hemoglobin in g\%}}{\text{hematocrit}} \times 100$$

An example of this calculation follows: The hemoglobin is 15 g%. The hematocrit is 40%.

$$MCHC = \frac{15}{40} \times 100 = 37.5\%$$

This measurement tells what percentage of the total volume of the red blood cell is occupied by hemoglobin. The concentration of the hemoglobin within the individual red cell is of considerable importance. The average normal value is 35%. Large erythrocytes will often have a normal MCHC, for a larger cell will contain more than the normal amount of hemoglobin. In true hypochromic anemias, the hemoglobin concentration is reduced, and values as low as 20 to 25% are not uncommon.

Precautions

It is essential to use only accurate data. The red blood cell count, the hematocrit results, and the hemoglobin values used must be accurate. It is also essential to check the appearance of the red blood cells in a well-stained blood film against the calculated indices. The calculations must correlate with the appearance of the red cells in the blood film,

PREPARATION OF SLIDES FOR THE LE TEST

The lupus erythematosus (LE) cell test is clinically important in the diagnosis of disseminated lupus erythematosus. The observation of an LE cell depends upon the reaction of an abnormal gamma globulin factor in the serum of a patient having this disease with the nucleus of a leukocyte. This reaction results in the formation of a swollen homogeneous mass of nuclear material which is phagocytosed by a normal granulocyte to produce the LE cell.

By traumatizing the white blood cells, the nuclear material is made more accessible to the LE factor. For this test, the blood from the patient is mashed through a sieve to provide the necessary trauma.

Procedure

1. Ten milliliters of venous blood is permitted to clot and remain at room temperature for 1 hour.
2. The clot is then mashed through a special sieve.
3. The clot fragments are centrifuged in a Wintrobe hematocrit tube at 1,000 rpm for 10 minutes. The buffy coat is removed, spread on a slide, and stained with Wright's stain.
4. The film is examined for the presence of LE cells by the pathologist or an experienced medical technologist.

EXAMINATION OF EXTRAVASCULAR FLUIDS

Examination of the various types of extravascular fluids, or body fluids, is done in various departments of the clinical laboratory, depending on what test is to be done and what type of fluid is to be examined. Cell counts are done on most body fluid specimens. For this reason, in many hospitals, the body fluid specimens are brought first to the hematology laboratory, and the specimen is either examined there or sent on from there to a specific department.

Many pathologic conditions may be associated with the fluid which accumulates in the various cavities of the body. The laboratory examination of the fluid may yield useful information regarding the formation and constituents of the fluid. The physician can also be alerted to the type of disease process present by the information obtained from the laboratory analysis of a patient's body fluid. Some of the body fluids examined in the laboratory are pleural, pericardial, peritoneal, synovial, and cerebrospinal fluids.

All body fluids, except synovial fluids, are to be received in the laboratory in a tube containing Sequestrene or balanced oxalate as an anticoagulant. The test for mucin done on synovial fluid needs no anticoagulant.

Body fluids should be considered contaminated, and all equipment must be decontaminated with 5% phenol after being used.

Since cell counts are done on many body fluid specimens, the specimen must be a fresh one. If the specimen is not fresh, cell disintegration will occur. No cell counts may be done on a clotted specimen; anticoagulants must be used to prevent coagulation of the specimen when a cell count is needed. Specific gravity tests must also be done on a clot-free specimen. Tests for mucin and protein, however, can be done on clotted specimens. When a glucose determination is ordered, the specimen must be immediately preserved with sodium fluoride to prevent glycolysis from taking place. Body fluid specimens to be cultured should be sent to the bacteriology laboratory. Specimens to be tested for a chemical constituent should be sent to the chemistry laboratory as soon as possible. Sometimes only one specimen is sent to the hematology laboratory, and several tests are required; the cell counts should always be done before other tests.

All body fluids are either transudates or exudates. Transudates are ultrafiltrates resulting from a difference in osmotic pressure across a membrane. Exudates are fluids which occur as a result of an inflammatory condition which leads to an increase in the permeability of a membrane. Generally, a transudate has a specific gravity below 1.018, a protein value of less than 2.5 g%, and very few cells. An exudate has a specific gravity above 1.018, a protein value greater than 2.5 g%, and many cells.

EXAMINATION OF BODY FLUIDS

In the hematology laboratory, the procedure followed in the examination of a body fluid (except cerebrospinal fluid) involves these observations: (1) the cell counts (red and white blood cells), (2) the specific gravity, (3) microscopic examination of a smear stained with Wright's stain, (4) the protein test (an Esbach quantitative protein determination can be run on these specimens), and (5) the mucin test. Cell counts and differential counts are done on cerebrospinal fluid by the hematology laboratory. For other tests ordered (such as glucose, protein, or chloride), the specimen is sent on to a specific department.

Procedure for Examination of Pleural, Pericardial, Peritoneal, and Synovial Fluids

1. The fluid is mixed by tipping the tube gently for 5 minutes. At least 1 ml of the specimen should be saved until all the tests are completed.

2. The red blood cell and white blood cell counts are done on whole, well-mixed fluid. This fluid is mounted on the counting chamber with a capillary pipet. Ten square millimeters is counted using the high-power objective ($43\times$). The cells are counted and classified as red blood cells or white blood cells, and the number of each per cubic millimeter is reported. Red cells and white cells are counted at the same time. If the

cell count is extremely high, dilutions may be made using the regular blood-diluting pipets. The diluent used is an isotonic solution of sodium chloride (saline solution). The dilution factor must be taken into consideration in the final calculations. Acetic acid cannot be used to destroy the red cells in order to count the white cells more easily, because acetic acid will precipitate the protein and this will obscure the field.

3. The specific gravity test is done on well-mixed fluid using the falling drop method. Copper sulfate solutions are used, ranging in specific gravity from 1.008 to 1.075. A capillary pipet containing the body fluid is held 1 cm above the copper sulfate solution, and one drop is allowed to fall from the pipet into the solution. If the specific gravity of the fluid is lower than that of the copper sulfate solution used, the drop will float. If the specific gravity of the body fluid is higher, the drop will sink.

4. Smears are prepared next. Even if a cell differential is not ordered, a smear is made to check the cell count. Three milliliters of well-mixed fluid is placed in a centrifuge tube and centrifuged for 15 minutes. The supernatant fluid is decanted and used for the protein determination. Four smears are made from the sediment, using an applicator stick to streak the sediment across the slide. The smears are dried immediately and stained with Wright's stain. Three hundred leukocytes are counted and classified as neutrophils, lymphocytes, eosinophils, and other cells (tissue cells). If any malignant cells appear to be present, the smears must be checked by the pathologist or an experienced medical technologist.

5. The protein test is done on the supernatant fluid (cell-free). An Esbach test can be run.[22] The centrifuged, cell-free body fluid is added to the special Esbach tube to the 1 mark and diluted to the 10 mark with deionized water. Esbach reagent is added to the R mark. The contents of the tube are mixed and allowed to stand at room temperature for 24 hours. At the end of 24 hours, the volume of the precipitate is read from the Esbach tube in grams per liter and then corrected for the dilution.

6. A qualitative test for mucin is done on the supernatant fluid.[23] One volume of deionized water and a few drops of 5% acetic acid are added to the fluid remaining. After 1 minute, a positive test is indicated by the appearance of a white precipitate or turbidity. The test is reported as positive or negative.

The mucin test using synovial fluids is done on the specimen after it has been centrifuged for 10 minutes. The supernatant fluid is decanted and used for the test. Two milliliters of 2% acetic acid is mixed with one milliliter of supernatant fluid to precipitate the mucin as a firm, rope-like clump. After 3 to 4 hours at room temperature, the precipitate is examined by agitating it with a stirring rod. Normal mucin remains firm and clotlike. Abnormal mucin may form a firm mass which becomes crumbly in 2 to 4 hours. The mucin clot is graded as 3+, firm; 2+, precipitate breaks up easily; 1+, small amount of precipitate; or 0, no precipitate.

EXAMINATION OF CEREBROSPINAL FLUID

Cerebrospinal fluid is more frequently tested than any of the fluids previously mentioned. This fluid fills the ventricles of the brain, the central canal of the spinal cord, and the subarachnoid spaces of the brain and spinal cord. It is formed in the ventricles and has many of the same characteristics as plasma, since most of its components are derived from the blood plasma. The only known function of the cerebrospinal fluid is a mechanical one that provides protection for the brain and spinal cord. The examination of the spinal fluid is important in the diagnosis of neurologic disorders, inflammatory diseases, and hemorrhage in the meninges.

The cerebrospinal fluid is obtained by puncturing one of the spaces between the lumbar vertebrae with a needle. There is a certain risk to the patient in this procedure, and, for this reason, the specimen is extremely precious and must be treated with the utmost care. Cerebrospinal fluid is also considered contaminated, and precautions must be taken to decontaminate all equipment used in connection with the specimen. Five percent phenol or seventy percent alcohol can be used for decontamination purposes. There is always the danger of spreading meningitis if cerebrospinal fluids are not handled properly. Cell counts on a spinal fluid specimen must be done as soon as possible after the spinal tap has been completed, since cells present will disintegrate within a short time. Tests for glucose in spinal fluid must also be performed immediately to prevent glycolysis. The use of sodium fluoride will slow down the glycolytic process. For the chemical tests ordered, the specimen shoud be sent to the chemistry laboratory.

The usual procedure for examination of a spinal fluid specimen by the hematology laboratory includes several observations. Some of them are (1) gross examination for abnormal color or presence of clots, (2) red blood cell count, (3) white blood cell count, and (4) examination of a smear stained with Wright's stain.

Procedure   *If you see yellow — be extra careful*

1. The spinal fluid is examined grossly for the presence of blood (a red or brown color), turbidity (cloudiness due to white blood cells), xanthochromasia (a yellow color), or clots.

2. The fluid is mixed by repeated inversions for 3 to 5 minutes.

3. For the red blood cell count, the well-mixed fluid is mounted from a clean, dry capillary pipet on both sides of a counting chamber. The cells are counted with the high-power objective in a total of 10 mm² (9 mm² on one side of the chamber and 1 mm² on the other side).

The red cells are small, round, yellow, and occasionally crenated. The percentage of crenated cells is reported in addition to the red cell count per cubic millimeter. Every red cell seen must be tallied, whether crenated or intact. If the spinal fluid is grossly bloody, it must be diluted using a white or red cell diluting pipet and Hayem's solution or isotonic saline solution. The count is reported in cells per cubic millimeter. The white blood cells will also be present in this preparation; they must therefore be separated from the red cells being counted.

4. For the white blood cell count, a capillary pipet is rinsed with glacial acetic acid. This pipet is carefully drained and the outside wiped. It is most important that no glacial acetic acid remain on the outside of the pipet because this would contaminate the specimen when the pipet is placed in it. This pipet is used to mount the spinal fluid in the counting chamber. The acid will destroy the red blood cells and emphasize the nuclei of the white cells. The white blood cells are counted in a 10-mm^2 area using the high-power objective. At the same time that the cells are being counted, they are classified into polymorphonuclear and mononuclear cells (the use of the glacial acetic acid enables this classification). When the cell count is above 100 white cells/mm^3, the cell differential is reported in percentage. The count is reported in cells per cubic millimeter.

5. When the white cell count is over 300 cells/mm^3, a differential count is done on a stained smear. The spinal fluid is centrifuged for 5 minutes at 3,000 rpm, and smears are made from the sediment. The smears are dried quickly and stained with Wright's stain. One hundred white blood cells are classified and reported in percent.

6. All equipment, pipets, tubes, and vials used in this procedure are put into phenol or alcohol. Every spinal fluid specimen must be treated with great caution.

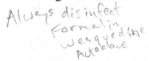

Always disinfect Formalin Wesqued the Autoclave

REFERENCES

1. G. Brickman, Blood from the Ear Lobe, *J. Lab. Clin. Med.*, 27:487, 1942.
2. J. Berkson, R. B. Magath, and M. Hurn, The Error of Estimate of the Blood Cell Count as Made with the Haemocytometer, *Am. J. Physiol.*, 128:309, 1940.
3. R. Biggs and R. L. Macmillan, The Errors of Some Hematologic Methods as They Are Used in Routine Laboratory, *J. Clin. Pathol.*, 7:269, 1948.
4. P. H. Bordewich, Electronic Counting of Blood Platelets, *Post grd. Med.*, 38:A44, 1965.
5. A. G. Hills, P. H. Farsham, and C. A. Finch, Changes in Circulating Leukocytes Induced by the Administration of Pituitary Adrenocorticotrophic Hormones (ACTH) in Man, *Blood*, 3:755, 1948.
6. G. W. Thorn, P. H. Farsham, F. T. G. Prunty, and A. G. Hill, Test

for Adrenal Cortical Insufficiency: Response to Pituitary Adrenocortico-
tropic Hormone, *J.A.M.A.*, 137:1005, 1948.
7. D. B. Huntsman, M. C. Dagget, and D. E. Holtkamp, Hinkleman's Solution as a Diluent for Counting Eosinophils, *Am. J. Clin. Pathol.*, 31:91,
1959.
8. T. C. Randolph, Blood Studies in Allergy: Direct Counting Chamber Determination of Eosinophils, *J. Allergy*, 5:96, 1944.
9. M. J. Stephens, Direct Eosinophil Counts, *Minn. Med. Tech.*, 14:3 1950.
10. Lot B. Page and Perry J. Culver, "A Syllabus of Laboratory Examinations
in Clinical Diagnosis," p. 58, Harvard University Press, Cambridge, 1960.
11. Maxwell Wintrobe, "Clinical Hematology," 5th ed., pp. 378–380, Lea
& Febiger, Philadelphia, 1961.
12. M. M. Strumia, A. B. Sample, and E. D. Hart, An Improved Microhematocrit Method, *Am. J. Clin. Pathol.*, 24:1016, 1954.
13. A. Westergren, The Technique of the Red Cell Sedimentation Reaction,
Am. Rev. Tuberc. Pulmonary Diseases, 14:94, 1926.
14. Wintrobe, *op. cit.*, p. 289.
15. W. W. Duke, The Relation of Blood Platelets to Hemorrhagic Disease:
Description of a Method for Determining the Bleeding Time and Coagulation Time and Report of Three Cases of Hemorrhagic Disease Relieved
by Transfusion, *J.A.M.A.*, 14:1185, 1910.
16. A. C. Ivy, P. F. Shapiro, and P. Melnick, The Bleeding Tendency in
Jaundice, *Surg. Gynecol. Obstet.*, 60:781, 1935.
17. R. I. Lee and P. D. White, A Clinical Study of the Coagulation Time
of Blood, *Am. J. Med. Sci.*, 145:495, 1913.
18. K. A. Evelyn and N. T. Malloy, Microdetermination of Oxyhemoglobin,
Methemoglobin, and Sulfhemoglobin in a Single Sample of Blood, *J. Biol.
Chem.*, 126:655, 1938.
19. E. J. King and M. Gilchrist, Determination of Hemoglobin by a Cyan-
Haematin Method, *Lancet*, 2:201, 1947.
20. Page and Culver, *op. cit.*, pp. 44–45.
21. J. Suess, D. Limentani, W. Dameshek, and M. J. Dolloff, A Quantitative
Method for the Determination and Charting of the Erythrocyte Hypotonic
Fragility, *Blood*, 3:1209, 1948.
22. Israel Davidsohn and Benjamin B. Wells, "Clinical Diagnosis by Laboratory Methods (Todd-Sanford)," 13th ed., p. 31, W. B. Saunders Company,
Philadelphia, 1962.
23. Page and Culver, *op. cit.*, p. 286.

BIBLIOGRAPHY

Biggs, R., and R. G. Marfarlane: "Human Blood Coagulation," Blackwell
Scientific Publications, Ltd., Oxford, 1962.
Brecher, G.: New Methylene Blue as a Reticulocyte Stain, *Am. J. Clin. Pathol.*,
19:895, 1949.
Cutler, J. W.: The Practical Application of the Blood Sedimentation Test
in General Medicine, *Am. J. Med. Sci.*, 183:643, 1932.

Hanauer, P.: Quality Control Methods in a Routine Hematology Laboratory, *Postgrad. Med.,* vol. 33, no. 5 (May), 1963.

Hawes, J. B.: A Study of the Reticulated Red Blood Cell by Means of Vital Staining Methods, *Boston Med. Surg. J.,* 161:493, 190?

Lillie, R. D.: Factors Influencing the Romanowsky Staining of Blood Films and the Role of Methylene Violet, *J. Lab. Clin. Med.,* 29:1181, 1944.

Quick, A. J.: "Hemorrhagic Diseases," Lea & Febiger, Philadelphia, 1957.

————, M. Stanley-Brown, and F. W. Bancroft: Determination of Prothrombin, *Am. J. Med. Sci.,* 190:501, 1935.

Rees, H. M., and E. E. Ecker: An Improved Method for Counting Platelets, *J.A.M.A.,* 80:621, 1923.

Wells, Benjamin B.: "Clinical Pathology," 3d ed., W. B Saunders Company, Philadelphia, 1962.

4

Urinalysis

INTRODUCTION

Of all the diagnostic procedures performed in the laboratory, the analysis of the urine is perhaps the most important. The urine samples are readily available, and many of the routine tests done are relatively simple to perform. The simplicity of the tests in no way means that they are unimportant or should be performed sloppily or in haste. The physician relies heavily on the laboratory findings of the urinalysis in diagnosing and treating many diseases. It cannot be overemphasized that it is extremely important in the urinalysis department, as well as in the other departments of the laboratory, to do careful, accurate work at all times. The life of the patient is often dependent on the accuracy of the laboratory personnel.

As an introduction to the study of urinalysis, the urinary system and the urine itself will be discussed. In general, urine can be considered a fluid composed of the wate materials of the blood. The urine is formed in the kidney and excreted from the body by way of the urinary system.

The urinary system consists of the kidney, ureters, bladder, and urethra (Fig. 4-1). The urine is actually formed in the nephron (working unit of the kidney), passed on to the bladder for temporary storage by way of the ureters, and then eliminated from the body by way of the urethra. The kidney functions as a means of eliminating waste materials from the body, but a better definition of this important organ is that it is the regulator of the extracellular fluid. The extracellular fluid is a water solution containing numerous dissolved substances; it consists of all the liquid in the body, outside the individual tissue cells. It includes the liquid part of the blood plasma, the lymph, and the interstitial fluid. The kidney regulates this extracellular fluid in such a way as to keep its composition

185

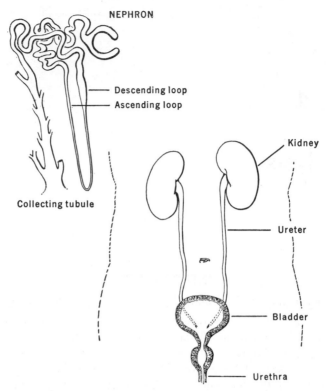

NEPHRON

Descending loop
Ascending loop

Kidney

Collecting tubule

Ureter

Bladder

Urethra

Fig. 4-1. Urinary system.

constant. This is very important, for the extracellular fluid is actually the environment of the individual body cells, and even slight changes in its composition may result in death. The kidney protects the extracellular fluid from changes in volume, acidity, composition, and osmotic pressure.

URINALYSIS DEFINED

The chemical or microscopic analysis of the urine is known as *urinalysis*. Several gross observations are also part of the urinalysis. The urinalysis is an important part of the initial examination of patients in all branches of medicine. It is made up of a number of different tests and observations. Some of these tests are actually chemical ones, while others are not. When the urinalysis is performed in an orderly fashion and the results are recorded accurately, the combination of observation and actual test results will provide the physician with a valuable picture of the patient's general health pattern. Many disorders of the body will be diagnosed with assistance from test results showing common abnormalities in the urine. The urinalysis is made up of three general parts: observations concerning physical properties (such as urine volume, color, transparency, odor, foam, pH, and specific gravity), simple chemical tests for abnormal constituents (such as sugar, protein, acetone, acetoacetic acid, bilirubin, and urobilinogen) and the microscopic examination of the urine sediment.

A urinalysis can give valuable information about the physiology or function of the kidney in general, an indication of possible renal infection at any point along the urinary tract, and information about the state of the body in general.

A typical routine urinalysis might include tests for, or observations of, the following:

Color
Transparency
Odor and foam
Specific gravity
pH
Sugar
Protein
Microscopic analysis of the sediment

Certain other tests are run when necessary either as indicated by results obtained from the above tests or if the laboratory director so instructs. These special tests include:

Quantitative test for sugar
Quantitative test for protein
Test for ketone bodies (acetone and acetoacetic acid)
Bilirubin test
Urobilinogen test
Hemoglobin (occult blood) test

COMPOSITION OF THE URINE

The actual composition of urine varies a great deal, depending on many factors. These include diet, metabolic rate, and the general state of the body. Urine is a complex aqueous mixture of various organic and inorganic substances. Most of these substances either are derived from the food eaten or are waste products from the body metabolism. Urine consists of approximately 96 percent water and 4 percent dissolved substances. These substances consist primarily of *urea* (the principal end product of protein metabolism), sodium chloride, sulfates, and phosphates. The substances present in *normal urine* may be divided into organic compounds and inorganic compounds. Some of these are:

Normal organic substances
  Urea
  Uric acid

Creatinine

Normal inorganic substances

As cations:

Sodium (Na^+)

Potassium (K^+)

Ammonium (NH_4^+)

As anions:

Chloride (Cl^-)

Phosphate ($PO_4^=$)

Sulfate ($SO_4^=$)

There are many *abnormal* substances that occur in urine in various conditions. It is important to know the relative amounts of these substances, because some of them occur even in normal urine in small amounts. These may exist as dissolved substances or as solids which are seen in the microscopic examination of the urinary sediment. Some of the more important substances that are considered *abnormal* in the urine are:

Acetone and acetoacetic acid	Glucose
Bile (or bilirubin)	Hemoglobin
Blood (red blood cells)	Protein
Casts	Spermatozoa
Cystine	Sulfonilamides
Fat	Urobilinogen
Epithelial cells (renal type)	White blood cells (or pus)

COLLECTION OF URINE SPECIMENS

The composition of urine in a random sample collected at any time during the day is likely to vary considerably, because the work of the kidney is so variable. It is not practical to collect an entire day's specimen (24-hour specimen), as it would take too long for any results to be ready for the physician; also, upon standing, many of the more important constituents found in the urine disappear or are altered. A 24-hour specimen is needed only when there is need to know the entire day's volume of urine output or when doing quantitative tests where the exact amount of urine must be known so that the exact amount of substance present may be reported.

Since a 24-hour collection is not necessary for a routine urinalysis, any random specimen that is passed during the day may be used. The first urine voided in the morning is usually recommended as most suitable. This is true primarily because the first morning specimen is the most concentrated specimen passed during the day. It is more concentrated because less fluid (or water) is excreted during the night while the same amount of solid or dissolved substance must be excreted if the kidney is to perform its function of maintaining the composition of the extracellular fluid. When testing for the presence of urine sugar, the best specimen to use is one voided 2 to 3 hours after a meal. This is the one exception to the recommended first morning specimen usually used for the other routine tests.

It is of prime importance that the containers used to collect the urine specimen be clean and dry. There are several types of containers which are suitable for this purpose. Glass jars, disposable paraffined containers, and plastic bags or jars are most often used.

PRESERVATION OF URINE SPECIMENS

If a fresh specimen of urine is left at room temperature for a period of time, the urine rapidly undergoes changes. It is for this reason that a good routine urinalysis should include the use of a *fresh specimen*. The decomposition of urine begins within half an hour after collection. The various laboratory tests to be done on a specimen of urine should be run within half an hour after collection, if possible; no longer than 1 or 2 hours should elapse before the tests are done unless the urine is preserved in some way.

Decomposition of urine involves primarily the growth of bacteria. At room temperature, bacteria reproduce rapidly. This bacterial growth results in a cloudy-looking specimen. Changes in pH also occur as a result of the bacterial growth. These changes interfere markedly with other tests. Other substances, namely, phosphates and urates, may precipitate out of solution, adding to the turbidity of the urine specimen.

Some of the other changes which occur upon prolonged exposure to room temperature are the following: the pH becomes alkaline because of the breakdown of urea by the bacteria to form ammonia; red blood cells, white blood cells and casts disintegrate; sugar decomposes, acetone evaporates, acetoacetic acid is converted to acetone; bilirubin is oxidized to biliverdin; and urobilinogen is oxidized to urobilin. It can be seen from these many changes that occur that it is most important that only fresh urine specimens be used in performing a reliable urinalysis.

If it is impossible to examine the urine specimen when fresh or if a 24-hour collection is required, the *urine must be preserved* in some manner. Various methods of preserving urine are available, most of which inhibit the growth of bacteria, thus preventing many of the alterations from occurring. One such method is refrigeration. If a chemical preservative is not added, the specimen may be kept 6 to 8 hours under refrigeration with no gross alterations occurring. Several chemical preservatives are available, one being toluene. This is a liquid which works by preventing the growth of bacteria. A thin layer of toluene is added, just enough to cover the surface of the urine. The toluene should be skimmed off or the urine pipeted from beneath it when the urine is examined. Toluene, or the commercially available product toluol, is the best all-around preser-vative, because it does not interfere with the various tests done in the routine urinalysis.

Another chemical preservative which is added to the urine is the crystal-line substance thymol. This too works to prevent the growth of bacteria. However, thymol may interfere with tests for urine protein and bilirubin. Formalin, a liquid preservative which acts by fixing the formed elements in the urinary sediment, may also be used. It may, however, interfere with the reduction tests for urine sugar and may form a precipitate with urea which interferes with the microscopic examination of the sediment.

In general, it should be remembered that a fresh urine specimen is best for urinalysis tests. It is the easiest to collect and will give the most satisfactory results.

OBTAINING THE URINE SPECIMEN

As stated previously, the specimen for urinalysis should be collected in a clean, dry container, and the specimen should be a fresh one. There are two ways to collect the specimen: a *freely voided* specimen may be used, or one may be obtained by *catheterization*. The preferred specimen for urinalysis is a freely voided one.

Occasionally it may be necessary to obtain a catheterized urine speci-men. These urine specimens are obtained by introducing a small tubular instrument called a catheter into the bladder, through the urethra, for the withdrawal of urine. This procedure should be avoided whenever possi-ble, as there is always a risk of introducing bacteria into an otherwise sterile bladder. This could initiate a urinary tract infection. Catheterized specimens are necessary when contamination by vaginal contents in female patients may alter the examination (especially during menstruation). It may also be necessary for obtaining urine specimens for bacteriologic examination when a sterile sample is needed. Under many conditions, however, a freely flowing voided specimen is satisfactory for bacteriologic cultures. Urine obtained by means of catheterization should be *handled very carefully* in the laboratory. Remember that it is an unpleasant proce-dure for the patient and it does involve some degree of risk.

CLASSIFICATION OF URINALYSIS TESTS

In the discussion of the actual laboratory procedures in the urinalysis department, there are three general categories of tests grouped according to their degree of accuracy: *screening tests, qualitative tests,* and *quanti-tative tests.* Most of the commercially available tests are in the screening test category, especially the dipstick tests and most tablet tests. These tests tell only if a substance is present or absent, and the results are reported as "positive" or "negative." For most screening tests, any random sample of urine can be used. As before, the first morning specimen is recommended for tests other than for urine sugar, a specimen obtained 2 to 3 hours following a meal being the preferred one for the urine sugar test.

Many of the tests used routinely in the laboratory are qualitative; they give a rough estimate of the amount of substance present. Results of qualitative tests are usually graded as negative, trace, 1+, 2+, 3+, or 4+. For most qualitative tests, the usual early morning specimen is preferred, the exception again being tests for sugar.

A quantitative test determines an accurate, or exact, amount of the substance which the test detects. These tests are much more time-consuming than the screening or qualitative tests, and for this reason they are not done routinely in the laboratory. The two most common quantitative tests performed in the urinalysis laboratory are those for sugar and for protein. The results of a quantitative test are usually reported in milligrams percent, grams percent, milliequivalents per liter, milligrams per 24 hours, grams per 24 hours, or milliequivalents per 24 hours. For all quantitative tests done in urinalysis, it is important to collect a complete 24-hour urine specimen. A preservative should be added to the container, and the specimens should be stored in the refrigerator until the test is done. The total volume of the 24-hour specimen is measured and the volume recorded; the urine is thoroughly mixed before a measured aliquot is withdrawn for analysis.

PHYSICAL PROPERTIES

The first part of a routine urinalysis usually involves an assessment of the various physical properties, such as volume, color, transparency, odor, and foam. Another physical property, specific gravity, is discussed later in this chapter. Observation of physical properties is probably the easiest part of any urinalysis. For this reason, physical properties are often considered unimportant, especially by the uninformed. This view, however, is unfounded. These simple observations are extremely useful both to the eventual diagnosis of the patient and to the laboratory personnel who perform the complete urinalysis. Such tests often give clues leading to findings in subsequent portions of the urinalysis. For example, if a urine specimen is cloudy and red, the presence of red blood cells will probably be revealed by the microscopic analysis of the urinary sediment. If red blood cells are not found, all parts of the urinalysis must be carefully rechecked for accuracy.

Certain tests are performed when abnormal physical properties are observed. For example, a chemical test for the pigment bilirubin is made when it is suspected on the basis of abnormal urine color. These are only two examples of several situations where the complete urinalysis may be evaluated by the laboratory for reliability before results are reported to the physician or where abnormal constituents are divulged in subsequent tests because abnormal physical properties were noted.

The final evaluation of urinalysis results will be described more completely after all parts of the routine urinalysis have been discussed. Physical properties are summarized in Table 4-1.

Table 4-1. Physical Properties of Urine

Physical Property	Report Description	Possible Cause	Procedure
Normal color........	Light straw Straw Dark straw Light amber Amber Dark amber	Urochrome, the chief pigment in normal urine with uroerythrin and urobilin	Mix urine and note color.
Abnormal color......	Pale	Dilute urine	Mix urine and note color.
	Dark yellow or brown-red	Concentrated urine	
	Yellow-brown or "beer-brown"	Bilirubin	
	Orange-red or red-brown	Urobilin (excreted colorless as urobilinogen)	
	Clear red	Hemoglobin	
	Cloudy red	Red blood cells	
	Dark red or "port wine"	Porphyrins	
	Clear dark reddish brown or "cola"	Myoglobin or myohemoglobin	
	Dark brown and black	Melanin, homogentisic acid and phenol poisoning	
	Milky white	Pus, phosphates, some urates, fat	
	Green, blue, orange	Drugs, medications, foodstuffs	
Transparency.......	Clear Hazy Cloudy Very cloudy Turbid	Mucin, phosphates, bacteria, urates, pus, blood, fat	Mix urine, hold up to light, and note transparency. Confirm cause under microscope.
Odor...............	Aromatic	Normal, volatile acids	Smell.
	Ammoniacal	Breakdown of urea by bacteria on standing	
	Putrid or foul	Urinary tract infection	
	Sweet or "fruity"	Ketone bodies	
Foam...............	White, small amount	Normal	On dark urine, stopper and shake. Note color and foam.
	Yellow, large amount	Bilirubin or bile pigments	

URINE VOLUME

Although a physical property, the actual measurement of urine volume is not part of a routine urinalysis. However, there are certain conditions when measurement of urine volume excreted in 24-hours is a valuable aid to clinical diagnosis. In normal persons with normal fluid intake, the average 24-hour urine volume is 1,200 to 1,500 ml.[1] The total volume of urine excreted in 24 hours must be measured when quantitative tests are performed, since urine volume enters into the calculation of results in these tests. The volume is usually measured in a graduated cylinder.

Under normal conditions, there is a direct relationship between urine volume and water intake. That is, if water intake is increased, the kidney will protect the body from excessive retention of water by eliminating a larger volume of urine than normal. Conversely, if water intake is decreased, the kidney will protect the body against dehydration by eliminating a smaller amount of urine. There are various situations which result in abnormal urine volumes. The term *polyuria* refers to the consistent elimination of an abnormally large volume of urine, over 2,000 ml/24 hours. *Diuresis* refers to any increase in urine volume, even if the increase is only temporary. *Oliguria* refers to the excretion of an abnormally small amount of urine, less than 500 ml/24 hours. The complete absence of urine formation is *anuria*. Finally, the excretion of urine at night is called *nocturia*. These terms merely describe abnormalities in urine volume. Each abnormality has several possible causes reflecting various abnormal conditions. It is the responsibility of the physician, with the aid of the routine urinalysis and other clinical or laboratory findings, to determine the actual cause and significance of volume changes.

URINE COLOR

Normal urine color varies considerably, even in a given person in a single day. There are numerous words that have been used to describe the range of normal color (few institutions will agree on exact terms). In general, it can be said that normal urine is some shade of yellow. The exact name that is attached is not as important as the recognition that the color is normal. So that the physician will understand that the color is normal, it is advisable that one institution use precise terms to define normal color. One such system is to describe the color as varying from straw to amber, straw indicating the lighter color, amber the darker. In this system all normal urine could be classified as being light straw, straw, dark straw, light amber, amber, or dark amber. Any other terms would indicate abnormal color.

It has been mentioned that urine color can vary considerably in one day. In general, the amount of color depends on the concentration of pigments in urine responsible for normal color. In other words, the intensity of color generally reflects concentration of the urine.

The more highly colored the urine, the greater the concentration of normal waste products due to diminished urine volume. Color, however, is not an adequate measurement of concentration. Specific gravity or osmolality values are preferred.

Normal urine color seems to be due to the presence of three pigments: urochrome, uroerythrin, and urobilin. Urochrome is a yellow pigment and is present in larger concentrations than the other two. Uroerythrin is a red pigment, and urobilin is an orange-yellow pigment.

The ability to recognize normal color is of course needed to ensure recognition of abnormal color. There are several abnormal colors which require special attention.

Pale *with high specific gravity indicates diabetes*

Pale urine suggests that the urine is dilute. The paleness results from large urine volume with corresponding low concentration of normal urine constituents, as in polyuria. Pale urine is often associated with diabetes mellitus or diabetes insipidus. In cases of diabetes mellitus, a pale greenish urine is characteristic. However, the large sugar content in diabetes mellitus results in a high specific gravity, unlike the low specific gravity characteristic of dilute urine.

Dark Yellow or Brown-red

As opposed to pale urine, the highly colored dark yellow or brown-red urine is indicative of a very concentrated urine with corresponding low urine volume. This is often seen in conditions associated with fever, where water is eliminated through sweat rather than the kidney.

Yellow-brown, or "Beer-brown" *Yellow foam when shaken) bilirubin / Turns green on standing § & jaundice.*

This is a very characteristic and alarming color to the experienced observer. It indicates the presence of bilirubin, a highly colored bile pigment related to the clinical condition jaundice if also present in the blood. Urine specimens containing bilirubin will foam considerably when shaken, and the foam will show a vivid yellow color. This is not true of other highly colored urine specimens. Whenever bilirubin is suspected, it is the responsibility of the laboratory worker to perform a chemical test for the detection of bilirubin. This is extremely important, for bilirubin may appear in the urine before clinical jaundice develops and detection will lead to early treatment of the condition, whatever the cause. Upon standing, urine containing bilirubin may become green as a result of the oxidation of bilirubin to biliverdin, a green pigment.

Orange-red, or Orange-brown *(takes this color upon standing) (check for this also, when testing for bilirubin)*
This color is very similar to that of urine containing bilirubin and is due to a related pigment, urobilin. In fact, urines which are tested for

bilirubin on the basis of color should also be tested for urobilinogen. When freshly voided, the pigment urobilin is present in a colorless form, urobilinogen. The urine slowly takes on color upon standing because of oxidation of urobilin to urobilinogen. If shaken, urine containing urobilin will not produce a colored foam.

Clear Red   Hemoglobinuria

Urine that is clear and red characteristically contains hemoglobin, the color pigment of red blood cells. The hemoglobin results from increased red blood cell destruction in the body (intravascular hemolysis) and will result from several causes. One possible cause is an incompatible blood transfusion reaction. The urine may be either bright red, red-brown, or even black as a result of the conversion of hemoglobin to methemoglobin. Urine showing this color should be tested chemically for the presence of hemoglobin.

Cloudy Red   Hematuria (red blood cells account for cloudiness)

This is similar to the clear red color. However, it is due to the presence of red blood cells, rather than merely hemoglobin; hence the cloudy appearance. It is important to differentiate hematuria (red blood cells in urine) from hemoglobinuria (hemoglobin in urine). This may be most easily done by observation under the microscope. However, if the urine is very dilute, red blood cells will lyse, resulting in hemoglobinuria. For this reason the specific gravity is important to the physician in determining whether the cause of red urine is hematuria or hemoglobinuria. The intensity of the red will depend on the number of red blood cells present, ranging from a smoky red or reddish brown urine to a highly colored cloudy urine specimen.

Dark Red, or "Port-wine"

This is characteristic of the presence of porphyrins in the urine.

Dark Reddish Brown, or "Cola"

This is characteristic of myoglobin or myohemoglobin, the form of hemoglobin contained in muscles. It is especially associated with cases of extensive muscle injury.

Dark Brown, or Black   (Takes this color upon standing)

This color may be due to melanin or homogentisic acid. In both cases the urine is colorless when voided and becomes black upon standing. Both are the result of serious conditions, and the color must not be overlooked. Melanin is associated with melanoma, a type of tumor. Homogentisic acid is associated with alkaptonuria, a result of an "inborn" error in the metabolism of tyrosine. Phenol poisoning may also result in an olive-green to black urine. Specific chemical tests for all these possible causes of black urine must be performed, since immediate diagnosis and treatment is imperative in each case. All these conditions are rarely encountered.

Miscellaneous

Various bizarre urine colors such as yellow, orange, red, pink, blue, green, and brown may result from such varied causes as vitamins, vegetables, fruits, certain chemicals, and dyes. These have very little clinical significance.

URINE TRANSPARENCY

When voided, urine is normally clear; most urines, however, will become cloudy when allowed to stand. If the specimen is cloudy when voided, it is usually of clinical significance and should not be disregarded.

The degree of cloudiness of the urine specimen is observed in a well-mixed urine specimen at the time of urinalysis. When cloudiness is noted, it must be accounted for in the microscopic analysis of the urinary sediment, since cloudiness must be due to solid materials that will be visible under the microscope.

As with color, there are numerous words which have been used in attempts to describe the degree of transparency in a urine specimen. Again, it is advisable that a particular institution use only one system of nomenclature. For example, the transparency may be said to vary from clear to hazy, cloudy, very cloudy, and finally turbid.

As mentioned previously, in virtually all urine specimens a certain amount of cloudiness will develop upon standing. This might well be due to the presence of *mucin,* or *mucous shreds,* in the urine. They are especially likely to solidify in urine stored under refrigeration and are of little clinical significance. Another substance commonly responsible for the development of cloudiness in urine is *amorphous phosphates.* These are especially likely to form in alkaline urine upon standing and are of no diagnostic significance. *Bacteria* are another common cause of cloudiness in urine specimens that have been allowed to stand. In this case, bacteria are not clinically significant. However, if the specimen is fresh or collected under sterile conditions such as catheterization, bacteria are of pathologic significance, indicating a urinary tract infection.

There are other causes of turbidity in urine specimens which may have pathologic significance. *Amorphous urates,* like amorphous phosphates, are often responsible for normal cloudiness in urine specimens. They appear as a white or pink cloud of material which settles out as the urine stands, especially if it is refrigerated. Unlike amorphous phosphates, the urates are characteristic of acid urines. The characteristic appearance is

[handwritten margin note: Fresh cloudy urine is usually of clinical significance. very alkaline—amorphous phosphates. very acid—amorphous urates. Mucous & bacteria & pus. Red blood cells. Fat]

often referred to as "brick dust" and is visible under the microscope. Amorphous urates may have pathologic significance when present in large numbers in various febrile conditions associated with highly concentrated urine, and also in some cases of gout and leukemia.

The occurrence of *white blood cells,* or *pus,* in urine is another abnormal cause of cloudiness. The white blood cells will be seen as white cloudiness in the urine and when present in large numbers will give the urine a "milky" appearance. Along with the white cells, bacteria will often be present, resulting in the urine's having a particularly foul odor. Both the bacteria and white blood cells should be confirmed in the microscopic analysis of the urinary sediment. Another cause of cloudiness, already mentioned under Urine Color, is the presence of *red blood cells.* These are especially pathologic, unless they are the result of vaginal contamination, and give the urine a characteristic "smoky red" or reddish brown appearance. They should be confirmed in the microscopic analysis of the sediment, and if present in very small numbers they will be noted only upon examination under the microscope. Finally, *fat,* although only rarely present, may be a pathologic cause of cloudiness in the urine specimen. In this case the urine has an "opalescent" appearance.

Again, it is stressed that most urine specimens show some cloudiness upon urinalysis, and the actual cause of cloudiness should be accounted for in the microscopic analysis of the urinary sediment.

URINE ODOR

It is obvious that normal urine has a characteristic, faintly aromatic odor. This is due to the presence of certain volatile acids. However, if allowed to stand, urine acquires a strong, *ammoniacal odor.* This is due to the breakdown of urea by bacteria (which are invariably present in the urine specimen), resulting in the formation of ammonia. This odor is important as an indication that the urine specimen is probably too old for the urinalysis to have clinical significance. That is, along with the breakdown of urea, various other decomposition reactions have occurred, resulting in the alteration or destruction of various components present at the time the urine was voided. Urine heavily infected with bacteria may have a particularly unpleasant order which may be described as *foul,* or *putrid.* This is also due to the action of bacteria on urea, forming ammonia, plus the decay of proteins also present in infection. Practically, it cannot be distinguished from the smell of "old" urine. Therefore, foul-smelling urine will indicate urinary infection only if the specimen is known to be fresh.

Another characteristic odor which is significant clinically is a so-called "fruity," or sweet, odor. This is due to the presence of acetone and aceto-acetic acid, especially as seen in cases of diabetic ketosis.

Finally, the ingestion of certain foodstuffs will result in characteristic urine odor. Probably the most obvious is the odor of asparagus. This is of no clinical significance.

URINE FOAM

Normal urine will foam slightly when stoppered and shaken, and the foam will be white. When certain bile pigments are present, especially bilirubin, the urine will foam significantly and show a vivid yellow color. This is a simple test for the detection of bilirubin, which should be performed on abnormally dark, or "beer-brown," urine specimens. However, it is not a confirmatory test, and all urine specimens suspected of bilirubin content should be tested with a chemical test whether the foam test is positive or negative.

pH

As mentioned previously, one function of the kidney is to regulate the acidity of the extracellular fluid. Some information about this function and other information, as well, may be obtained by testing the urinary pH.

The pH is the unit that describes the acidity or alkalinity of a solution. In ordinary terms, acidity refers to the sourness of a solution, while alkalinity refers to the bitterness of that solution. Lemon juice is an example of a sour, or acid, solution; baking soda (sodium bicarbonate) is a bitter, or alkaline, substance in solution. In chemical terms, acidity refers to the hydronium ion (H_3O^+) concentration of a solution, and the alkalinity of a solution refers to its hydroxyl ion concentration. These concentrations are usually expressed in terms of pH.

All solutions can be placed somewhere on a scale which ranges from 0 to 14. There are some solutions which are neither acid nor basic. These solutions are neutral and are placed at 7 on the pH scale. Water is an example of a neutral solution; i.e., the pH of water is 7. Water is neutral because the concentration of hydronium ions are equal to the concentration of hydroxyl ions. Any solution which has an equal number of hydronium and hydroxyl ions is neutral and has a pH of 7.

As stated previously, the acidity of a solution refers to the hydronium ion concentration. A solution with more hydronium ions than hydroxyl ions is an acid solution. On the pH scale an acid solution has a value ranging from 0 to 7. The farther it is from 7, the greater the acidity. For instance, solutions of pH 2 and pH 5 are both acid solutions; however, a solution of pH 2 is more acid than a solution of pH 5. In simpler terms, a solution of pH 2 is more sour than a solution with a higher pH value. For example, lemon juice has a pH of about 2.3, while orange juice is about 3.5.

An alkaline solution has a pH value greater than 7. It can be anything from 7 to 14; the farther it is from 7, the greater the alkalinity, or the more bitter the solution.

CLINICAL IMPORTANCE

Regulation of the pH of the extracellular fluid is an extremely important function of the kidney. The normal pH of blood is about 7.4 and normally varies no more than ±0.05 pH units. If the blood pH is from 6.8 to 7.3, marked acidosis will be seen clinically; if from 7.5 to 7.8, marked alkalosis. Anything less than 6.8 or greater than 7.8 will result in death. The carbon dioxide produced as a result of normal metabolism results in a tremendous amount of acid, which must be eliminated from the blood and extracellular fluid or death will result. This acid is normally eliminated from the body by the lungs and the kidneys.

Because the kidney is generally working to eliminate excess acid, the pH of urine is normally between pH 5 and 7, with a mean of 6. The kidney is capable of producing urine ranging from pH 4.5 to 8.0. Although the kidney is essential in controlling the pH of blood and extracellular fluid, measurements of urinary pH are of little clinical value in obtaining information about this role. However, the routine urinalysis does include a measurement of urinary pH for the following reasons:

1. Freshly voided urine usually has a pH value of 5 or 6. However, on standing at room temperature, urea is converted to ammonia by bacterial action. The production of ammonia raises the hydroxyl ion concentration, resulting in an alkaline urine specimen. Therefore, unless it is known that a urine specimen is fresh, an alkaline pH probably indicates an "old" urine specimen.

2. Alkalinity of a freshly voided urine may indicate a urinary tract infection due to the presence of large numbers of bacteria. In addition, white cells are probably present.

3. The urinary pH will give a clue to chemical consituents found in the microscopic analysis of the urinary sediment.

4. If the urine specimen is dilute and alkaline, various formed elements, such as casts and red blood cells, will rapidly dissolve.

5. Persistently acid urine may be seen in a variety of metabolic disorders, especially diabetic acidosis resulting from an accumulation of ketone bodies in the blood.

6. Persistently alkaline urine may be seen in some infections, in metabolic disorders, and with the administration of certain drugs.

7. It is sometimes necessary to control the urinary pH in the management of kidney infections, in cases of renal calculi (or stones), and during administration of certain drugs. This is done by regulating the diet; meat diets generally result in acid urine and vegetable diets in alkaline urine.

METHODS OF MEASURING URINE pH

Blue and Red Litmus Paper

Blue and red litmus paper will only indicate if a solution is acid or basic. Blue litmus will turn red in an acid solution, while red litmus will turn blue in a basic solution. However, this test is not sensitive enough to be of use in a routine urinalysis.

Combistix Dipsticks (Ames Co., Elkhart, Indiana)

Combistix is a commercial dipstick test for urine protein, glucose, and pH. Other dipsticks make use of the same pH indicator system. These indicators are methyl red and bromthymol blue. They are accurate from pH 5 to 9 with a series of colors ranging from orange to blue which are matched against reference color charts.

Nitrazine Paper

Nitrazine paper makes use of a universal pH indicator, namely, sodium dinitrophenolazo-naphthol disulfonate, which has a range from pH 4.5 to 7.5. There is a color change from yellow to blue as the pH value increases. The color is easily matched against reference color charts.

Procedure Using Nitrazine Paper

1. Tear off 1 in. of Nitrazine paper.
2. Dip paper in urine, briefly.
3. Compare paper with permanent color scale as soon as the color stabilizes. This will take only a few seconds.
4. Report result as acid, 5, 6, 7, or alkaline.

NOTE: Most Nitrazine paper is manufactured with color charts ranging from pH 3 or 4 to pH 9. However, Nitrazine paper has an accurate range of only 4.5 to 7.5. For this reason, only results which compare with colors 5, 6, and 7 are accurate. If the moistened paper compares with a color less than 5, the result should be reported as acid. If the moistened paper compares with a color greater than 7, the result should be reported as alkaline.

SPECIFIC GRAVITY

As mentioned previously, the kidney is a regulator of the volume, acidity, composition, and osmotic pressure of the extracellular fluid. A measurement of the specific gravity of urine is one means of assessing the ability of the kidney to regulate the composition and osmotic pressure of the extracellular fluid.

Urine is a mixture of various substances dissolved and suspended in water. In normal urine, these dissolved substances are primarily urea and sodium chloride. A determination of urine specific gravity is useful as a measure of the amount of dissolved substances present in a solution.

More technically, specific gravity defines the relationship of the weight of a solution to the weight of an equal volume of water. It is the ratio of the density of a solution to the density of pure water. Density defines the relationship of mass or weight of a substance to volume in terms of mass per unit volume. Since the density of a solution varies with temperature, temperature must be specified in determining the specific gravity of a solution. More completely, the specific gravity of a solution may be defined as the weight of one volume of solution at given temperature divided by the weight of an equal volume of water at the same temperature.

From this definition it should be obvious that the specific gravity of water is always 1.000. (Since specific gravity is a ratio, it has no units.) The specific gravity of urine should always be reported to the third decimal place to have clinical significance.

To illustrate, assume that 1 liter of pure water at room temperature if found to weigh 996.5 g. To calculate the specific gravity of any solution, divide the weight of that solution by the weight of an equal volume of water. In this case, 996.5 g divided by 996.5 g equals 1.000, which is the specific gravity of water.

It has been stated that the specific gravity of a solution is a measure of the dissolved substances present in a solution. To illustrate this, assume 20 g of sodium chloride is added to the 1 liter of water weighed in the preceding example. Assume that there is no change in volume, although this is not strictly true. The weight of this solution of sodium chloride in water will now be 996.5 g plus 20 g, or 1,016.5 g. To calculate the specific gravity of this solution of sodium chloride, divide the weight of the sodium chloride solution by the weight of an equal volume of water. Therefore 1,016.5 g divided by 996.5 g equals 1.020; i.e., the specific gravity of this particular sodium chloride solution is 1.020.

It is now possible to apply this information to the specific gravity of urine. Remember that urine is merely a solution of various substances dissolved in water. These dissolved substances are primarily urea and sodium chloride. However, there are several other dissolved substances which are normally present in urine. In addition to this, there are several abnormal substances which will increase the specific gravity of urine when they are present. In order to determine the specific gravity of a urine specimen, assume that 1 liter of urine weighs 1,008.5 g. In addition, assume that 1 liter of water at the same temperature weighs 996.5 g. The specific gravity of the urine specimen should then be 1,008.5 g divided by 996.5 g, or 1.012.

Of course it would be extremely time-consuming to determine the specific gravity of each urine specimen in the manner which has been described, especially since the number of specific gravity determinations in a single day will vary from 1 to 100 or more, depending on the individual laboratory, and specific gravity determinations are only part of a routine urinalysis. Therefore, a less time-consuming method must be available. The method most frequently used involves the use of a device called a *urinometer*. A urinometer is a type of hydrometer. A hydrometer is a floating instrument devised to determine the specific gravity of liquids. This floating device is weighted with mercury on the bottom and has an air bulb and a graduated stem above. The device is weighted with sufficient mercury to float at the 1.000 graduation when placed in deionized water, (Fig. 4-2).

CLINICAL APPLICATION

Clinically, the specific gravity of urine may be used to obtain information about two general functions: the state of the renal epithelium and the state of hydration of the patient. If the kidney is performing adequately, it is capable of producing urine with a specific gravity ranging from 1.003 to 1.030 or higher.[2] If, however, the renal epithelium is not functioning adequately, it will gradually lose the ability to concentrate and to dilute the urine. The specific gravity of the protein-free glomerular filtrate is 1.007. Without any active work on the part of the kidney this will increase to 1.010 as a result of simple diffusion as the filtrate passes through the kidney tubules. Thus, if the kidney has completely lost its ability to concentrate and dilute the urine, the specific gravity will remain at 1.010. If it is known that the kidney is functioning adequately, the state of hydration may be reflected by the specific gravity. For example, if the urine is consistently very concentrated, dehydration is implied.

The normal value for urinary specific gravity in healthy individuals on a normal fluid intake ranges from 1.015 to 1.025.[3] Since the specific gravity is a reflection of the amount of dissolved substances present in solution, the specific gravity varies inversely with urine volume. This is logical, since a fairly constant amount of waste is produced each day. Therefore, if the urine volume is increased because of increased water intake, the amount of waste produced remains constant, and the specific gravity of the urine will decrease. In other words, if the urine volume is high, the specific gravity is low, and vice versa, assuming that the kidney is functioning normally. With an individual on a restricted fluid diet, the normal kidney is capable of concentrating urine to a specific gravity of about 1.030 or more. If placed on a very high-fluid diet, the normal kidney is capable of diluting the urine to about 1.003. Since fluid intake is normally decreased at night and since a constant amount of waste products is eliminated at all times, the first urine specimen passed in the morning is normally a more concentrated specimen and should have a specific gravity of at least 1.020 if the kidney is functioning normally.[3] It is for this reason that the first morning urine collection is preferred for the routine urinalysis. Since the urine is more concentrated at this time, small amounts of abnormal urinary constituents are more likely detected. Or, if a urine specimen is very dilute, as seen by a very low specific gravity, it is unlikely that abnormal constituents would be in sufficient concentration to be detected.

Two frequently observed cases where specific gravity does not vary inversely with urine volume are diabetes mellitus and certain types of nephritis. With diabetes mellitus abnormally large urine volume associated with abnormally high specific gravity is observed. This is due to the presence of large amounts of sugar, a dissolved substance which raises the specific gravity of the urine. In certain types of nephritis there is a combination of low specific gravity and low urine volume. This is probably due to the inability of the renal epithelium either to excrete normal amounts of water or to concentrate the waste products. As mentioned previously, the specific gravity in these cases may eventually be "fixed" at about 1.010.

OTHER MEASUREMENTS OF SOLUTE CONCENTRATION: OSMOLALITY AND REFRACTIVE INDEX

Although measurement of specific gravity has been the most convenient way of measuring urine solute concentration, it is not the only such measurement available. Two other measurements of solute concentration are osmolality and refractive index. Measurement of osmolality is actually preferred as a means of determining solute concentration; however, such measurements are not practical in routine urinalysis. Osmolality may be determined by measuring the freezing point of a solution, since the freezing point is depressed in proportion to the amount of dissolved solids present. With normal persons on normal diet and fluid intake, the urine will contain about 500 to 850 mOsm/kg of water. Refractive index of a solution is also related to the content of dissolved solids present. Measurement of refractive index of urine has recently become feasible and extremely convenient with the development of a clinical refractometer.* This device requires only a few drops of urine (unlike the minimum 15 ml of urine necessary with the urinometer), and results correlate well with urinometer readings. Although the device measures refractive index of solutions, scale readings of the instrument have been calibrated in terms of specific gravity. Probably the major obstacle to universal use of this instrument is its cost in comparison with the urinometer. However, it is rapidly gaining in popularity.

* Temperature-compensated hand refractometer (TS Meter), American Optical Company, Buffalo, N.Y.

THE URINOMETER

As mentioned previously, the specific gravity of a urine specimen is usually measured with the urinometer. The urinometer is a glass float weighted with mercury, with an air bulb above the weight and a graduated stem on the top (Fig. 4-2). The urinometer is weighted so as to float at the 1.000 graduation in deionized water when placed in a glass urinometer cylinder or appropriate-sized test tube. It is important that the cylinder, or test tube, be of the correct size, so that the urinometer can float freely. The specific gravity of the urine is read directly from the graduated scale in the urinometer stem.

Calibration

In order to obtain correct specific gravity readings in urine, the urinometer must be calibrated. That is, it should be weighted so as to read exactly 1.000 in pure water. This is essential for reliable results. There are basically two methods which may be used to test the urinometer calibration:

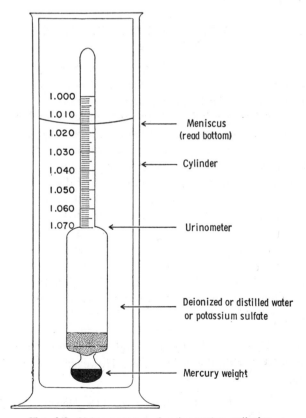

Fig. 4-2. Urinometer and urinometer cylinder.

by reading the specific gravity value from the scale in deionized or distilled water, or by taking the reading from the urinometer in a solution of known specific gravity.

1. Calibration in deionized or distilled water. In this case a reading is obtained in deionized or distilled water following exactly the same procedure as in urine. The reading on the urinometer scale should be exactly 1.000. If it is not, a correction must be applied to all values obtained from urine specimens with the urinometer. For example, suppose that the urinometer actually reads 1.002 in deionized water. The specific gravity of water is 1.000. Therefore 1.002 minus 1.000 results in a urinometer correction of 0.002. In this case, the apparent reading is greater than it should be. Therefore, 0.002 must be subtracted from subsequent urine specific gravity readings. In the case of a urine specimen with the apparent specific gravity 1.037, this value minus 0.002 results in the corrected specific gravity of 1.035 for the urine specimen.

2. Calibration in potassium sulfate of specific gravity 1.015. Any solution of a known specific gravity can be used to check the urinometer. However, the solution most commonly used is a solution of potassium sulfate with a specific gravity of 1.015. This solution may be prepared by diluting 20.29 g of potassium sulfate to 1 liter in deionized water. A reading is obtained in the known solution following exactly the same procedure as in urine or water. The reading on the urinometer scale should be exactly 1.015. If not, a correction must be applied to all readings in the urine specimens using the particular urinometer being calibrated. For example, suppose that the urinometer actually reads 1.012 in the potassium sulfate solution. The correction is now 1.015 minus 1.012, or 0.003. In this case, the reading is less than it should be. Therefore, 0.003 must be added to all urine specimen specific gravity readings. Using the same urine specimen as the preceding example, the apparent reading in this case would be 1.032. This value plus the correction 0.003 results in the actual specific gravity of 1.035.

Few urinometers read exactly 1.000 or 1.015 in water or potassium sulfate, respectively. Therefore, it is necessary to calibrate each urinometer before it can be used with accuracy. In addition, the correction can change from day to day. Therefore, it is necessary to calibrate the urinometer each day before urine specific gravity readings are determined.

Temperature Corrections

By definition, the specific gravity of a solution is dependent on temperature. Urinometers are calibrated to read 1.000 in water at a given temperature. If the urine specimen is either warmer or cooler than the urinometer calibration temperature, the result will be inaccurate. For precise work 0.001 should be added to the urinometer reading for each 3°C that the urine specimen is above the calibration temperature, and 0.001 should be subtracted from the urinometer reading for each 3°C below the calibration temperature.

Most urinometers have been calibrated at 60°F, which is 16°C. The calibration temperature is stated on each urinometer. Since room temperature is approximately 18 to 22°C, it is acceptable to report the specific reading directly from the scale if the reading is made when the urine specimen is at room temperature. However, a significant error will result if the reading is taken from a urine specimen which has been refrigerated. The temperature of a refrigerated urine specimen is 4°C. The difference between 16 and 4°C is 12°. Twelve divided by three equals four. The temperature correction in this case is then 4 times 0.001, or 0.004. Assuming that a urine specimen reads 1.015 at 4°C, the actual specific gravity for this specimen is 0.015 minus 0.004, or 0.011. Instead of applying this correction to urine specimens which have been refrigerated, the urine specimen is merely allowed to warm to room temperature before specific gravity is determined.

Correction for Abnormal Dissolved Substances

As mentioned previously, specific gravity represents the amount of dissolved substances present in urine. In determining specific gravity of a urine specimen, the clinician is interested in assessing the kidneys' ability to concentrate and dilute normal waste products. In other words, the concentration of normally appearing waste products is desired. In certain instances specific gravity of urine specimens might be artificially elevated because of the presence of abnormal urine constituents such as glucose, giving the impression that the kidney is adequately concentrating the urine when in reality it is not. For this reason it is important to know how to correct for the presence of abnormal substances such as glucose.

Each gram of glucose present per 100 ml of urine will raise the specific gravity 0.003. Urine specimens of persons with diabetes mellitus often contain large amounts of glucose, often 3 or 4 g of glucose/100 ml of urine. This would represent a considerable error in the apparent specific gravity as seen in the following example:

Assume that the apparent specific gravity of a urine specimen is 1.020. However, it is determined that this urine contains 4 g glucose/100 ml of urine. Therefore, the specific gravity is elevated 4 times 0.003, or 0.012, because of the presence of glucose. The actual specific gravity of this specimen in terms of normal urine constituents is 1.020 minus 0.012, or 1.008.

In the preceding example the urinary specific gravity was lower than normal. However, in the case of most diabetics, urinary function is normal in spite of the large sugar content. For this reason, it is common to find diabetic urine specimens with specific gravity values well above 1.030, even up to 1.060. When values above 1.030 are discovered, diabetes is often suspected, and the medical laboratory technician should expect to find indications of large amounts of sugar in the urine. This is not to say, however, that all specimens with abnormally high specific gravity readings contain sugar.

It is not usual for the laboratory to correct specific gravity readings for the presence of sugar when laboratory results are reported. Rather, the clinician will be aware that the specific gravity is elevated because of the presence of sugar and take this into account in his assessment of kidney function. If results are corrected by the laboratory, it is imperative that this be noted on the report form and values both before and after correction be noted.

Another abnormal substance which will raise the specific gravity of a urine specimen is protein. Protein too will raise the specific gravity 0.003 for every gram per 100 ml of urine. However, unlike glucose, 1 g of protein/100 ml represents an extremely large amount of protein and is seldom seen. Therefore, it is generally unnecessary to correct the urine specific gravity when protein is present unless the amounts of protein present are extremely large.

Procedure

1. Check the cleanliness of the urinometer cylinder. Clean the urinometer cylinder at the end of each day or laboratory period, following the standard procedure for chemically clean glassware. A dirty cylinder will result in a thin, hard-to-read meniscus.

2. Calibrate the urinometer in deionized water or potassium sulfate before use each day. Follow the same procedure as with urine (see Steps 3 to 8).

3. Fill the test tube to about 1 in. from the top with well-mixed urine. (Be sure that the test tube is the correct size for the urinometer, i.e., that the urinometer is able to float freely. All tubes should be of the same size and filled to the same level with urine.)

4. Remove any bubbles from the top of the urine with gauze or filter paper.

5. Grasp the urinometer stem at the top and insert slowly. Avoid wetting the stem above the water line, as excessive wetting of the stem will cause the urinometer to be depressed, and this will result in an inaccurate reading. Twirl the urinometer slightly as it is inserted, and note the reading as soon as it comes to rest. Be sure that the urinometer floats freely away from the sides of the container while reading results.

6. Observe the following requirements when reading the specific gravity:

   a. Urinometer must be clean.

   b. No bubbles around the urinometer.

    c. Avoid wetting the stem above the water line.

    d. Urinometer must float freely about 1 in. off the bottom of the container.

    e. Read on a flat level surface.

    f. Read urinometer at the bottom of the thick meniscus.

    g. Keep the eye at the same level in relation to the urinometer for each reading.

    h. Recalibrate the urinometer each day in deionized water or standard potassium sulfate.

7. Apply the appropriate correction to the results when necessary, and report the corrected specific gravity.

8. Rinse the urinometer in fresh water, and dry the stem before proceeding to the next specimen.

9. When all determinations are complete, clean the urinometer and cylinder. Store the clean urinometer floating in fresh deionized water in the cylinder.

SUGAR

Although a test for sugar in the urine should be included in every routine urinalysis, determinations for urinary sugar are not necessarily included to obtain information about the state of the kidney or urinary tract. Rather, the occurrence of sugar in the urine indicates that the disease diabetes mellitus should be suspected, and tests for urine sugar are commonly used for the diagnosis and management of this disease.

The particular type of sugar that is present in the urine in cases of diabetes mellitus is *glucose,* which is also called *dextrose.* Any condition in which the sugar glucose is found in the urine is termed *glycosuria* (also, *glucosuria*), which comes from the Greek words for glucose and urine. Although the condition diabetes mellitus is suspected in cases of glycosuria, the occurrence of glycosuria is not diagnostic of the condition, since there are many other causes. For example, glycosuria may be seen after eating large amounts of sugar or foods containing sugar, in cases of acute emotional strain where glucose is liberated by the liver for energy, and after exercise. Glycosuria may also be found associated with pregnancy, certain types of meningitis, hypothyroidism, certain tumors of the adrenal medulla, and some brain injuries, to name a few conditions.

In addition to this, certain abnormal conditions are characterized by the presence of sugars other than glucose in the urine. One such disease that it is imperative to diagnose is galactosuria, the presence of the sugar galactose in the urine. For this reason, it is often desirable to include methods which test for sugar in general, rather than those specific for glucose in the routine urinalysis.

Test for sugar in general, not just glucose.

Although there are various causes of glycosuria, the occurrence of glucose in the urine is not normal. The blood glucose concentration normally varies between 65 and 100 mg% (Nelson-Somogyi method). After a meal this may increase to 120 to 160 mg%. Normally all glucose in the blood is filtered into the glomerular filtrate, and normally all the filtered glucose is reabsorbed back into the blood. Therefore, glucose is not normally found in the urine. If, however, the blood glucose concentration becomes greater than a given level for any person (usually 170 to 180 mg%), any additional glucose will not be reabsorbed back into the blood and will be eliminated from the body in the urine.

The lowest blood glucose concentration that will result in glycosuria is termed the *renal threshold*. The actual renal threshold will vary somewhat from person to person. Any condition in which the renal threshold for glucose is exceeded will result in glycosuria; the most common such condition is diabetes mellitus. In grossly simplified terms, diabetes mellitus is a deficiency of the hormone insulin, which has the effect of lowering the blood glucose concentration. As a result of a deficiency of insulin, the blood glucose concentration exceeds the renal threshold, and glucose is spilled over into the urine. It should then be obvious that tests for diabetes mellitus will also include tests of the blood glucose level, in addition to tests for the presence of urinary glucose.

Virtually all *tests for urine sugar* may be classified as one of two types: (1) nonspecific tests for sugars in general which are based on the ability of glucose to act as a reducing substance and (2) specific tests for glucose which are based on the use of the enzyme glucose oxidase.

Tests which are based on the reducing ability of glucose are not specific for glucose. In these tests, the glucose is merely acting as a reducing agent, and any compound with a free aldehyde or ketone grouping will give the same reaction. Glucose is not the only reducing substance which may be found in urine. Nonglucose reducing substances (NGRS) which may be found include uric acid, creatine, galactose, fructose, lactose, pentose, homogentisic acid, ascorbic acid, chloroform, and formaldehyde. All these substances (including glucose) have the ability to reduce a heavy metal from a higher to a lower oxidation state. Usually copper (II) ions are reduced to copper (I) ions. Since this is an oxidation-reduction reaction, the reducing substance is oxidized to a higher oxidation state. In the case of glucose acting as the reducing agent, glucose is oxidized to gluconic acid. A positive reaction is indicated by a color change which varies in intensity in proportion to the amount of reducing substance present in the urine specimen. In other words, these are basically qualitative tests, and the results may be graded as negative, trace, 1+, 2+, 3+, and 4+, depending on the intensity of color formation, giving a rough estimate of the amount of reducing substance in the original specimen.

[handwritten margin note: means that insulin isn't storing glucose + constantly exceeds the blood so it spills out in the urine. so the renal threshold]

Commonly used nonspecific tests for urine sugar which will be described in detail are Benedict's qualitative test and the Clinitest tablet test (Ames Co.).

Although these nonspecific tests are often thought of as testing for glucose, it must be remembered that this is not true. Nonspecific tests will give the same reaction with any reducing substance that may be present in the urine, either naturally or as a contaminant. In cases where the presence of a reducing sugar other than glucose is suspected in the urine, a nonspecific test must be performed. For example, in the detection of galactosuria, an inherited metabolism error which will result in mental retardation if not treated immediately, one of the nonspecific tests must be used. For this reason, although the specific tests for glucose are commonly used as screening tests for the presence of glucose, all specimens obtained from pediatric patients should be tested with a nonspecific method, in addition to the specific screening test for glucose.

In case of the presence of a nonglucose reducing substance as indicated by a negative test specific for glucose coupled with a positive nonspecific test for reducing substances, the nonglucose reducing substance must eventually be identified. The appropriate method which should be used to identify the nonglucose reducing substance may be obtained by referring to one of the many standard texts of laboratory procedures.

Tests which are specific for glucose are all based on the enzyme glucose oxidase. An enzyme is often described as a biologic catalyst, a substance which must be present before a chemical reaction will occur. The enzyme glucose oxidase, as is true of most other enzymes, is absolutely specific. It will react only in the presence of glucose. It will not react with any other substance. The basic reaction for tests using glucose oxidase is diagramed below:[4]

Step 1: Glucose (in urine) $+ O_2$ (from air) $\xrightarrow[\text{glucose oxidase}]{}$

$$\text{gluconic acid} + H_2O_2$$

Step 2: $H_2O_2 +$ reduced form of dye $\rightarrow$

oxidized form of dye (indicated by color change from reduced form)

$$+ H_2O$$

The glucose oxidase, peroxidase, and reduced form of the oxidation-reduction indicator are all impregnated on a dip strip or paper strip. The different products commercially available differ in the actual oxidation-reduction indicator employed and substance that the reactants are impregnated upon.

Examples of specific tests for urinary glucose which will be described in detail are Tes-Tape (Eli Lilly Co., Indianapolis, Indiana) and Clinistix (Ames Co.). The Ames company manufactures various other dipstick tests which employ the Clinistix for urinary glucose in addition to tests for other substances such as protein, ketones, blood, and pH impregnated upon the same dipstick.

Although the intensity of color formation is said to be related to the amount of glucose present in the original specimen, the reliability of grading color intensity is questionable.[5] Therefore, specific tests for glucose should merely be considered to be screening tests, and the results should be reported only as positive or negative for glucose.

Since the specific tests for urine glucose are so simple, taking from only 10 to 30 seconds to obtain a result, it is common practice to use these tests as an initial screening procedure for all urine specimens. Tests which show positive reactions should then be retested with one of the qualitative nonspecific tests for urine sugar to give an estimate of the actual amount of glucose present. Since the specific tests using glucose oxidase are generally more sensitive to the presence of glucose, it is also possible to find a positive reaction with the specific test and a negative reaction when retesting with the qualitative test because of the presence of very small amounts of glucose. Again, it must be remembered that the nonglucose reducing substances will not be detected with the specific tests for glucose; therefore, certain situations, such as testing urine specimens obtained from infants and children under sixteen, require the use of the nonspecific test for reducing substances.

Occasionally it is necessary to determine exactly how much sugar is present in a given urine specimen. In this case, the qualitative result is not sufficient, but a quantitative result is required. Results obtained from quantitative urine sugar determinations are typically reported in terms of grams per 24 hours of urine excretion. For these tests a complete 24-hour urine collection is required. The total volume of the specimen must be measured and the specimen preserved with a suitable chemical preservative which will not interfere with the reaction employed to test the specimen. Two methods which are often used are Benedict's quantitative method and the Somogyi method for quantitative urine sugar. The exact procedure may be obtained by referring to one of the many texts of clinical laboratory procedures. Both these methods are based upon the reducing ability of glucose and make use of the reduction of copper (II) ions to copper (I) ions.

A. BENEDICT'S QUALITATIVE TEST[6-8]

Principle

This is a nonspecific test for urine sugar based upon the reducing ability of glucose or any nonglucose reducing substance which may be present in the urine specimen. It is a basically qualitative test where the amount of color formation is proportional to the amount of reducing substance present in the specimen, and results are graded as negative, trace, 1+, 2+, 3+, and 4+.

The test is based upon the ability of glucose (or any nonglucose reducing substance) to reduce the blue-colored copper (II) hydroxide [$Cu(OH)_2$] present in Benedict's qualitative reagent in the presence of heat to copper (I) oxide (Cu_2O), which is yellow or red. A positive reaction is graded as a change in color ranging from blue to green, yellow, orange, and finally red. The overall reaction is diagramed below:

$$CuSO_4 + 2NaOH \rightarrow Cu(OH)_2 + Na_2SO_4$$

(bluish)

$$\downarrow \text{heat}$$

CuO

Rapid reaction (occurs (black)

as if one step) $\downarrow$ reducing substance (e.g., glucose)

Cu_2O + oxidized form of reducing substance

(yellow   (e.g., gluconic acid)

to red)

The above reaction may be shortened to:

$$2Cu^{++} + \text{reducing sugar (e.g., glucose)} \xrightarrow[\text{heat}]{\text{alkali}}$$

$$Cu_2O + \text{oxidized sugar (e.g., gluconic acid)}$$

The copper (II) ions are supplied in Benedict's qualitative reagent in the form of copper sulfate. In the presence of a strong alkali this is converted to $Cu(OH)_2$. The heat is supplied by means of a boiling-(100°C-) water bath. The reaction may be stopped at any time by removing the source of heat. This is done by cooling the test tubes in a cold-water bath after exactly 5 minutes of boiling. The time of boiling is critical (since the reaction has not necessarily reached completion after 5 minutes) if results are to be graded accurately. However, the time of cooling is not critical. The tubes are merely brought back to room temperature and the results read when convenient.

Benedict's Qualitative Reagent

Dissolve 17.3 g $CuSO_4 \cdot 5H_2O$ in 100 ml of deionized water. Dissolve 173 g of sodium citrate ($Na_3C_6H_5O_7 \cdot 2H_2O$) and 100 g of anhydrous sodium carbonate (Na_2CO_3) in 700 ml of deionized water. Add these reagents to the water slowly with constant swirling. It may be necessary to apply heat in order to dissolve the reagents completely. When cool, combine the two solutions, and dilute volumetrically to 1 liter with deionized water. This reagent keeps indefinitely.

Procedure

1. Measure exactly eight drops of well-mixed urine into a test tube.
2. Add 5 ml Benedict's qualitative reagent.
3. Place in a boiling-water bath for exactly 5 minutes. Both the time and temperature of the water bath are critical.

4. Remove from the boiling-water bath, and immediately cool to room temperature in a cold-water bath for approximately 10 minutes.

5. A positive reaction depends upon the presence of a fine yellow, orange, or brick-red precipitate. The test is then graded on the basis of the color of the *mixed* solution.

6. Grade results according to the following critera:

Negative—either no change in the blue color of the reagent or the occurrence of a white or green precipitate from phosphates in the urine; also, an alteration of the color of the reagent without any precipitate formation.

Trace—slight amount of yellow precipitate with a greenish blue to bluish green mixed solution. (Represents less than 0.5 g% of sugar.)

1+—moderate amount of yellow precipitate with green, often referred to as apple-green, mixed solution. (Approximately 0.5 g% of sugar.)

2+—large amount of yellow precipitate with a yellowish green, often called muddy green, mixed solution. (Approximately 0.75 g% of sugar.)

3+—large amount of yellow precipitate with greenish yellow, or muddy orange, mixed solution. Some blue color remains in the supernatant. (Approximately 1.0 g% of sugar.)

4+—large amount of yellow to red precipitate with reddish yellow to red mixed solution. More important than the color of the mixed solution, no blue remains in the supernatant. (Approximately 2.0 or more g% sugar.)

NOTE: Tests for ketone bodies should routinely be performed on all 3+ and 4+ Benedict's qualitative reactions. In addition, tests for ketone bodies should be performed routinely on all urine specimens from pediatric patients.

B. CLINITEST TABLET TEST (AMES CO.)[9,10]

Principle

This is a basically qualitative, nonspecific test for urinary sugar. The principle of the Clinitest is essentially the same as Benedict's qualitative test: the ability of glucose to reduce copper (II) ions to copper (I) ions in the presence of heat and alkali. The Clinitest tablet may be thought of as a solid form of Benedict's qualitative reagent. In addition, the Clinitest tablet contains anhydrous sodium hydroxide, which results in moderate boiling when added to dilute urine in addition to giving off heat in its reaction with citric acid. In other words, the heat for the reaction is also supplied in the tablet, making a boiling-water bath unnecessary. Aside from this, the reaction of Clinitest is analogous to Benedict's reaction. Results are also graded as negative, trace, 1+, 2+, 3+, or 4+ by comparison with a permanent color chart supplied with the tablets. Colors are comparable to those described for Benedict's qualitative test.

Contents of the Tablet

The Clinitest tablet contains copper sulfate, citric acid, sodium bicarbonate, and anhydrous sodium hydroxide.

Precautions

Observe the precautions on the literature supplied with the Clinitest tablets. The bottle must be kept tightly closed at all times to prevent absorption of moisture and kept away from direct heat and sunlight, in a cool, dry place. The tablets normally have a spotted bluish white color. If not stored properly they will absorb moisture or deteriorate from heat, turning dark blue or blackish. In this condition they will not give reliable results.

Procedure

Follow directions supplied with the Clinitest tablets.

1. Place five drops of urine in a test tube, and add 10 drops of water.
2. Add one Clinitest tablet.
3. Watch while boiling takes place, but do not shake.
4. Wait 15 seconds after boiling stops, then shake the tube gently, and compare the color of the solution with the color scale.
5. Grade results as negative, trace, 1+, 2+, 3+, or 4+.
6. It is important to watch the solution carefully while it is boiling. If at this time the solution passes through orange to a dark shade of greenish brown, it indicates that more than 4+ sugar is present, and this should be recorded as 4+ without reference to the color scale.

C. CLINISTIX DIPSTICK TEST FOR GLUCOSE (AMES CO.)[11,12]

Principle

This is a specific test for glucose based upon the use of the enzyme glucose oxidase, which is impregnated on a dipstick. In the presence of glucose, glucose oxidase will oxidize glucose to gluconic acid and at the same time reduce atmospheric oxygen to hydrogen peroxide. The hydrogen peroxide which is formed will, in the presence of the enzyme peroxidose, oxidize the reduced form of orthotolidine to the oxidized form of the indicator. A positive reaction is seen as a change of color from red to blue. Although there will be some gradation in the intensity of blue color formation, this is merely a screening test, and results should be reported as positive or negative. The overall reaction is summarized below:

$$\text{Glucose} \xrightarrow[\text{glucose oxidase}]{\text{oxygen}} \text{gluconic acid} + H_2O_2 \xrightarrow[\substack{\text{reduced ortho-}\\\text{tolidine (red)}}]{\text{peroxidase}}$$

$$\text{oxidized orthotolidine (blue)} + H_2O$$

Clinistix is more sensitive to the presence of glucose than either Benedict's test or the Clinitest tablets and will detect 0.1 g% of glucose or less in the urine. For this reason, it is possible to find urine specimens that react positively upon screening with Clinistix and negatively when tested with the Benedict or Clinitest methods. Of course, since Clinistix is specific for glucose while Benedict's and Clinitest are nonspecific, a urine specimen containing a nonglucose reducing substance will give a negative Clinistix reaction, while Benedict's and Clinitest reactions will be positive.

Contents of the Dipstick

The Clinistix dipstick contains glucose oxidase, peroxidase, and orthotolidine.

Precautions

Observe the precautions on the literature supplied with the Clinistix strips. The reagent strips must be properly moistened. The test area must be completely moistened; however, excessive contact with the specimen will result in dissolution of the reagents from the strip. In addition, results must be read within 10 seconds, or false-positive results may be obtained.

Procedure

Follow directions supplied with the strips.
1. Rapidly dip the test end of the strip in the urine.
2. Read results after exactly 10 seconds for the presence of any purple color.
3. Record the results as positive or negative only. If the test area remains red, the result is negative. A positive result is indicated by the appearance of a purple color in the test area.

D. TES-TAPE TEST FOR GLUCOSE (ELI LILY CO.)[10]

Principle

Tes-Tape is also a screening test specific for glucose. The principle of the test and reaction is virtually identical with Clinistix with the exception of the actual oxidation-reduction indicator employed and the material the reagents are impregnated upon. In the case of the Tes-Tape, the reagents are impregnated upon a tear strip of special paper, and the indicator is yellow in its reduced form and green to blue in its oxidized form. Therefore, a positive reaction is the appearance of a green to blue color. Like Clinistix, Tes-Tape is more sensitive to the presence of glucose than are the Benedict's or Clinitest methods and will detect 0.1 g% of glucose or less.

Contents of the Tear Strip

The Tes-Tape is impregnated with glucose oxidase, peroxidase, and an oxidation reduction indicator in its reduced form.

Precautions

Observe the precautions in the literature supplied with the product.

Procedure

Follow the manufacturer's directions.

1. Tear off approximately $1\frac{1}{2}$ in. of tape.
2. Dip part of the tape into the urine specimen; remove it immediately.
3. Wait for 30 seconds; then observe for the appearance of any green color.
4. Record the results as positive or negative only. If the test area remains yellow after 30 seconds, the result is negative. If any green coloration is present at this time, the result is positive.

PROTEIN

One of the most important and indispensable portions of the routine urinalysis is a test for urinary protein. In the detection and diagnosis of renal disease, probably the most significant single finding is that of urinary protein. The presence of protein will also be correlated with certain findings in the urinary sediment, as part of the eventual diagnosis. Therefore, the inclusion and correct performance of tests for urinary protein are essential. In cases of renal disease, it is essential that the diagnosis be made and treatment started as soon as possible in order to prevent extensive and permanent renal damage.

The occurrence of protein in the urine is an abnormal condition, probably the most important pathologic condition found in a routine urinalysis. The finding of protein in the urine should be referred to as *proteinuria*. Previously it was referred to as "albuminuria"; however, this is a poor term. Proteinuria is preferable, since the protein which is present in the urine is derived from the plasma proteins and is made up of the same proteins as occur in the plasma, mainly albumin and globulin.

An explanation of how proteinuria occurs involves a consideration of normal urine formation. In this light, remember that the glomerular filtrate, the initial stage of urine formation, is merely an ultrafiltrate of blood plasma, consisting in essence of blood plasma without the larger protein molecules and certain fatty substances. If for any reason the glomerular capsule is damaged, it can allow the larger protein molecules passage, resulting in protein in the urine. In other words, one cause of protein in the urine might be increased permeability of the glomerulus.

It has been stated that protein is not a normal part of the glomerular filtrate. This is not completely true. A very small amount of protein normally does find its way into the glomerular filtrate. However, in normal situations, all of this protein is reabsorbed back into the blood through the renal convoluted tubules. Although the concentration of protein that normally filters into the glomerular filtrate is extremely small and only $\frac{1}{180}$ of the glomerular filtrate is eliminated from the body as urine (the rest is reabsorbed), the failure to reabsorb any protein from this large volume of glomerular filtrate will result in fairly large amounts of protein in the urine. In other words, another cause of proteinuria might be termed decreased reabsorption of protein by the renal tubular cells. It is usually impossible to say which of these mechanisms is responsible for the occurrence of proteinuria; it is most likely a combination of the two. The important consideration is that there is proteinuria and that it indicates the presence of some sort of renal disease.

Although when proteinuria is discovered renal disease must be suspected, the actual diagnosis of the particular situation is the responsibility of the physician. He will depend upon the laboratory technician to detect any protein that is present and then make a diagnosis based on additional tests and the amount of protein excreted per day as determined by quantitative urine protein tests. The results of the microscopic analysis of the urinary sediment and the patient's particular case history will also be considered. Because of the severity of kidney disease, it cannot be stressed too much that the laboratory technician must become proficient in performing tests for urine protein.

There are certain cases where transient and small amounts of protein may occur in normal persons. This is particularly true in young adults after excessive exercise or exposure to cold, or in so-called "orthostatic proteinuria," which occurs when the patient is engaged in normal activity but which disappears when he is lying down. In general, the proteinuria associated with renal disease is consistent, while that found in normal persons is transient.[13] In determining the actual cause of the proteinuria it will often be necessary to perform a quantitative determination employing a 24-hour urine collection to determine exactly how much protein is lost. Tests for orthostatic protein are made on urine collections obtained when the patient is at rest and after he has been engaged in activities involving walking and standing, but not sitting. The actual methods to be used will be determined by the physician or particular laboratory.

The occurrence of proteinuria must also be correlated with the microscopic examination of the urinary sediment in order for the physician to arrive at a diagnosis. There is a correlation between the presence of casts in the urinary sediment and proteinuria, since casts are made of precipitated protein. Bacterial infections of the kidney will often show the presence of white blood cells and bacteria in the urinary sediment in addition to protein in the urine. In these cases the amount of protein excretion is usually fairly small. When white blood cells and bacteria are found in the urinary sediment without the occurrence of urinary protein, it probably means the existence of a lower urinary tract infection without renal involvement.[14,15]

As previously indicated, the implications of protein in the urine are extremely serious. Extensive renal destruction is incompatible with life, and any renal destruction is permanent. Therefore, prompt diagnosis and treatment are vitally important. In addition, the loss of protein from the blood plasma will result in severe water balance problems, since the osmotic pressure of the blood is largely dependent on the concentration of plasma proteins. This is readily seen in the edema which is often associated with various kidney disorders.

Tests for urinary protein may be placed in one of two major categories. These are (1) tests which are based on the precipitation of protein by chemicals or coagulation by heat and (2) tests which are based on the use of the so-called "protein error" of pH indicators. There are numerous tests which fit into these two categories; none is necessarily a better method, and the particular test which is used will depend on the individual laboratory situation and volume of work. Most important is to learn the general principle, which can then be applied to the particular test which you will finally use in practice.

In the various tests which make use of precipitation of protein, the protein is either precipitated out of the urine specimen by means of a chemical, which is usually a strong acid, or the protein is coagulated out of solution with heat. The results are read in terms of the amount of precipitate or turbidity that is formed in a test tube or by the size of a ring of contact between reagents. The amount of turbidity or precipitation is roughly proportional to the amount of protein present in the urine specimen; therefore, these roughly qualitative results are generally graded as negative, trace, 1+, 2+, 3+, or 4+. The tests which depend on the coagulation of protein by means of heat depend on the fact that protein is most insoluble at the isoelectric point of the protein molecule. At the isoelectric point, protein will readily precipitate out when heat is applied. The isoelectric point of the proteins found in urine has a pH of approximately 5; therefore, these tests will in some way adjust the pH of the test solution and urine to a pH of 5.

Since results in the tests based on the precipitation of protein are determined by the presence of either turbidity or a precipitate, it is important that the urine be perfectly clear, or free from particles, before the test is performed. For this reason, the various tests will include a step to clear the urine specimen. Since any protein will be in complete solution, this is usually done by filtering the urine specimen and then testing the clear filtrate or by centrifuging the urine specimen and testing the clear supernatant for the presence of protein. If the urine is centrifuged, the solid material left after collecting the supernatant is tested by observation under the microscope, since this constitutes the urinary sediment. It has already been mentioned that findings in the urinary sediment will often correlate with the presence of protein in the urine.

One normal urine constituent which may interfere with the various precipitation tests for urinary protein by giving false-positive results is mucin. Interference by mucin may be avoided by acidifying the urine with acetic acid to precipitate the mucin, next filtering to remove the precipitated mucin, and finally testing the clear filtrate. More simply, however, interference may be avoided by adding sufficient sodium chloride or other salt to raise the specific gravity to a level that will keep the mucin in solution.

As mentioned, there are several methods available to get a rough estimate of the amount of protein present in a urine specimen which are based on the precipitation of protein. Among them are Roberts' test and Heller's test, both of which are ring, or contact, tests; Exton's sulfosalicylic acid test, and the analogous commercial product, Bumintest, (Ames Co.); and the many tests which make use of acetic acid, salt, and heat variously called the heat and acetic acid test, salt and acetic acid test, and Purdy's test.

The second category of tests for urine protein are those tests involving the use of pH indicators, which are substances which have characteristic colors at specific pH's. However, at a fixed pH, certain pH indicators will show one color in the presence of protein and another color in the absence of protein. This phenomenon is referred to as the *protein error of indicators*. This phenomenon, often a problem in the laboratory, is made of use when testing for urine protein. Here, the pH of the urine is held constant by means of a buffer. By maintaining a constant pH, any change of color of the indicator will now indicate the presence of protein.

The tests for urine protein which make use of the protein error of indicators are all commercial tests. They are available in either tablet or dipstick form, either alone or in combination with other dipstick tests. In general, these tests are less sensitive to the presence of protein than are the various precipitation tests and will not allow even a rough estimation of the amount of protein present in the urine specimen. All results should be reported merely as positive or negative for protein. In addition, all positive specimens should be retested with a method based on the precipitation of protein.

Since the tests using the pH indicators are less sensitive to protein than are the various precipitation methods, it would be possible to miss very small amounts of protein in a routine urine specimen if the method used to screen all urine specimens were based upon the use of protein error of indicators. For this reason, many laboratories continue to test all urine specimens for protein with the more complicated and older methods which involve the precipitation of protein.

Not all the numerous tests which have been developed for the detection of urinary protein will be described in this book. The various methods will be readily found in texts of clinical laboratory procedures. The procedures described here were chosen only because they show methods involving slightly different principles and have been found workable in teaching reasonably large groups of students.

A. HEAT AND ACETIC ACID TEST[16]

Principle

There are several variations of heat and acetic acid tests. This particular variation differs from most in that it uses a boiling-water bath rather than a burner flame as a source of heat. The boiling water bath facilitates the testing of large numbers of urine specimens at one time.

The test is based upon the precipitation of protein with acetic acid and heat. The acetic acid is present to adjust the pH to the isoelectric point of protein. Since proteins are most insoluble at their isoelectric point, they will readily precipitate out of solution when heat is applied. The salt is present in order to prevent the precipitation of mucin by raising the specific gravity. Precipitated mucin would be indistinguishable from protein and give false-positive results.

The amount of protein that is precipitated is roughly proportional to the amount of protein in the urine specimen. Therefore, results should be graded and reported as negative, trace, 1+, 2+, 3+, or 4+.

Reagent

Dissolve 150 g of sodium chloride in water. Add 50 ml glacial acetic acid. Dilute to 1 liter with water.

Procedure

1. Centrifuge an aliquot of urine. (Use exactly 10 ml of urine if sediment is to be used for microscopic analysis.)

2. Decant the supernatant into a second test tube with one motion. (Leave exactly 1 ml for microscopic analysis.)

3. Check the supernatant for clarity. If centrifuging did not clear the urine, make a note of this, or set up a blank for comparison in reading final results.

4. To the supernatant add approximately ⅓ vol. of the salt and acetic acid reagent. Mix.

5. Place the mixture in a boiling-water bath for 5 minutes.

6. Cool to room temperature in a cold-water bath, and allow the precipitate to settle for a short time.

7. Grade and report the results as follows:

Negative—clear solution or, if turbid before boiling, no increase in turbidity (less than 10 mg% of protein)

Trace—faint turbidity throughout solution (50 mg%)

1+—small amount of precipitate filling less than one-fourth of the solution (0.25 g%)

2+—moderate amount of precipitate filling from one-fourth to one-half of the solution (0.5 g%)

3+—heavy precipitate filling from one-half to three-fourths of the solution (1 g%)

4+—coagulation of the entire solution or precipitate filling greater than three-fourths of the solution (2 to 3 g%)

B. BUMINTEST TABLET TEST (AMES CO.) AND EXTON'S SULFOSALICYLIC ACID TEST[17] NOT USED ANY MORE

Principle

These analogous tests are based upon the precipitation of protein with sulfosalicylic acid. In the case of Bumintest, the reagent is supplied in the form of a tablet which contains sulfosalicylic acid and sodium bicarbonate. The sodium bicarbonate causes rapid dissolution of the tablet by its effervescent interaction with water. Exton's reagent is a 5% solution of sulfosalicylic acid in conjunction with sodium sulfate. In both cases the free sulfosalicylic acid in the working reagent serves to precipitate any protein in the specimen.

In both cases, a positive reaction is the presence of turbidity. The amount of cloudiness, or turbidity, that is formed is roughly proportional to the amount of protein in the original specimen. Therefore, grade results as negative, trace, 1+, 2+, 3+, or 4+. Since results depend on the degree of turbidity, it is important to begin with a urine specimen that is free from any turbidity. Use either a filtered or centrifuged urine specimen.

Working Bumintest Reagent

Dissolve four Bumintest tablets in 30 ml of deionized water. This produces a 5% solution of sulfosalicylic acid. It is ready for use when effervescence subsides, and it is stable indefinitely.

Exton's Sulfosalicylic Acid Reagent

Dissolve 200 g of sodium sulfate in approximately 750 ml of deionized water. If necessary, heat to dissolve. Add 50 g of sulfosalicylic acid, and dilute to exactly 1,000 ml with deionized water.

Procedure

1. Place equal parts of the reagent solution and cleared urine in a test tube. (Use at least 10 drops of each.)
2. Shake the test tube gently, and note the degree of turbidity by looking through light against a dark background.
3. Grade and report results as follows:

Negative—no turbidity or no increase in turbidity
Trace—barely perceptible turbidity
1+—distinct turbidity but no granulation
2+—turbidity with granulation but no flocculation
3+—turbidity with granulation and flocculation
4+—clumps of precipitate or tube of solid precipitate

C. ALBUTEST TABLET TEST (AMES CO.)[18]

Principle

This is a commercial tablet test for urinary protein based on the phenomenon of protein error of indicators. The tablet consists of the pH indicator bromophenol blue in conjunction with a salicylate buffer in an absorbant cellulose base. The salicylate buffer provides a hydrogen ion concentration of a pH of approximately 3. At this pH, bromophenol has a yellow color, while at this same pH in an increasing concentration of protein the indicator will show a green to blue color. However, the test is not sensitive enough to give even a rough estimate of the amount of protein present, and results should be reported merely as negative or positive.

Procedure

1. Observe precautions in the literature supplied with the tablets.
2. Place the tablet on a clean surface (paper or gauze), and put one drop of urine on the tablet.
3. After the urine has been absorbed, add two drops of water, and allow penetration before reading results.
4. Observe the tablet for appearance of a green or blue color, and report results as positive or negative:

Positive—appearance of a green to blue spot on the tablet surface after the addition of water
Negative—the original color of the tablet not materially changed at the completion of the test

D. ALBUSTIX DIPSTICK TEST (AMES CO.)[15]

Principle

This test for urinary protein is very similar to Albutest. It too is based upon protein error of indicators; however, the reagents are slightly different from those used in Albutest and are impregnated on a dipstick rather than in a tablet. The test area of the dipstick consists of the pH indicator tetrabromophenol blue and a citrate buffer. The citrate buffer provides a hydrogen ion concentration of a pH of approximately 3. At this pH, tetrabromophenol blue has a yellow color, whereas at this same pH in the presence of protein the indicator will show a green to blue color. Again results cannot be graded but are reported merely as negative or positive for protein. There are several other commercial dipstick tests which include the Albustix test for urine protein along with tests for other urinary constituents.

Procedure

1. Observe precautions on the material supplied with the product.
2. Dip the yellow test end of the stick in urine.
3. Immediately observe the test area for the appearance of a green to blue color, and report results as positive or negative:

Negative—the original color of the stick is not materially changed at the completion of the test.

Positive—the yellow end of the test stick changes immediately to a yellow-green to blue-green color depending on the amount of protein in the urine.

KETONE BODIES

Tests for the ketone bodies are not part of every routine urinalysis. Rather, these tests are performed when ketone bodies are indicated on the basis of other findings in the routine urinalysis or when specifically requested.

The so-called ketone bodies (also called acetone bodies) are a group of three related substances: acetone, acetoacetic acid (or diacetic acid), and β-hydroxybutyric acid. Their similarity of structure is shown in Fig. 4-3. These ketone bodies are normal products of fat metabolism. However, they are not normally detectable in the blood or urine.

In fat catabolism (i.e., breakdown for energy), acetoacetic acid is produced first. The acetoacetic acid is further converted either to β-hydroxybutyric acid or to acetone. All three ketone bodies are utilized by muscle tissue as a source of energy and are eventually converted to carbon dioxide and water. When normal amounts of fat are utilized by the body, the

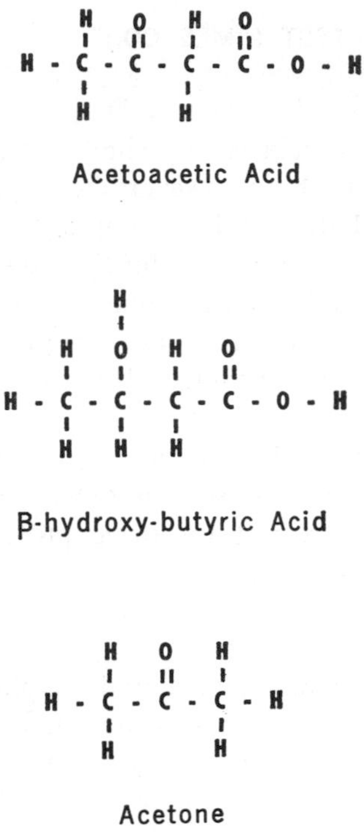

$$
\begin{array}{ccccccc}
H & & O & & H & & O \\
| & & \| & & | & & \| \\
H - C & - & C & - & C & - & C & - O - H \\
| & & & & | \\
H & & & & H
\end{array}
$$

Acetoacetic Acid

$$
\begin{array}{c}
H \\
| \\
H \quad O \quad H \quad O \\
| \quad | \quad | \quad \| \\
H - C - C - C - C - O - H \\
| \quad | \quad | \\
H \quad H \quad H
\end{array}
$$

β-hydroxy-butyric Acid

$$
\begin{array}{c}
H \quad O \quad H \\
| \quad \| \quad | \\
H - C - C - C - H \\
| \quad\quad | \\
H \quad\quad H
\end{array}
$$

Acetone

Fig. 4-3. The ketone bodies.

muscles are able to use the entire ketone production as an energy source. However, if more fat than normal is metabolized by the body, muscles are unable to utilize all the ketone bodies that result. The clinical result is increased concentration of ketones in the blood (ketosis) accompanied by increased concentration of ketones in the urine (ketonuria).

Whenever fat (rather than carbohydrate) is used as the major source of energy, ketosis and ketonuria may result. The two outstanding causes of ketone accumulation are diabetes mellitus and starvation. In diabetes mellitus, the body is unable to use carbohydrate as an energy source. It attempts to compensate by resorting to fat catabolism, which results in accumulation of the ketones. In cases of starvation, the body is depleted of any stored carbohydrate and must resort to fat as an energy source. The same situation may result in cases of severe liver damage. Most carbohydrate is stored as liver glycogen. In liver damage, there is no stored glycogen; hence, the body again must resort to fat for energy. Finally, the existence of a ketogenic diet will result in ketone accumulation. A ketogenic diet is one which is high in fat and low in carbohydrates— more specifically, a diet containing more than 1.5 g of fat/1.0 g of carbohydrate.

The physiologic effects of ketone accumulation (ketosis and ketonuria) are quite serious. The substances acetoacetic acid and β-hydroxybutyric acid are both organic acids. Their presence will contribute excess hydrogen ions to the blood, resulting in acidosis. As mentioned under pH, acidosis is an extremely serious condition and will definitely result in death if allowed to continue. Therefore, the body will attempt to compensate for excess acid in the blood by elimination of acid through the urine. The kidney is capable of producing urine with a pH as low as 4.5. As a result of this compensation, the occurrence of ketones in the urine is associated with low urinary pH. Before the use of insulin in treatment of diabetes mellitus, acidosis was the cause of death in two-thirds of all cases. In the treatment of diabetes mellitus, it is important to control the amount of insulin so that ketosis and acidosis will not occur. A typical urine specimen from an uncontrolled diabetic will be pale and greenish, will contain a large amount of sugar, will have a high specific gravity and a low pH, and will contain ketone bodies.

Another physiologic effect of ketosis concerns the substances acetone and acetoacetic acid. Both have been found to be toxic to brain tissue when present in increased concentrations in the blood. Of the two, acetoacetic acid is the most toxic. Hence, ketosis might result in permanent brain damage.

When ketones do accumulate in the blood and urine, they do not occur in equal concentrations. Acetone is present in the smallest concentration, with five to fifteen times more acetoacetic acid than acetone. β-Hydroxybutyric acid is present in the greatest concentration; usually there is two to four times more β-hydroxybutyric acid than acetoacetic acid.[19] However, most of the tests which are used in testing for ketosis and ketonuria are most sensitive to the presence of acetoacetic acid. Since β-hydroxybutyric acid is present in the greatest concentration, it would seem ideal to test for it. However, there are no simple laboratory tests available for this substance. Most tests react with acetone, acetoacetic acid, or both. The most commonly used test is Rothera's test or its various modifications which make use of the reagent nitroprusside. These tests are often referred to as tests for acetone; however, they are all significantly more sensitive to the presence of acetoacetic acid than to acetone. There is one test which is specific for acetoacetic acid, Gerhardt's test. This test, however, is positive only in the presence of large amounts of acetoacetic acid, indicating severe ketonuria.

It was mentioned that in the normal formation of ketone bodies, acetoacetic acid is produced first and β-hydroxybutyric acid and acetone are produced from it. Similarly, if a urine specimen containing all three ketone bodies is allowed to stand after voiding, a definite change will occur. This time the β-hydroxybutyric acid and acetoacetic acid will be converted to acetone. Since it is volatile, acetone will eventually disappear from the urine specimen. Practically, this means that urine should be tested for ketone bodies when fresh, or a false-negative result may be obtained. Heat will accelerate this conversion; therefore, refrigeration should be used to help to preserve the urine if it cannot be tested immediately.

It has been stated that tests for ketone bodies are not actually part of the routine urinalysis. However, they should be included whenever urine specimens are found to contain sugar (e.g., on 3+ or 4+ Benedict tests), on urine specimens from patients under sixteen years of age, and when requested by the physician.

Descriptions of actual tests for ketone bodies[20] in urine specimens follow.

A. ROTHERA'S TEST

Rothera's test is a roughly qualitative test for acetone and acetoacetic acid. Although it is often thought of as a test for acetone, it is actually more sensitive to the presence of acetoacetic acid. A very sensitive test, it will detect acetoacetic acid at a dilution of 1:125,000. Acetone will be detected at a dilution of 1:10,000. The test is based upon a reaction between acetoacetic acid or acetone with sodium nitroprusside in an alkaline solution with the formation of a reddish purple color.

REAGENTS

1. Rothera's reagent. Pulverize 7.5 g of sodium nitroprusside, and mix with 200 g of ammonium sulfate.
2. Concentrated ammonium hydroxide.

PROCEDURE

1. Place 1 g of Rothera's reagent in a test tube.
2. Add 5 ml of well-mixed urine. Mix thoroughly.
3. Carefully overlay the solution with 1 ml of concentrated ammonium hydroxide.
4. Observe the interface for the presence of a reddish purple ring within 1 or 2 minutes. (A brown color is of no significance.)
5. Grade and report results as follows:
Negative—a brown ring at the interface or no color formation.
Trace—delayed appearance of a faint pinkish purple ring.
2+—a narrow dark purple ring.
4+—a wide dark purple ring appearing rapidly.

B. ACETEST TABLET TEST (AMES CO.)[21]

Acetest is another roughly qualitative test for acetone and acetoacetic acid based on a color reaction with sodium nitroprusside. The principle is virtually identical to that of Rothera's test. In addition, it can be used to test whole blood, plasma, or urine. Urine specimens must meet the same requirements for analysis as with Rothera's test.

Contents of the Tablet

The Acetest tablet contains sodium nitroprusside with aminoacetic acid (glycine), disodium phosphate, and lactose.

Precautions

Observe the precautions in the literature supplied with the product.

Procedure

Follow the manufacturer's directions.

1. Place the tablet on a clean surface, preferably a piece of white paper.

2. Place one drop of urine on the tablet.

3. Read the results at 30 seconds, comparing the color of the tablet with the color chart provided by the manufacturer.

If acetone and acetoacetic acid are present, the tablet will show a color varying from lavender to deep purple. Report the results as negative, small, moderate, or large, as the manufacturer directs.

C. KETOSTIX DIPSTICK TEST (AMES CO.)[22]

Ketostix is another test for acetoacetic acid and acetone based on a color reaction with sodium nitroprusside. It is virtually identical to Acetest; the reagents are impregnated on a cellulose dipstick rather than in tablet form. Ketostix may be used to test urine, serum, or plasma. It is more sensitive to acetoacetic acid than to acetone. Urine specimens must meet the same requirements for analysis as with Rothera's test.

Contents of the Dipstick

These are similar to Acetest. The primary reagent is sodium nitroprusside once again.

Procedure

Follow the manufacturer's directions.

1. Dip the test end of the dipstick briefly into urine, serum, or plasma, or pass the test end of the dipstick through the urine stream.

2. Exactly 15 seconds after moistening the stick, compare the color of the test area with the color chart supplied by the manufacturer. Positive colors will range from lavender to deep purple. Report the result as negative, small, moderate, or large, as indicated on the color chart.

D. GERHARDT'S TEST[20]

Gerhardt's test is specific for acetoacetic acid; however, it is capable of detecting only large amounts of acetoacetic acid. Since it detects only very large amounts of acetoacetic acid, any specimen giving a positive

Gerhardt's test result must also give a positive reaction with the various tests using nitroprusside.

Gerhardt's test is used as a means of determining the severity of ketosis.* If positive, it indicates that severe ketosis exists and treatment must be started immediately. For this reason, Gerhardt's test should be performed whenever a positive reaction is found using any of the nitroprusside tests.

Principle

Acetoacetic acid will react with a 10% solution of ferric chloride and form a "Bordeaux red" color. However, the same Bordeaux red color will be produced from an interaction between salicylates and ferric chloride. For this reason, whenever a Bordeaux red color develops when ferric chloride is added to urine, the presence of acetoacetic acid or salicylates must be confirmed. As mentioned previously, acetoacetic acid will convert to acetone in the presence of heat. Gerhardt's test is specific for acetoacetic acid; it will not react with acetone. Therefore, to confirm the presence of acetoacetic acid, heat the test solution by boiling it. After boiling, the Bordeaux color will not be present if acetoacetic acid was present in the urine. However, salicylates are unaffected by heat. Therefore, the Bordeaux red color will remain after boiling if the original specimen contained salicylates.

Reagent

The reagent used is a 10% ferric chloride solution (W/V).

Procedure

1. Place 5 ml of urine in a test tube. Add 10% ferric chloride dropwise until the precipitate of ferric phosphate dissolves.

2. If acetoacetic acid or salicyates are present, a red-brown to Bordeaux red color will develop.

3. To confirm the presence of acetoacetic acid, divide the test solution in half and boil one portion for 5 minutes. If acetoacetic acid is present, the solution color will disappear or become lighter after boiling because of conversion of acetoacetic acid to acetone. If the color remains unchanged after boiling, salicylates are present.

4. Report results as positive or negative for acetoacetic acid.

---

* Rather than perform Gerhardt's test, a measure of the severity of ketosis may be obtained by diluting the original specimen giving a "large" value with Ketostix or Acetest until a "moderate" reaction is obtained. If, for example, the specimen required a 1:3 dilution for a "moderate" reaction, the result would be reported as "large—1:3 dilution moderate."

TWO BY-PRODUCTS OF RED BLOOD CELL DESTRUCTION: BILIRUBIN AND UROBILINOGEN

Individual red blood cells do not exist indefinitely in the body, rather they are degraded after approximately 120 days. As part of red blood cell degradation, the heme portion of the hemoglobin molecule is converted to the bile pigment bilirubin by the R-E cells. Bilirubin, as mentioned previously, is a highly colored vivid yellow pigment. An increase, for any of various reasons, in the concentration of bilirubin in the blood indicates the presence of jaundice. Although it it useful in the bile, bilirubin is a waste product which must eventually be eliminated from the body. When formed by the R-E cells, bilirubin is not soluble in water. For this reason, the bilirubin molecule is normally carried through the bloodstream linked to plasma protein, primarily to albumin. This water-insoluble form of bilirubin is often referred to as *free bilirubin*.

Bilirubin is normally excreted from the body by the liver, through the intestine. It is excreted by the liver rather than by the kidney because free bilirubin linked to protein cannot pass through the glomerular capsule. When free bilirubin reaches the liver, it is converted to a water-soluble product by the Kupffer cells of the liver. It is made soluble by conjugation with glucuronic acid and some other hydrophilic substances to form bilirubin glucuronide.

Water-soluble bilirubin is often referred to as *conjugated bilirubin*. Being water-soluble, conjugated bilirubin can be eliminated from the body by way of the kidney or the intestine. Normally, conjugated bilirubin is excreted by the liver into the bile and eliminated from the body through the intestine.

In the intestine, most of the bilirubin is converted to urobilinogen. Bilirubin is reduced to urobilinogen by the action of certain bacteria which make up the intestinal flora. Urobilinogen is actually a group of colorless chromogens, all of which are referred to as urobilinogen. Approximately one-half of the urobilinogen which is formed in the intestine is absorbed into the portal blood circulation and returned to the liver. In the liver, most of the urobilinogen is excreted into the bile once again and returned to the intestine.

A very small amount of urobilinogen escapes this liver clearance and is therefore excreted from the body by way of the urine. This represents only about 1 percent of the urobilinogen produced in 1 day. Urobilinogen in the intestine is either eliminated from the body unchanged or oxidized to the colored compound urobilin. Incidentally, urobilin is the substance which gives the feces its normal color. The net effect is that, in normal circumstances, 99 percent of the urobilinogen formed from bilirubin is eliminated by way of the feces.

From this it should be clear that urine normally contains only a very small amount of urobilinogen and no bilirubin. Both are abnormal urinary constituents. However, there are several varied and serious conditions where either of or both these substances are found in the urine. Tests for urobilinogen and bilirubin are not part of the routine urinalysis. However, they are also included on the basis of other urinary findings. Urine should be tested for both these substances, not merely one or the other.

BILIRUBIN

Jaundice is a condition which occurs when the serum bilirubin concentration becomes greater than normal and there is an abnormal accumulation of bilirubin in the body tissues. The causes of jaundice are numerous and must be discovered as soon as possible in order to initiate prompt and proper treatment. In general, the various types of jaundice may be placed in one of two broad categories, retentive and obstructive or regurgitative jaundice. Retentive jaundice is associated with overproduction of bilirubin due to excessive hemolysis of red blood cells. With retentive jaundice, the liver functions normally, conjugating and eliminating bilirubin in the normal manner, but because of the large bilirubin production the liver is unable to clear free bilirubin from the blood, and jaundice results. In retentive jaundice, bilirubin will not be found in the urine, since the liver excretes all the conjugated bilirubin by way of the intestine. Regurgitative jaundice results when the liver conjugates bilirubin but is unable to excrete it or when conjugated bilirubin is regurgitated back into the bloodstream because of obstruction of the bile flow into the intestine. In regurgitative jaundice, bilirubin is typically found in the urine, since it has been conjugated but is not able to reach the intestine. Because of liver involvement in jaundice, tests for bilirubin are liver function tests.

Tests for urine bilirubin are not part of a routine urinalysis. However, a chemical test for bilirubin should be included in the urinalysis when indicated on the basis of urine color or when requested by the physician. Since bilirubin is a highly colored yellow pigment, urine containing bilirubin will typically show a "beer-brown" color and produce a yellow foam when shaken. If only small amounts of bilirubin are present, these signs may be lacking, or the urine may appear only slightly darker than normal. In addition, bilirubin is not stable in solution but will be oxidized to biliverdin. Biliverdin is a green pigment; therefore, urine containing biliverdin will show a green color. In other words, urine containing bilirubin will show a typically beer-brown color when voided and will change to a green color upon standing. The various tests for bilirubin will not be positive in the presence of biliverdin; therefore, the urine must be examined when fresh.

Several methods are available for the detection of bilirubin in urine.[23] One of the oldest laboratory methods known is the *foam test* for bilirubin.

This was used by the early Greeks to help determine the cause of jaundice. However, this method of simply shaking the urine and looking for the presence of a yellow foam is not sufficient today. Several chemical tests for bilirubin are available. *Smith's test* involves the use of tincture of iodine diluted with nine times its volume of alcohol. This reagent is overlaid on the urine, and the interface is observed for the presence of an emerald-green ring. *Gmelin's test* makes use of fuming nitric acid. There are various methods of combining the urine and nitric acid in this test. Results involve a play of colors; green and violet are associated with the presence of bilirubin. Two other tests which will be discussed in detail are Harrison's test and Ictotest.

A. HARRISON'S TEST[24]

Principle

The Harrison's tests for bilirubin depends upon the precipitation of bilirubin with barium chloride and subsequent oxidation of bilirubin to biliverdin with Fouchet's reagent. The formation of biliverdin results in a green color on the barium chloride which constitutes a positive reaction. The barium chloride used to precipitate the bilirubin from the specimen may be provided in several ways. In this particular modification of Harrison's test, the barium chloride is supplied on thick filter paper which has been soaked in a saturated solution of barium chloride. Barium chloride tablets are available commercially. The same procedure is performed directly on the surface of the commercially prepared tablet. Harrison's test is sensitive to 0.1 to 0.2 mg% of bilirubin.

Reagents

1. Fouchet's reagent. Dissolve 25 g of trichloroacetic acid in 100 ml of distilled water. Add 10 ml of 10% ferric chloride.
2. Barium chloride paper. Soak thick filter paper (Schleicher & Schuell number 470) in saturated barium chloride. Dry and cut into small strips.

Procedure

1. Hold a strip of barium chloride paper perpendicularly in urine for a few seconds.
2. Place one or two drops of Fouchet's reagent on the saturated area.
3. Look for the appearance of a green color, which constitutes a positive reaction.
4. Report results as positive or negative according to the following criteria:
Negative—the formation of any color except green, or no color formation
Positive—the appearance of a green color

B. ICTOTEST TABLET TEST (AMES CO.)[25]

Principle

Ictotest is typical of various tests which use the diazo reagents of sulfanilic acid, napthylamines, and others to demonstrate the presence of bilirubin as azobilirubin. The tablets are supplied with a special mat. Urine is placed on the mat, the liquid portion is absorbed, and the bilirubin remains on the outer surface of the mat. The tablet contains the reactive ingredients. When bilirubin is present, there is a chemical coupling of bilirubin with p-nitrobenzene diazonium p-toluene sulfonate resulting in a blue or purple color. Other ingredients in the tablet provide proper pH and ensure solution of the tablet when water is added, so that the reaction can take place. Ictotest is sensitive to 0.05 to 0.1 mg% of bilirubin in urine.

Contents of the Ictotest Tablet and Mat

The Ictotest tablet contains p-nitrobenzene diazonium p-toluene sulfonate (bilazo), sulfosalicylic acid, and sodium bicarbonate. The mats are absorbent asbestos cellulose.

Precautions

Observe the precautions in the literature supplied by the manufacturer. Be sure to use the special mat provided. Either side may be used. Be sure to observe results within 30 seconds, since a confusing pink color may appear after 30 seconds.

Procedure

1. Place five drops of urine on either side of the special test mat supplied with the reagent tablets.
2. Place the tablet in the center of the moistened area.
3. Flow two drops of water on the tablet.
4. Observe the mat around the tablet for the appearance of a blue to purple color within 30 seconds.
5. Report results as positive or negative according to the following criteria:

Negative—the mat shows no blue or purple within 30 seconds. Ignore any color which forms after 30 seconds or a slight pink or red that may appear.

Positive—the mat around the tablet turns blue or purple within 30 seconds. Ignore any color change on the tablet itself.

UROBILINOGEN

As previously described, urobilinogen is a by-product of red blood cell degradation resulting from intestinal reduction of bilirubin. Increased destruction of red blood cells results in increased production of urobilinogen and may be accompanied by large amounts of urobilinogen in the urine. When increased red cell destruction does not exist, tests may be considered liver function tests. One of the first mechanisms impaired in a damaged liver is the ability to remove urobilinogen from the blood circulation and excrete it through the intestine. Loss of the ability to excrete urobilinogen by the liver results in removal of it by the kidney with urobilinogen in the urine. Since inability to excrete urobilinogen is one of the first functions lost in liver disease, tests for urine urobilinogen are useful for the early detection of liver damage.

Normally, 1 percent of the total urobilinogen production is excreted with the urine and 99 percent in the feces. However, there are certain conditions in which urobilinogen is completely absent from the urine and the feces. When there is destruction of the normal intestinal bacterial flora, urobilinogen cannot be produced. Urobilinogen is also absent if the liver does not conjugate bilirubin or with bilary tract obstruction resulting in the failure of conjugated bilirubin to reach the intestinal tract.

Tests for urobilinogen are not part of the routine urinalysis; however, urine should be tested for urobilinogen when this is requested by the physician or whenever the presence of urobilinogen is suspected on the basis of abnormal urine color. Urine containing urobilinogen will often show a characteristic orange-red or orange-brown color due to the presence of urobilin. Whenever tests for bilirubin are performed, a test for urobilinogen should also be included.

It is particularly necessary to use a fresh urine specimen when tests for urobilinogen are required, since urobilinogen is an unusually unstable substance and is rapidly oxidized to urobilin. This oxidation takes place so readily that most urine specimens which contain urobilinogen will show an abnormal color due to partial oxidation to urobilin. The presence of urobilinogen and that of urobilin have the same clinical significance; however, they give different chemical reactions, and urine is more frequently tested for urobilinogen. Hence, the absolute necessity of a fresh urine specimen.

Another substance somewhat related to urobilinogen is porphobilinogen. As mentioned previously, urobilinogen is a by-product of the degradation of red blood cells. The porphyrins consist of a group of compounds which are utilized in the synthesis of the hemoglobin molecule. The heme portion of hemoglobin is a type of porphyrin, namely, ferroprotoporphyrin 9. In normal individuals various porphyrins are eliminated from the body in the urine and feces mainly as corproporphyrin I with a small amount of coproporphyrin III. However, there are certain errors of porphyrin metabolism in which there is an increased excretion of other porphyrins in the urine. These conditions are collectively called *porphyrias*. A complete discussion of these conditions will not be attempted here. However, certain types of porphyrias are associated with the presence of porpho-bilinogen in the urine. Ehrlich's aldehyde test, which is described here as a test for urobilinogen, will also react with porphobilinogen.

EHRLICH'S QUALITATIVE ALDEHYDE REACTION FOR UROBILINOGEN AND PORPHOBILINOGEN[26-30]

Principle

Ehrlich's aldehyde reaction occurs with urobilinogen (and porphobilino-gen) but not with urobilin. Therefore, absolutely fresh urine is necessary for this test. In the presence of Ehrlich's reagent, urobilinogen will give a characteristic "cherry-red" color. This color will be enhanced in the presence of saturated sodium acetate. However, porphobilinogen will give the same cherry-red color with Ehrlich's reagent and sodium acetate; there-fore it must be distinguished from urobilinogen. In addition certain intermediate Ehrlich-reactive compounds will give the same color and must also be distinguished. In order to distinguish urobilinogen, porpho-bilinogen, and intermediate Ehrlich-reactive compounds, the test solution is extracted with the organic solvents chloroform and butanol. Urobilino-gen is soluble in both organic solvents, porphobilinogen is not soluble in either organic solvent, and intermediate Ehrlich-reactive compounds are soluble in butanol but not soluble in chloroform (Table 4-2).

In addition, fresh urine should be cooled to room temperature before the test is carried out to prevent the so-called "warm aldehyde" reaction. This is because normal urine contains a chromogen (probably indoxyl) which gives a weak Ehrlich reaction at body temperature.

Reagents

1. Ehrlich's reagent. Combine 0.7 g of *p*-dimethylaminobenzaldehyde, 150 ml of concentrated hydrochloric acid, and 100 ml of deionized water.
2. Saturated sodium acetate in deionized water.
3. Chloroform.
4. Butanol.

Procedure

1. Place 1 vol (approximately 3 ml) of urine in a test tube. Add an equal volume of Ehrlich's reagent. Mix well by inversion.
2. Add 2 vol of saturated sodium acetate, and mix. A red or deep pink (cherry-red) color is a positive result and indicates the presence of urobilinogen, porphobilinogen, or other Ehrlich-reactive compounds. If the test is positive at this stage, split the colored solution into two parts, and continue with Step 3.
3. Add a few milliliters of chloroform to one portion of the colored solution and shake vigorously. Observe whether or not the color is com-

Table 4-2. Results of Ehrlich's Qualitative Aldehyde Reaction

Result	Ehrlich's Reagent plus Sodium Acetate	Chloroform Extract	Butanol Extract
Negative............................	No pink color		
Urobilinogen........................	Pink	Pink	Pink
Porphobilinogen.....................	Pink	Colorless	Colorless
Intermediate Ehrlich compounds.......	Pink	Colorless	Pink

pletely extracted into the lower chloroform layer. Extract the colored solution with chloroform as many times as is necessary. If the color is due to urobilinogen, it will be extracted into the chloroform layer. Color due to porphobilinogen or intermediate Ehrlich-reactive compounds is not soluble in chloroform.

4. If the color is not extracted by chloroform, extract the other portion of the colored solution with a few milliliters of butanol to distinguish porphobilinogen from intermediate Ehrlich-reactive compounds. Color due to urobilinogen will be extracted into the butanol.

5. Report results as follows:

Positive or negative for urobilinogen
Positive for porphobilinogen
Positive for both urobilinogen and porphobilinogen (very rare)

Do not report the finding of intermediate Ehrlich-reactive compounds.

SCHLESINGER'S TEST FOR URINE UROBILIN[31]

Principle

Urobilin is an oxidation product of urobilinogen. Urobilin is a colored compound, whereas urobilinogen is colorless. Both compounds have the same clinical significance when present in urine; however, they give different chemical reactions.

Reagent

The reagent used in this test is a saturated alcohol solution of zinc acetate.

Procedure

1. Mix equal parts of urine and alcohol-zinc acetate in a test tube and filter.

2. Examine the filtrate for green fluorescence by examining the tube from above as the solution is passed through the direct rays of a fairly strong light.

3. Report as positive or negative.

QUANTITATIVE DETERMINATION OF URINE UROBILINOGEN

Quantitative determinations of urine urobilinogen are very similar to Ehrlich's qualitative aldehyde reaction. With the quantitative determination the reagents are measured volumetrically, and the degree of color formation is measured with a photometer. One difference between this and other quantitative tests is related to the freshness of the specimen. Because urobilinogen is so rapidly oxidized to urobilin, it is impossible to employ a complete 24-hour urine collection. Rather, a complete 2-hour collection is used. A specimen collected between 1 P.M. and 3 P.M. is preferred, since excretion of urobilinogen is highest during this period. The test must be performed within ½ hour of collection because of the instability of urobilinogen. In addition, specimens must be protected from sunlight and other sources of intense heat. Therefore, they are collected in brown bottles and stored under refrigeration.

HEMOGLOBIN IN URINE AND FECES[32-37]

Although the clinical significance of hemoglobin in urine is different from that of its presence in feces, its chemical detection in both will be discussed in this section. The various tests covered, although said to be tests for hemoglobin, will react also with red cells and with myoglobin.

It is clinically significant, too, to differentiate between red cells and hemoglobin in the urine. Since tests for hemoglobin are positive in the presence of both free hemoglobin and red cells, it would seem that the main differentiation between hematuria and hemoglobinuria is the finding of red blood cells in the microscopic analysis of the urinary sediment. However, the absence of red cells with the presence of hemoglobin in the urine does not necessarily mean that the hemoglobin was originally free urinary hemoglobin. Red blood cells rapidly lyse in urine, especially in urine with a specific gravity of 1.006 or less, or in alkaline urine. For this reason urine should be absolutely fresh when examined for the presence of red cells. In addition, the specific gravity and pH of the urine will be useful in differentiating between hematuria and hemaglobinuria.

Tests for hemoglobin in stool specimens are often referred to as tests for "occult blood." This is because hemoglobin may be present in the feces as evidenced by positive chemical tests for blood and yet not be detected by the naked eye. In other words, occult blood is hidden blood and requires a chemical test for its detection. Occasionally there will be enough blood present in the feces to result in a tarry black or even bloody-appearing specimen. However, even these specimens should be tested chemically for hemoglobin, or occult blood. The detection of occult blood in the feces is extremely useful in the early diagnosis of gastric carcinoma and ulcers.

Numerous tests are available for the detection of hemoglobin (or blood) in both urine and feces. Most of these tests are based upon the same general principles and reaction. They all make use of peroxidase activity in the heme portion of the hemoglobin molecule. The reagents most commonly used are gum guaiac, benzindine, or orthotolidine. They all involve the presence of hydrogen peroxide or a suitable precursor. Peroxidase activity of the hemoglobin molecule will result in the liberation of oxygen from hydrogen peroxide. This oxygen will cause the oxidation of gum guaiac, benzidine, or orthotolidine to colored oxidation products which are usually blue or green.

These reactions are summarized below:

$$\text{Hemoglobin} + \text{hydrogen peroxide} \xrightarrow{\text{peroxidase}} \text{oxygen}$$
$$\text{Oxygen} + \text{gum guaiac, benzidine, or orthotolidine} \rightarrow$$
$$\text{blue or green oxidation products}$$

The various reagents which are commonly used in testing for hemoglobin have varying degrees of sensitivity. Of the three, orthotolidine is the most sensitive to the presence of hemoglobin, benzidine is less sensitive than orthotolidine, and gum guaiac is least sensitive. However, all these tests are based on peroxidase activity of the heme portion of the hemoglobin molecule. For this reason, other substances with peroxidase activity will also give positive reactions in the tests for occult blood.

Interfering substances which may give false-positive reactions include substances with peroxidase activity of dietary origin, such as iron, meat, and fat, in the feces. In addition, false-positive results may be obtained from copper, bismuth, bromides, iodides, formalin, or white cells or bacteria with peroxidase activity. Consideration of positive reactions with interfering substances is important in determining the reliability of the various tests for occult blood. In general, the more sensitive the test is to hemoglobin, the less reliable, since it will be more likely to react with interfering substances. For this reason, gum guaiac is the most reliable of the three tests mentioned, while orthotolidine is the least reliable. In fact, gum guaiac is the only test which is routinely negative in normal persons who have been on normal diets. With the benzidine and orthotolidine tests, the patient must be placed on a meat-free diet to avoid false-positive reactions before the test can be interpreted. Therefore, the gum guaiac test is the one most often used as a screening test for occult blood in feces. If the gum guaiac test is negative and the patient has been on a meat-free diet, the feces may be further tested with the more sensitive benzidine test.

Filter paper tests for blood in feces using gum guaiac and benzidine are described below. Both these tests may also be used to test urine for hemoglobin. When urine is to be tested, it should be centrifuged in order to remove white blood cells and bacteria, which will give false-positive results due to peroxidase activity. In addition, centrifuging the urine will remove intact red blood cells, so that only free hemoglobin in the urine will be measured.

Various commercial tests, both tablet and dipstick tests, have been developed to test both urine and feces for the presence of hemoglobin. These tests usually use the more sensitive orthotolidine as the color reagent. However, these commercial tests have been adjusted so that they will not give the false-positive reactions typical of orthotolidine tests. When these tests are used, the manufacturer's directions should be followed and the literature consulted for possible reactions with interfering substances.

A. GUM GUAIAC FILTER PAPER TEST

Reagents

1. Glacial acetic acid.
2. Three percent hydrogen peroxide. Dilute 10 ml of 30% hydrogen peroxide to 100 ml with deionized water. Store in the refrigerator.
3. Three percent gum guaiac in ninety-five percent ethanol. Dilute 3 g of gum guaiac to 100 ml with 95% ethanol. Store in the refrigerator.
4. Working reagent. Combine 1 part gum guaiac and 1 part hydrogen peroxide. Prepare fresh daily.

Procedure

1. Hands, equipment, and working area must be clean and free from traces of blood.
2. Mix the specimen as thoroughly as possible.
3. Spread a small amount of feces on a filter paper.
4. Add two drops of glacial acetic acid.
5. Add four drops of the working guaiac-peroxide reagent.
6. Observe, grade, and report results as follows:

Negative—no blue color
Small—faint blue color forming slowly
Moderate—clear blue color appearing almost immediately but never intense
Large—intense blue color forming immediately

B. BENZIDINE FILTER PAPER TEST

Reagents

1. Three percent hydrogen peroxide as prepared for the gum guaiac test.

2. Benzidine reagent. Combine 1 g of benzidine dihydrochloride, 30 ml of deionized water, 20 ml of glacial acetic acid, and 50 ml of 95% ethanol. Store in the refrigerator.

Procedure

1. Hands, equipment, and working area must be clean and free from traces of blood.
2. Mix the specimen as thoroughly as possible.
3. Spread a small amount of feces on a piece of filter paper.
4. Add three drops of benzidine reagent and mix with the feces.
5. Add three drops of 3% hydrogen peroxide.
6. Observe, grade, and report results as follows:

Negative—no blue color

Small—faint blue color forming slowly

Moderate—clear blue color appearing almost immediately but never intense

Large—intense blue color forming immediately

Both the gum guaiac and benzidine filter paper tests may be used to test urine as well as feces. Centrifuge the urine specimen, and use three drops of clear supernate in place of feces on the filter paper.

C. CONTROLS

Since there are several causes of both false-positive and negative reactions in the various tests for occult blood, it is essential that both positive and negative controls be included. *Positive controls* consist of the reagents normally employed, plus blood and filter paper. Whole blood is substituted for feces, and the procedure is performed as usual. If the control is adequate, the reaction should be equivalent to a large amount of blood present in feces. If not, new working reagents should be prepared and the control repeated. The positive control is used to check the reagents for false-negative reactions. *Negative controls* consist of the reagents normally employed and filter paper only. No specimen is used; rather, the test is performed as usual but on clean filter paper. In this case the result should be negative. If not, make new working reagents, or use different filter paper. The negative control is used to check both the reagents and the filter paper for false-positive results.

D. HEMASTIX REAGENT STICKS (AMES CO.)[38]

Hemastix is a commercial test for hemoglobin, red blood cells, and myoglobin in urine. It is based upon the oxidation of orthotolidine by peroxidase activity of the hemoglobin molecule. In this case the oxygen liberated by peroxidase activity is derived from cumene hydroperoxide. The sticks seem to be quite specific for hemoglobin, red cells, and myo-

globin and do not give false positives unless in reaction with highly contaminated urine as a result of bacterial peroxidases. It has been found
negative in up to 1,000 mg% of potassium iodine.[39] The test is more
sensitive to free hemoglobin than to intact red blood cells and may not
react when only a few intact red cells are present with no free hemoglobin.

Contents of the Sticks

Hemastix reagent sticks contain:

Orthotolidine
Cumene hydroperoxide
Citrate buffers

Procedure

1. Dip the test end of the Hemastix into well-mixed urine.
2. Exactly 1 minute after moistening the dipstick, compare with the
color chart provided by the manufacturer.
3. Report the results as negative, small, moderate, or large depending
on the amount of blue color formation at 1 minute.

URINARY SEDIMENT

The urinary sediment refers to all solid materials suspended in the
urine specimen. Very few urine specimens are absolutely clear, and even
those which appear clear to the naked eye have some solid material suspended in them. In addition, many urine specimens obviously contain
varying degrees of solid material as evidenced by the degree of cloudiness:
hazy, cloudy, very cloudy, or turbid. Any amount of cloudiness which
is visible to the naked eye must be accounted for in a microscopic analysis
of the urinary sediment. Even the supposedly clear urine will be found
to contain important solid materials when examined under the microscope.
All these solid materials may be identified only under the microscope,
and a microscopic examination of the urinary sediment is essential to any
routine urinalysis. In fact, it may be the most important part of the
urinalysis.

When the urinary sediment is to be examined, only a portion of the
urine is used, rather than a well-mixed specimen. The sediment is concentrated before examination in order to ensure detection of less numerous
constituents. In order to concentrate the sediment, a well-mixed, measured
portion of urine is centrifuged. Upon centrifuging, the solid material will
settle to the bottom. It is then possible to decant the clear supernatant
and examine a portion of the concentrated sediment under the microscope
(the supernatant may be further tested for chemical constitutents, as for
example, urinary protein). The various parts of the sediment are not
only identified but counted in order to give qualitative results. For these

results to have any meaning, a constant amount of urine must be centrifuged and a constant volume of supernatant urine removed. Urine is therefore centrifuged in a graduated centrifuge tube. Results in this section describing the microscopic examination of the sediment are based on centrifuging exactly 10 ml of urine and removal of exactly 9 ml of supernatant, leaving 1 ml of sediment for examination under the microscope. The actual volume used may vary in different laboratories but must be consistent within each laboratory.

What actually constitutes the urinary sediment consists of a great variety of material. Some of the various constituents are normal, while others are abnormal and represent serious conditions. It is important to learn to identify both the normal and the abnormal constituents. In general, the normal constituents are more obvious and easily seen under the microscope, and must be recognized so that they do not obscure the presence of the less obvious but more serious constituents. Recognition of the abnormal constituents is extremely important in the diagnosis and treatment of various renal diseases. They will often give information about the state of the kidney and the urinary tract. In addition, the microscopic analysis of the sediment will help confirm and account for various findings in other portions of the routine urinalysis. For example, protein in the urine is often associated with the presence of casts in the sediment.

In general, the various constituents may be classified as belonging to the organized or the unorganized sediment. The organized sediment is the biologic part. This includes the red blood cells, white blood cells, epithelial cells, casts, bacteria, yeast, and fungi. Casts are long cylindrical structures which result from the solidification of material within the lumen of the kidney tubules. The organized sediment is the more important portion, the red and white blood cells and casts being of primary importance. Unfortunately, these are also the most difficult to detect. The unorganized sediment is the chemical portion. It consists of the various crystals of chemicals and amorphous material. In general, the unorganized sediment is not as important. However, there are certain abnormal crystals which do have pathologic significance. In addition, the unorganized sediment sometimes is such a large part of the total sediment that it tends to obscure the more important parts, which must be searched for with great care.

URINE SPECIMEN REQUIREMENTS

As is most often the case, the ideal specimen for microscopic analysis of the urine sediment is a fresh, first morning specimen. A first morning specimen is preferable, since it is the most concentrated and therefore even small amounts of abnormal constituents are more likely to be detected. In addition, the various formed elements are less likely to disintegrate in the more concentrated urine.

A fresh urine specimen is particularly important for reliable results upon microscopic analysis. If the urine cannot be examined shortly after voiding, it should be refrigerated. If it must be kept in the refrigerator for more than a few hours, a chemical preservative should be added. Formalin may be used as a preservative which will "fix" the various formed elements. However, formalin will interfere with various chemical tests. Other preservatives, such as toluene, may be used to prevent bacterial contamination. None of the preservatives, however, is completely satisfactory, and fresh collections are definitely preferred.

Various changes that may occur as the urine stands include the following: Red blood cells become distorted because of the lack of an isotonic solution. They will either swell or become crenated and therefore will be difficult to recognize, and will finally disintegrate. White blood cells will also disintegrate in hypotonic solutions. Casts too will disintegrate, especially as the urine becomes alkaline, since they must have sufficient acidity and solute concentration in order to exist. In addition, various other components which are found only in acid urine will disappear as the urine becomes alkaline. The increase in alkalinity is due to the growth of bacteria and production of ammonia. Finally, bacteria will multiply rapidly, obscuring various components.

In addition to being fresh and a first morning collection, the urine for microscopic examination should be clean and free of external contamination. This is sometimes a problem with female patients, since vaginal contamination will result in misleading results due to the presence of epithelial cells, red blood cells, and white blood cells originating from the vagina. For this reason, it is sometimes necessary to obtain the specimen by catheterization; however, this procedure should be avoided whenever possible.

In discussing the urinary sediment, it is useful to divide the types as follows: red blood cells, white blood cells, casts, crystals (abnormal and normal), and miscellaneous structures.

RED BLOOD CELLS

Red blood cells are a formed element which make up part of the organized urinary sediment. They are abnormal urinary constituents, and their presence is always of pathologic significance. The condition in which red blood cells are found in urine is termed *hematuria*. Often, the clinician will want to distinguish between hematuria and hemoglobinuria (the occurrence of free hemoglobin in urine). This may be done by observing the existence of red blood cells under the microscope. However, red blood cells lyse so easily in urine that the specimen must be absolutely fresh when this distinction is attempted. In addition the lysis may occur within the urinary tract, yet not be intravascular.

Hematuria may be the result of bleeding at any point along the genital urinary tract and may be seen with almost any disease of the urinary tract. In order to determine the cause of hematuria, the clinician will try to determine the site of bleeding. This involves various information, both laboratory and clinical. Part of this information will depend upon other findings in the microscopic urine analysis in addition to other portions of the routine urinalysis. For example, bleeding in the nephron (or kidney) itself will often be accompanied by red cell casts. This is an extremely serious situation; therefore, red cell casts must be looked for carefully when red cells occur. The occurrence of hematuria without accompanying protein and casts usually indicates that the bleeding has occurred in the lower genitourinary tract.[40]

As is true of most of the important constituents of the urine sediment, red blood cells are not obvious or easy to find under the microscope. Rather, detection of red blood cells requires careful examination. They must be searched for with great care, using the high-power (44×) objective. The light must be reduced, or they will be missed. Their detection also requires continual refocusing with the fine adjustment of the microscope. The correct illumination and focusing technique come with practice and require experience.

In absolutely fresh urine red blood cells will be unaltered or intact and appear much as they do in diluted whole blood. They show a characteristic bluish-green sheen, are intact biconcave disks which are especially apparent as they roll over, have a generally smooth appearance as opposed to the granular appearance of white blood cells, and measure about 7 μ in diameter (Fig. 4-4). However, red blood cells rapidly undergo morphologic changes in urine specimens and are rarely observed as described. This is due to the fact that urine is rarely an isotonic solution with red blood cells. In other words, the solute concentration within the red blood cells is rarely the same as the solute concentration of urine. The urine may be more or less concentrated than blood, with the following changes as a result:

When the urine is hypotonic or dilute as evidenced by a low specific gravity, the red blood cells will appear *swollen* and *rounded* because of diffusion of fluid into the red blood cell. If the urine is hypertonic or concentrated (high specific gravity), the red cells will appear *crenated* and *shrunken* (Fig. 4-4). This is due to loss of fluid from the red blood cells into the urine. When crenated, the red cells have little spicules, or projections, which cause confusion with white blood cells. However, a crenated red blood cell is significantly smaller than a white blood cell and has a generally smooth, rather than granular, appearance. Finally, when the urine is dilute and alkaline, the red blood cells will often appear as *shadow,* or *ghost, cells* (Fig. 4-4). In this situation the red cells have burst and released the hemoglobin. All that remains is the faint colorless cell membrane, a ghost, or shadow, of the original cell. This form is often

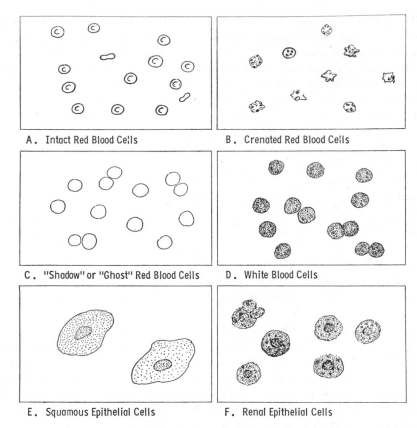

A. Intact Red Blood Cells   B. Crenated Red Blood Cells

C. "Shadow" or "Ghost" Red Blood Cells   D. White Blood Cells

E. Squamous Epithelial Cells   F. Renal Epithelial Cells

Fig. 4-4. Cells found in urine.

seen in old urine specimens. Eventually even these ghosts will disappear as the cell completely disintegrates.

It has been mentioned that red blood cells are not particularly easy to detect in a urine specimen. In addition, they are often confused with other structures that are found in the urine sediment. Red blood cells are often confused with *white blood cells*. However, the white blood cell is larger and has a generally granular appearance plus a nucleus (Fig. 4-4). If a morphologic differentiation is impossible, a drop of 2% acetic acid may be added to a new preparation or introduced under the coverslip. Acetic acid will lyse red blood cells and at the same time stain (or accentuate) the nuclei of white blood cells.

Yeast may also be confused with red blood cells in urine. However, yeast cells generally are smaller than red cells, are spherical rather than flattened, and show considerable variation in size (Fig. 4-7). Although red cells may vary in size, this variation is from specimen to specimen, rather than variation within a given specimen. Yeast cells, however, show considerable size variation within one urine specimen. In addition, since yeast reproduces by budding, the occurrence of buds or little outgrowths should identify yeast.

Bubbles or *oil droplets* are also confused with red blood cells, especially by the inexperienced. These show considerable variation in size, are extremely refractile or reflective, and are obvious under the microscope (Fig. 4-7).

The presence of red blood cells can be confirmed chemically by one of the chemical tests for hemoglobin. This is because both red blood cells and free hemoglobin will give the same chemical reaction.

Red blood cells that are present in the urinary sediment should be reported by grading as occasional, 1+, 2+, 3+, or 4+. Criteria for grading will be given under Laboratory Procedure: Microscopic Examination of the Urinary Sediment.

WHITE BLOOD CELLS

White blood cells are another formed element which make up part of the organized urinary sediment. Unlike red blood cells, the presence of a few white blood cells in urine is normal. More than an occasional white blood cell (over five per high-power field) is considered abnormal. The presence of large numbers of white blood cells in the sediment indicates inflammation at some point along the genitourinary tract. The inflammation may be due to a bacterial infection or other causes. Therefore, the presence of white cells is often associated with bacteria, but either bacteria or white cells can be present without the other. In bacterial infection, ingested bacteria are often seen within the white blood cell.

The condition in which increased numbers of white cells are found in urine is termed *pyuria*. Pyuria may cause clouding of the urine, and when this is severe enough, the urine will have a characteristic milky white appearance. Under the microscope the white cells may appear singly or in clumps. They may be mononucleated or polynucleated.

White blood cells too must be searched for with the high-power objective, reduced light, and continual refocusing using the fine adjustment. Typical white cells are about 10 to 12 μ in diameter (about twice the size of red cells); however, this size difference may not be obvious. White cells show thin cytoplasmic granulation and have a nucleus. Even if the nucleus is not distinct, the center of the cell appears granular as opposed to the generally smooth red cell (Fig. 4-4). White cells are not nearly as fragile as red cells, although they will disintegrate in old alkaline urine specimens. Various stages of disintegration may be observed in a single urine specimen.

As with red cells, other structures may be mistaken for white cells. Most often they are confused with *red cells* and *epithelial cells*. White cells are generally larger than red cells, appear granular, and have a nucleus. A 2% solution of acetic acid may be used to aid in identification. *Epithelial cells* may also be confused with white cells. There are several very different morphologic types of epithelial cells. In general, the epithelial cell is larger than the white cell and has a proportionately smaller nucleus. The nucleus is generally more distinct, and there is more cytoplasm surrounding the nucleus (Fig. 4-4). Epithelial cells will be described under Miscellaneous Structures.

White blood cells should be reported by grading the number present as occasional, 1+, 2+, 3+, or 4+. Criteria for grading will be given under Laboratory Procedure: Microscopic Examination of the Urinary Sediment.

CASTS

Casts make up another portion of the organized urinary sediment. They are at once the most difficult portion to discover and of the greatest importance. Both their importance and name derive from the manner in which they are formed. Casts are formed in the actual lumen of the kidney tubules by a solidifying of material in the tubule. They are important in that anything that is contained within the tubule is flushed out in the form of the cast. Thus a cast represents a biopsy of an individual tubule. In other words, anything contained within the cast must have been present in the tubule, so that the cast provides a means of examining the content of the kidney tubule. It is believed that casts may be formed at any point along the nephron either by precipitation of protein or by a grouping together (conglutination) of material within the tubular lumen.

Before casts can form within the renal tubules, certain conditions must exist. Since the cast is made up of protein, there must be a sufficient concentration of protein within the tubule. In addition the pH must be low enough to favor precipitation, and there must be a sufficient concentration of solutes.[41] Since these conditions are most likely to exist in the distal tubules, it is felt that cast formation is more likely in the distal rather than the proximal convoluted tubules. For the same reasons, casts are not likely to be found in dilute alkaline urine, since these conditions do not favor cast formation. It also means that the urine must be examined when fresh, for as it becomes alkaline as a result of aging, casts will disintegrate.

Since casts represent a biopsy of the kidney, they are extremely important clinically. Casts often contain various substances such as red blood cells, white blood cells, epithelial cells, and bacteria. These inclusions are not normally present within the renal tubule; they represent an abnormal situation. The formation of casts implies at least a temporary blocking of the renal tubules in order to allow the cast formation. Although a few hyaline casts (made merely of precipitated protein) are normal, considerable numbers of casts always indicate renal damage. The number of hyaline casts may increase in mild irritations of the kidney associated with fever.

Since casts are extremely difficult to see, they must be searched for carefully with reduced light and the low-power (10×) objective. They are both searched for and graded using low power but must be identified as to type by means of the high-power objective. The refractive index of the cast is nearly the same as for glass, resulting in an image very difficult to see under the microscope. As might be imagined from the shape of the tubular lumen, casts are cylindrical bodies and have rounded ends. To be identified as a cast, the outline should be an even and definite line, and the structure should have two rounded ends. Although they will vary somewhat in size, casts should have a uniform diameter (about seven or eight times a red cell diameter) and be several times longer than wide.

Structures similar to casts and seen in the urine sediment are *cylindroids*. These structures are similar to casts in every respect except that, rather than being a cylinder with two rounded ends, the cylindroid has one end which tapers to a point, or a tail. The exact mechanism of formation and site or origin of cylindroids is not known, but they seem to occur in conjunction with hyaline casts and are considered to have the same significance clinically. Cylindroids are often confused with strands of mucus, and care must be taken to avoid this mistake.

Classification of casts is not always simple. Classification in the laboratory is done mainly on the basis of morphologic groupings: hyaline, finely granular, coarsely granular, waxy, cellular, or fatty. However a given urine specimen may contain more than one morphologic type, and a given cast may show more than one type; e.g., one end may be hyaline, while the other end is cellular. A most complete classification on the basis of composition and origin has been proposed by Lippman.[42] This system is especially useful in relation to understanding cast formation but is not completely practical for use in the laboratory, where only morphologic classification is possible. The following classification is based on morphologic features but incorporates material proposed by Lippman. Lippman proposes only three main cast group types on the basis of composition and origin which he terms hyaline, epithelial, and blood casts. These together with their subdivisions in effect present the same groupings as the morphologic classification used here.

Hyaline Casts

Hyaline casts are colorless, homogeneous, nonrefractile, semitransparent structures (Fig. 4-5). This type of cast is the most difficult to discover under the microscope. Hyaline casts result from precipitation of protein within the lumen of kidney tubules. Since they are believed to result from a gel formation, the cast will include any material that may be present

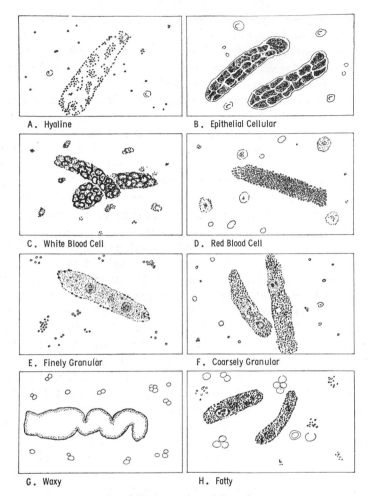

Fig. 4-5. Casts found in urine.

such as cells or cellular debris. Hyaline casts are soluble in water and even more soluble in slightly alkaline solution. Therefore, hyaline casts are more likely to be found in more concentrated and acid urine and may not form in cases of advanced renal failure with the inability to concentrate the urine or maintain the normal acid pH.[43] In addition, hyaline casts will dissolve as the urine stands and becomes alkaline, so that fresh urine specimens are essential for detection. Lippman further classifies hyaline-type casts according to their inclusions as hyaline cellular, hyaline coarsely granular, hyaline finely granular, and hyaline fatty casts.

Cellular Casts

These casts contain intact white cells, red cells, or epithelial cells. They are further named on the basis of the actual type of cell present: white blood cell cast, red blood cell (or blood) cast, and epithelial cast (Fig. 4-5). A truly cellular cast results from a clumping, or conglutination, of cells rather than precipitation of protein. Cellular casts are more easily detected under the microscope than hyaline casts, since the cells give definite structure unlike homogeneous solidified protein.

Epithelial cell casts represent a more serious situation than the presence of hyaline casts. They result from a clumping of epithelial cells which line the renal tubules and therefore represent a destruction or desquamation of the renal tubule. These tubular epithelial cells are responsible for the work done by the kidney, and such kidney damage is irreversible. Often the epithelial cast is seen to consist of two rows of epithelial cells implying tubular desquamation. However, the cells may also vary in size and shape and not show a regular pattern. Lippman notes that the epithelial cell cast does not remain constant once formed but undergoes a series of changes. These changes are due to cellular disintegration, since the cast remains within the kidney as a result of decreased urine flow (stasis). Therefore, Lippman views a series of epithelial-type casts as beginning with the cellular and degenerating to coarsely granular, finely granular, and finally waxy casts. In this view, the waxy-type cast represents the most serious situation, a sufficient period of blockage of renal flow for the slow disintegration of cells to a homogeneous mass, the waxy cast. All these various types often are seen in the same urine specimen.

Red blood cell casts, or blood casts, may also be thought of as resulting from the clumping, or conglutination, of cells, this time red cells. There is disagreement concerning the composition and origin of blood casts. They are often divided into two types: the red blood cell cast and the true blood cast. The red blood cell cast is thought to be composed of a solid mass of conglutinated red cells with no stroma visible between the packed cells. The true blood cast shows a completely homogeneous matrix with no cell margins discernible. Both types of blood casts have a characteristic orange-yellow color which is unlike anything else seen in the urinary sediment. Lippman feels that red blood cell casts are formed by the clumping of red blood cells which disintegrate, as did the epithelial cell cast, to form the true blood cast. The true blood cast would then be analogous to the waxy cast. When seen in large number, blood casts are usually associated with glomerulitis, most commonly glomerulonephritis. As seen before, when red cells are found in urine, the occurrence of red cell casts helps determine the site of bleeding.

Finely Granular Casts

These are casts which contain many fine granules. They look much like hyaline casts; however, the presence of fine granules make them more distinctive, or easier to find. They usually are grayish or pale yellow (Fig. 4-5). Lippman describes two types of finely granular casts: hyaline finely granular casts and finely granular epithelial-type casts.

Coarsely Granular Casts

Coarsely granular casts appear to contain degenerated epithelial or blood cells and other debris in the form of large granules. They tend to be darker than finely granular casts in addition to being shorter and more irregular in outline (Fig. 4-5). The darker color and larger granules make them easier to find than either the hyaline or finely granular casts. Again, Lippman describes two types of coarsely granular casts. The hyaline coarsely granular cast is primarily a hyaline-type cast containing large granules of cellular debris present in the tubule at the time of cast formation. The coarsely granular epithelial-type cast is described by Lippman as the first stage of the in vivo disintegration of the epithelial-type cast. These differences are not usually possible to identify morphologically but seem logical in terms of origin.

Waxy Casts

Waxy casts appear most like hyaline casts and may be mistaken for them; however, they are much more significant clinically. The waxy cast appears to be made of wax; hence the name. It is homogeneous, as is the hyaline cast, but is yellowish and more refractile. Waxy casts tend to be wider than hyaline casts and usually have irregular broken ends (Fig. 4-5). As mentioned previously, Lippman feels that waxy casts are the final step in the distintegration of epithelial casts and are especially serious since they imply renal stasis, or blockage, in order to form.

Fatty Casts

Fatty casts, as the name implies, contain droplets of fat. Fat droplets are highly refractile under the microscope (Fig. 4-5). They will stain bright orange with Sudan III stain. Fatty casts are very serious, since they result from fatty degeneration and desquamation of the renal tubular epithelium, as seen in cases of nephrosis. Such fat droplets may be contained within either hyaline- or epithelial-type casts. They are often seen along with "oval fat bodies," which are renal epithelial cells which have degenerated by being filled with fat and sloughed off into the urine.

Broad and Narrow Casts

Broad and narrow casts are not types of casts in the sense previously used. Rather, they may be any type of cast with a description of the diameter included. Since casts are formed within the distal convoluted tubules of the nephron and since the tubular diameter is fairly constant, there is normally little variation in cast diameter. *Narrow casts* probably result from swelling of the tubular epithelium with a narrowing of the tubular lumen. They are not particularly important. *Broad casts* are much more serious. The diameter of broad casts is several times greater than normal. The broad diameter is felt to result from their formation in the collecting tubules (several nephrons empty into common collecting tubules), which have a greater diameter than the tubules of the nephron. Cast formation in the collecting tubules must result from urinary stasis in the group of nephrons feeding a single collecting tubule. If not, the fluid pressure would be far too great for cast formation to occur. This represents serious stasis. Broad casts can be of almost any type, but, because of the degree of stasis, most tend to be of the waxy type.

Structures Confused with Casts

The difficulty in finding casts under the microscope has been stressed. In addition to the failure to notice casts when they do exist, the inexperienced observer tends to confuse other structures with casts. As previously noted, *cylinderoids* are similar to hyaline casts except that one end is elongated and tapering, rather than rounded. They have the same significance as simple hyaline casts and are often seen with these.

Mucous threads also may be confused with casts. The refractive index is similar to that of hyaline casts; however, these are long ribbonlike strands with undefined edges and pointed or split ends. They also appear to have longitudinal striations.

Rolled squamous epithelial cells may also be mistaken for casts. In this case squamous epithelial cells have rolled into a cigar shape. However, they have pointed ends rather than rounded and are shorter, and a single round nucleus may be discovered with careful focusing.

Bits of *hair or threads* of material fibers are also mistaken for casts by the beginner. However, these are extremely refractile structures which have nothing in common with the appearance of protein microscopically. Likewise, *scratches* on the glass slide or coverslip may be mistaken for casts at first. Again, they are much too definite and obvious to be important. Finally, *hyphae of molds* are sometimes mistaken for hyaline casts. This is similar to the mistaking of yeast for red blood cells. Again, the hyphae are much more refractile. They are also jointed and branching structures which can be observed upon closer examination.

CRYSTALS AND AMORPHOUS MATERIAL

Crystals and amorphous precipitates of certain chemicals make up the unorganized urinary sediment. These materials are obvious under the microscope. Because they are so striking, there is a natural tendency to pay considerable attention to them. However, they are the most insignificant part of the urinary sediment and deserve little attention. In the past, great emphasis was placed upon identification of these materials. However, it is generally preferable to search carefully for more pathologic constituents and note only briefly the occurrence of crystals.

Most urine specimens will contain some crystalline material when voided. As urine specimens stand, especially when refrigerated, most become cloudy because of the precipitation of amorphous material. In addition, as urine stands, various crystals precipitate out of solution. Both crystals and amorphous materials have little significance. Normal crystals and amorphous materials should be learned and identified, however, for the following reasons:

First, the presence of large numbers of crystals or amorphous material will obscure the presence of such important structures as red blood cells, white blood cells, or casts. These more important structures must be searched for with extreme care when crystals and amorphous materials are present. Secondly, the precipitation of certain crystals will accompany kidney stone formation (lithiasis). This is one reason for the attention that was formerly given to urinary crystals. Finally, there are certain chemicals (such as cystine, leucine, and tyrosine) which may crystalize in urine and indicate serious metabolic disorders.

Also, administration of sulfonamide drugs may cause the formation of sulfonamide crystals, especially in acid urine. The formation of various sulfonamide crystals within the kidney may result in blockage of renal output and severe renal damage. This problem is no longer as prevalent as when the sulfonamide drugs were first introduced; the identification of such crystals is therefore losing importance. In any case, it is necessary to recognize the various normal crystals, so that when abnormal crystals are encountered, they will not be overlooked.

Normal crystals should be identified and reported merely as few or many seen per low-power field. Normal crystals are reported merely on the basis of microscopic examination and do not require chemical tests. Abnormal crystals should be reported by grading the number according to the criteria given under Laboratory Procedure: Microscopic Examination of the Urinary Sediment and in Table 4-3. Further, abnormal crystals cannot be reported on the basis of microscopic evidence alone but require confirmatory chemical tests. These chemical tests will not be described but may be found in any standard clinical laboratory text. Identification of normal urinary crystals and amorphous material is further simplified by the fact they occur in either acid or alkaline urine. Therefore the pH of the urine should always be known when microscopic examination is made. Also, it must be remembered that it is the shape rather than the size that is characteristic of chemical crystals.

Normal Crystals of Acid Urine { amorphous urates / Uric acid / Calcium oxalate

Amorphus Urates

This is the amorphous material found in acid urine. *Amorphous* means without shape, or form. The urates show a characteristic yellowish red shapeless granulation (Fig. 4-6). When present in sufficient numbers mi-

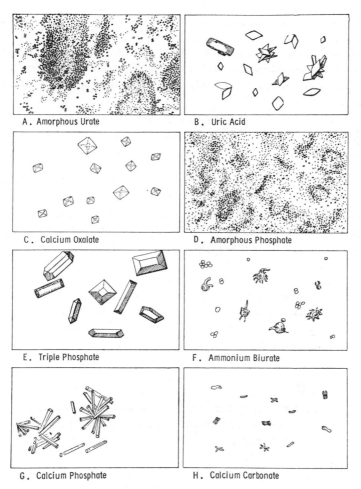

A. Amorphous Urate

B. Uric Acid

C. Calcium Oxalate

D. Amorphous Phosphate

E. Triple Phosphate

F. Ammonium Biurate

G. Calcium Phosphate

H. Calcium Carbonate

Fig. 4-6. Normal crystals.

croscopically, the urates will form a characteristic fluffy pink precipitate often called "brick dust."

Uric Acid

These crystals have a variety of shapes and colors. Typically they are yellow or reddish brown, much like the chemically related amorphous urates. The most typical shape is the "whetstone." Other shapes include rhombic plates or prisms, somewhat oval forms with pointed ends ("lemon-shaped"), wedges, rosettes, and irregular plates (Fig. 4-6). They are usually recognized by color, but some, especially the rhombic plates, may appear colorless.

Calcium Oxalate

Calcium oxalate crystals have a characteristic "envelope" appearance. They vary somewhat in size but are typically small, colorless, glistening octahedrals (Fig. 4-6). Less frequently they may appear in a dumbbell shape.

Normal Crystals of Alkaline Urine

Amorphous Phosphates

The amorphous material found in alkaline urine is amorphous phosphate. Generally, the phosphates have a finer or more lacy precipitate than the amorphous urates and are colorless (Fig. 4-6). Phosphates are the most common cause of turbidity in alkaline urine and are seen as a fine white precipitate microscopically.

Triple Phosphates

Triple phosphates are colorless crystals and commonly show great variation in size from tiny to relatively huge crystals microscopically. They have a characteristic "coffin-lid" shape which is impossible to ignore (Fig. 4-6). Less commonly, they occur in a fern form.

Ammonium Biurate

Ammonium biurate is the alkaline counterpart of uric acid and amorphous urates in urine. They are characteristically "thorn apples," or spherical objects with radial or concentric striations and long prismatic spicules (Fig. 4-6). They are yellow.

Calcium Phosphate

Calcium phosphates are colorless crystals. They may occur as flat plates (which are often mistaken for epithelial cells) or as slender wedge-shaped crystals which occur singly or in rosettes (Fig. 4-6).

Calcium Carbonate

Calcium carbonate crystals are tiny colorless granules typically occurring as "dumbbells" but also singly (Fig. 4-6).

Abnormal Urinary Crystals

Normal crystals of urine may be reported on the basis of microscopic examination alone. However, abnormal crystals should not be reported without the use of confirmatory chemical tests. The following description of abnormal crystals is superficial, and if the occurrence of such crystals is suspected, a more detailed text must be consulted both for microscopic appearance and confirmatory chemical procedures.

Cystine

Cystine crystals appear as colorless, refractile, hexagonal plates.

Tyrosine

Tyrosine crystals appear as fine needles arranged in sheaves which are usually black in color.

Leucine

Leucine crystals appear as yellow, oily-appearing spheres with radial and concentric striations. Leucine and tyrosine crystals usually appear together.

Cholesterol

Cholesterol crystals appear as large, flat, hexagonal plates with one or more corners notched out.

Hippuric Acid

Hippuric acid crystals appear as brownish needles or prisms.

Sulfonamides

Various sulfonamides appear in several and various forms depending upon the particular form of the drug. They include the following:

1. *Sulfanilamide* is rarely seen. It occurs as large colorless needles, frequently in sheaves or rosettes.

2. *Sulfapyridine* occurs as colorless arrowheads or whetstones; also, as brown needles in large conglomerate masses or rosettes.

3. *Sulfathiazole* occurs as brownish shocks of wheat with central binding or rosettes with radial striations; also, as colorless diamond and hexagonal plates, sometimes in rosettes.

4. *Sulfadiazine* is the most dangerous form of the drug in urine. It occurs as colorless to greenish brown shocks of wheat with eccentric binding and rosettes with radial striations, sometimes covered with needlelike processes.

5. *Sulfaguanidine* appears as colorless needles grouped as shocks of wheat with eccentric binding; also, as rectangular plates with slight bulging in the long axis.

6. *Sulfamethylthiazole* occurs as colorless to greenish brown needles clumped in the shape of a fan.

MISCELLANEOUS STRUCTURES

There are various structures which may occur in the urinary sediment which have not yet been described. These will be classified as miscellaneous structures and should be identified and reported as few or many present.

Epithelial Cells

The various structures that make up the urinary system consist of several layers of epithelial cells except for the single-layered tubules of the nephron. The epithelial cells of the multilayered organs are continually sloughed off into the urine and replaced by cells originating from deeper layers. Therefore, urine will always contain some epithelial cells.

The outer layer of cells which are normally replaced are of the *squamous epithelial* type. These are very large flat cells, made up of a thin layer of cytoplasm and a single distinct nucleus (Fig. 4-4). They are large enough to be seen easily under low power and sometimes roll into cigar shapes which are mistaken for casts. This type of epithelial cell is of little significance and should be reported only if present in large numbers. As the epithelial cell layers become deeper, the cells become thicker and rounder-looking, more and more like white blood cells.

There are several intermediate forms of epithelial cells varying from the squamous to the *renal epithelial cells* which line the nephron tubules. The occurrence of renal epithelial cells in urine is important, for it implies destruction of renal tubules, as did the presence of the epithelial-type cast. However, identification of renal epithelial cells cannot be made on the basis of microscopic evidence alone, since they resemble both white blood cells and deeper layers of cells lining the urinary system. Morphologically, renal epithelial cells closely resemble white blood cells but are typically larger, with a single distinct nucleus (Fig. 4-4). When present they are often seen in association with casts. The presence of epithelial casts will help confirm their identification, and when renal cells are suspected, casts should be searched for with great care.

Oval Fat Bodies

Oval fat bodies are renal epithelial cells which are filled with fat droplets (Fig. 4-7). They indicate a serious pathologic condition. The fat droplets are highly refractile and may be stained with Sudan III stain. The use of polarized light may also be useful for indicating the presence of cholesterol esters in the fat. Oval fat bodies are often seen along with fat droplets and fatty casts in the urinary sediment.

Fat Globules

Fat may be found in the urinary sediment as highly refractile droplets of various sizes. Fat will stain orange or red with Sudan III stains. Most commonly, fat arises from extraneous sources such as unclean collection utensils or oiled catheters. However, fat droplets are occasionally present

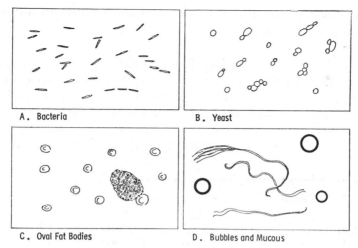

Fig. 4-7. Miscellaneous structures found in urine.

as the result of degenerative tubular diseases. In this case they are seen in association with oval fat bodies and fatty casts. Polarized light is useful in identification of significant fat content.

Bacteria

Under normal conditions the urinary tract is free of bacteria. However, most urine specimens will contain at least a few bacteria, due to contamination when the urine is voided. Bacteria multiply rapidly as urine is allowed to stand at room temperature. In specimens which are obtained (by catheterization) and kept under sterile conditions, the presence of bacteria may indicate a urinary tract infection. In this case, they are likely to be associated with the presence of white blood cells, although this is not always true. The presence of bacterial infection should be confirmed by bacteriologic culture and examination. Bacteria are easily recognized morphologically. They are extremely small, only a few microns long. They may be either rods or cocci and may occur singly or in chains (Fig. 4-7). They are often motile, which helps in their identification. Bacteria are most often seen in alkaline urine and may be confused with amorphous material at first, but this will not be a problem as experience in observation is gained.

Yeast

Yeast cells are occasionally seen in urine, especially the urine of females and of diabetic patients. They are associated with the presence of sugar in urine. Sugar is the energy source for yeast cells, which grow and multiply rapidly when it is present. For this reason yeast cells are often discovered in the urine of diabetics along with high sugar content, low pH, and ketones.

Yeast cells are often mistaken for red blood cells. They are generally smaller than red cells and show considerable size variation even within a given specimen. They have a typically ovoid shape, lack color, and have a smooth and refractile appearance. The most distinguishing characteristic is the presence of little buds, or projections, from the yeast cell due to their manner of reproduction (Fig. 4-7).

LABORATORY PROCEDURE: MICROSCOPIC EXAMINATION OF THE URINARY SEDIMENT

1. Pour exactly 10 ml of well-mixed urine into a graduated centrifuge tube, and centrifuge for 5 to 10 minutes.
2. Decant 9 ml of clear supernatant urine leaving exactly 1 ml (±0.1 ml) to ensure consistency in grading results.
3. Resuspend the sediment for examination by mixing thoroughly.
4. Transfer a drop or two of well-mixed sediment to a clean, labeled glass slide. The size of the drop is important. The fluid should completely fill the area under the coverslip but without overflowing the area or causing the coverslip to float.
5. Carefully place a coverslip over the sediment, taking care that no bubbles appear. If bubbles appear, a new preparation must be made on a clean slide. Bubbles are confusing and make grading impossible, since they prevent random distribution of the various substances to be graded.
6. Place the preparation on the microscope stage, and focus and adjust the light using the low-power objective. Systematic examination is important. No preparation should be observed longer than 3 minutes, or drying will occur, making identification inaccurate. First, look for the various substances that are identified and graded under low power. Then change to high power, refocus and readjust the light, and search for the various substances that are graded and identified under high power. All gradings are based on the average number of structures seen in a minimum of 10 microscopic fields. To ensure accurate results prepare two separate portions of sediment, and count the structures seen in five microscopic fields in each preparation. (Of course, the first portion should be prepared and observed before the second is prepared.) In order to obtain a meaningful average, observe and count structures in the four quadrants and center of each preparation. Describe separately the various structures searched for under low and high power. Casts and cells are most important; search for these most carefully, observing the less important crystals and miscellaneous structures almost in retrospect.

a. Using the low-power (10X) objective, search for:

(1) *Casts*

Search for casts and grade these under low power. Since they tend to roll to the edges of the coverslip, search for them around all four edges of the preparation, and then search the center. When a cast is discovered using low power, change to high power to identify it. Grade casts as negative, occasional, 1+, 2+, 3+, or 4+ on the basis of the average number of casts seen in a minimum of 10 low-power fields (Table 4-3). If more than one type of cast is found in a single specimen, identify and grade each type separately.

(2) *Crystals and amorphous material*

Many crystals and much amorphous material can be seen and identified under low power, although some require high power to be seen. Look for these structures in the same way as for casts. Report normal crystals as few or many seen per low-power field. Confirm abnormal crystals first by means of a chemical test, and then grade them on the average number seen in a minimum of 10 low-power fields (Table 4-3).

(3) *Miscellaneous structures*

Various miscellaneous structures can be seen and are reported as few or many with the low-power objective. They should be noticed as casts are searched for.

Table 4-3. Grading System for the Urinary Sediment*

Constituent	Negative	Occasional	1+	2+	3+	4+
RBC/hpf	0	Less than 4	4–8	8–30	Greater than 30, less than packed	Packed field
WBC/hpf	0	Less than 5	5–20	20–50	Greater than 50, less than packed	Packed field
Casts/lpf	0	Less than 1	1–5	4–10	10–30	Greater than 30
Abnormal crystals/lpf	0	Less than 1	1–5	4–10	10–30	Greater than 30

* This grading system applies to a microscope field viewed with the usual 10X eyepiece and the 10X and 44X objective lenses. The approximate diameters of such a field under low and high power are 1.5 and 0.35 mm, respectively. A correction should be applied when a microscope with a different-sized field is used in order to maintain consistency in the reporting of results.

b. Using the high-power $(44\times)$ objective, search for:

(1) *Red blood cells*

Search for red cells and grade them under high power. Grade them as negative, occasional, 1+, 2+, 3+, or 4+ on the basis of the average number seen in a minimum of 10 high-power fields (Table 4-3).

(2) *White blood cells*

Search for white cells and grade them under high power. Grade them as negative, occasional, 1+, 2+, 3+, or 4+ on the basis of the average number seen in a minimum of 10 high-power fields (Table 4-3).

(3) Identify casts, and search for smaller crystals and amorphous material.

(4) *Miscellaneous structures*

Look for the various miscellaneous structures which can only be seen with the high-power objective. Identify and report these structures as few or many.

REFERENCES

1. Israel Davidson and Benjamin B. Wells, "Clinical Diagnosis by Laboratory Methods (Todd-Sanford)," 13th ed., p. 23, W. B. Saunders Company, Philadelphia, 1963.
2. Robert M. Kark, James R. Lawrence, Victor E. Pollak, Conrad L. Pirani, Robert C. Muehrcke, and Homero Silva, "A Primer of Urinalysis," 2d ed., p. 10, Hoeber Medical Division, Harper & Row, Publishers, Incorporated, New York, 1963.
3. C. J. Watson and Ellis S. Benson, "Outlines of Internal Medicine," pt. V, 10th ed., p. 548, Wm. C. Brown Company, Dubuque, Iowa, 1962.
4. Kark et al., *op. cit.,* p. 38.
5. Lot B. Page and Perry J. Culver, "A Syllabus of Laboratory Examinations in Clinical Diagnosis," rev. ed., p. 305, Harvard University Press, Cambridge, Mass., 1960.
6. Philip B. Hawk, Bernard L. Oser, and William H. Summerson, "Practical Physiological Chemistry," 13th ed., p. 826, McGraw-Hill Book Company, New York, 1954.
7. Page and Culver, *op. cit.,* p. 306.
8. Watson and Benson, *op. cit.,* p. 568.
9. Kark et al., *op. cit.,* pp. 36–38.
10. Page and Culver, *op. cit.,* pp. 306–307.
11. Kark et al., *op. cit.,* pp. 38–40.
12. Page and Culver, *op. cit.,* pp. 305–306.
13. Kark et al., *op. cit.,* pp. 20–21.
14. *Ibid.,* p. 23.
15. Richard W. Lippman, "Urine and the Urinary Sediment," 2d ed., pp. 8–9, Charles C Thomas, Publisher, Springfield, Ill., 1957.

16. Watson and Benson, *op. cit.*, p. 566.
17. Davidsohn and Wells, *op. cit.*, p. 31.
18. Kark et al., *op. cit.*, p. 28.
19. Page and Culver, *op. cit.*, p. 309.
20. Watson and Benson, *op. cit.*, p. 570.
21. Kark et al., *op. cit.*, pp. 42–44.
22. *Ibid.*, p. 44.
23. Davidsohn and Wells, *op. cit.*, pp. 37–38.
24. M. Z. Barakat, S. K. Shehab, and M. M. El-Sadr, New Tests for Bile and Detection of Bile in Serum and Urine, *Clin. Chem.*, 3:135, 1957.
25. Kark et al., *op. cit.*, pp. 47–48.
26. S. Schwartz, M. H. Berg, I. Bossenmaier, and H. Dinsmore, Determination of Porphyrins in Biological Materials, *Methods Biochem. Anal.*, 8:221, 1960.
27. S. Schwartz, M. Keprios, and R. Schmid, Experimental Porphyria. II. Type Produced by Lead, Phenylhydrazine, and Light, *Proc. Soc. Exptl. Biol. Med.*, 79:463, 1952.
28. Watson and Benson, *op. cit.*, p. 578.
29. C. J. Watson, I. Bossenmaier, and R. Cardinal, "Acute Intermittent Porphyria," *J.A.M.A.*, 175:1087, 1961.
30. C. J. Watson and S. Schwartz, "A Simple Test for Urinary Porphobilinogen," *Proc. Soc. Exptl. Biol. Med.*, 47:393, 1941.
31. Watson and Benson, *op. cit.*, p. 574.
32. *Am. J. Digest. Disease*, 15:23–26, January, 1948.
33. O. E. Hepler, P. Wong, and H. D. Pihl, "Comparison of Tests for Occult Blood in Feces," *Am. J. Clin. Pathol.*, 23:1263, 1953.
34. Kark et al., *op. cit.*, pp. 51–56.
35. A. I. Mendeloff, "Selection of a Screening Procedure for Detecting Occult Blood in Feces," *J.A.M.A.*, 152:798, 1953.
36. Page and Culver, *op. cit.*, pp. 374–379.
37. Watson and Benson, *op. cit.*, pp. 586–590
38. Kark et al., *op. cit.*, p. 55.
39. *Ibid.*, p. 56.
40. *Ibid.*, p. 67.
41. Lippman, *op. cit.*, p. 11.
42. *Ibid.*
43. *Ibid.*, p. 20.

5

Blood Banking

INTRODUCTION

Blood banking is unlike any other field of clinical laboratory investigation. Although accuracy is always important in the laboratory, it is absolutely essential in blood banking. Even the smallest error can directly result in the death of the patient from a hemolytic transfusion reaction. As R. R. Race says in the preface to "Techniques in Blood Grouping" by Dunsford and Bowley, "Blood group tests are different from most laboratory tests used in medicine in a vital way—the reported result must be correct, for the wisest physician cannot protect his patient from the consequences of a blood grouping error."[1]

This chapter is meant only as a very general introduction to the subject of blood banking. It is definitely not sufficient preparation for work in blood-banking laboratories. It is hoped that this introduction to the subject will help the student to be aware of his inadequacy in this field. Specific blood-banking procedures will not be presented; only principles will be discussed. There are several excellent texts available in the field of blood banking; however, most of them seem complex (even unintelligible) to the person who has no background in this area. In this respect too it is hoped that this chapter will be of help to the student. Probably the best single reference in the area in a practical sense is the American Association of Blood Banks manual.[2] This indispensible reference will be found in any licensed blood bank and is constantly consulted by the regular blood bank staff.

To carry out blood-banking procedures a thorough knowledge of the principles involved, recognition of the many difficulties that may be encountered, and exactness of technique are essential. Shortcuts must never be taken. Everyone working in a given blood bank must use exactly the same technique. Also, an elaborate system of safeguards must be established and thoroughly understood by all personnel. These safeguards and checks may seem repetitive but are essential. When an incompatible transfusion reaction does occur, it is usually due to a breakdown of, and/or failure to observe, the established system.

Complete and permanent records must be kept of every sequence of the many steps involved in finally administering a unit of blood. These records must be completely legible and permanent. Since blood banking is an area where medicolegal problems are apt to occur, records must be meticulously kept to have legal validity. Results and observations are always recorded directly on the permanent record, never recopied, as recopying will invariably result in error at some time.

GENERAL INFORMATION ABOUT BLOOD

Whole human blood consists of two major portions, solid and liquid. The solid portion consists primarily of the formed elements: red blood cells, white blood cells, and platelets. This makes up approximately 45 percent of the total blood volume. The liquid portion consists of the plasma, which makes up approximately 55 percent of the total volume. The blood volume of normal adults is approximately 5 to 6 liters, or 10 to 12 pt. In blood banking a *unit* of blood is often referred to. For practical purposes a unit of blood may be considered one pint.

Of course, infused blood, or that blood which is administered by means of transfusion, must be anticoagulated blood. However, the portion of blood that is used for blood bank procedures such as typing and crossmatching must be clotted blood. If anticoagulated blood is used, there is a chance that small fibrin clots may be present in the plasma which may be incorrectly interpreted as a positive result. Therefore, laboratory blood bank tests employ red cells and serum (the liquid remaining after blood has been allowed to clot), not red cells and plasma.

HISTORICAL INTEREST IN TRANSFUSIONS

The importance of blood to life has been realized from the earliest times. By observation early men must have realized that if a person lost enough blood, because of an injury of some sort, he would die. This may be evidenced by the rituals of various primitive groups. It was often felt that by giving the blood of one person to another, various characteristics of the donor could be given to the recipient. The discovery of the circulation of blood by Harvey in 1616 did much to advance interest in transfusion of blood. One early transfusion was attempted by Denis in 1667, in which lamb's blood was transfused into a man. At first the transfusion seemed to benefit the man, who was given a total of three such transfusions. However, after the third transfusion of lamb's blood the man suffered a reaction and died. In general, it was found that it is impossible to transfuse the blood of one species of animal into another, whether from animal to man, man to animal, or animal of one species to animal of another species. Transfusions were also attempted within the same species of animal, from man to man and from one species of animal to another of the same species. These seemed to work about half the time, but far too often the result was death.

INTRODUCTION TO BLOOD GROUPS

It is now known that the incompatibility of the various transfusions was due to the presence of certain factors on red cells. It seems that each species of animal, man included, has a certain factor that is unique to that species and present on the red cells of all members of that species. Therefore, if the red cells of sheep, for example, are introduced into the blood system of man, man will produce an anti-sheep substance in his blood. This anti-sheep substance will destroy any sheep red cells which are subsequently introduced. This cell destruction is what is meant by an incompatible transfusion reaction, and it will result in the death of the recipient.

It is also known that certain factors are common to some members of a given species but not to all members of that species. Therefore, if blood containing a certain factor is transfused into a recipient whose red cells do not contain that factor, the recipient will form an anti-factor which will result in an incompatible transfusion reaction.

So far, this seems rather simple. Why all the difficulty in blood banking? All that is necessary is to find what factor is present on the red cell and transfuse only blood containing that factor. The principle is correct, but there are innumerable factors which may be present on any person's red blood cells. The various factors that are known have been grouped into units referred to as *blood group systems*. A partial list is:

ABO	Kidd	Lutheran	Kell
Rh	P	Ii	Xg^a
Lewis	Diego	MNS_s	Duffy

More systems are being discovered all the time. The actual factor or factors that exist on a person's red cells within a given blood group system represent his type for that system. The number of possible types within one system varies with the system. In the ABO system there are six possible types plus additional types determined by less frequent subgroups. The more complex Rh-Hr system has 110 possible types. Taking all systems and type combinations into account, there are over 500 billion different types of blood possible. In essence, each person has a unique blood type.[3]

At this point it would seem that blood transfusion is impossible, since no two persons should have exactly the same type of blood. Fortunately, only certain factors are likely to give problems in transfusion (i.e., incompatible transfusion reactions), although there is always the possibility that an unknown or untested-for factor may occur that will result in such a reaction. The factors most likely to cause reactions are located within the ABO and Rh-Hr blood group systems and must be tested for whenever blood is administered. Other factors are routinely tested for indirectly through crossmatching and antibody screening techniques.

Thus far, only the terms "factor" and "anti-factor" have been used. These are not scientific terms. What has been called a "factor" is actually an *antigen* in blood banking. The "anti-factor" is an *antibody*. When a person is given an antigen not present on his red blood cells, he produces an antibody in his plasma which will react with the foreign antigen. This is evidenced by destruction of the red cell containing the foreign antigen.

INHERITANCE OF BLOOD GROUPS

All the factors or antigens present on a person's red cells are inherited. Each antigen is controlled by a *gene,* which is the unit of inheritance. In other words, antigens, or factors, are inherited as genes. If the gene for a particular antigen is present, that antigen will be found on all that person's red blood cells.

Each cell (except for mature red cells) consists of two basic parts: the cytoplasm and the nucleus. If the nucleus is observed under the microscope at approximately the time of cell division, several long, threadlike structures will be visible. These structures are referred to as *chromosomes*. Each species has a given number of chromosomes. Human beings have 46 chromosomes contained within the cell nucleus. In addition, the chromosomes may be seen to occur in pairs. Human beings have 23 chromosome pairs. The paired chromosomes are similar in size and shape and have their own distinct and specific functions. Each chromosome of a chromosome pair is derived, or inherited, from each parent. Chromosomes occur in pairs in all cells of the body except the sex cells. In other words human cells contain 23 pairs of chromosomes except for the sex cells (sperm and ovum), which contain 23 single chromosomes.

Since the gene is the unit of inheritance, it must also be located within the nucleus. Genes are exceedingly small particles which when associated in linear form make up the chromosome. They are too small to see under the microscope but together are visible as the chromosome. Genes are now thought to be made up of deoxyribonucleic acid (DNA). Each trait that is inherited is controlled by the presence of a specific gene. The genes responsible for a particular trait always occur at exactly the same point or position on a particular chromosome. The position of a gene on its chromosome is referred to as its *locus*. A particular gene will always have the same locus; however, not much is known of the actual locus of genes for traits which are inherited. Most of the knowledge of gene loci concerns those genes which are located on the sex chromosomes. However, if genes for different inherited traits are known to be carried on the same chromosome, they are said to be *linked*. The closer the loci of the genes, the closer the linkage is said to be.

Inherited traits are somewhat variable within a species. For example, people have different-colored eyes. It is known that eye color is inherited. Therefore, each possible eye color must be the result of a gene for that color. Blue-eye genes are responsible for blue eyes, and so on. The various possibilities of genes for a particular trait are referred to as *alleles* for that trait. Since a person has only two genes (one pair) for any given trait, his cells will have only two alleles. However, the number of possible alleles for any trait varies with the trait. When a person has identical alleles for a given trait he is said to be *homozygous* for that trait. For example, a person with blue eyes carries two blue-eye genes and is homozygous for blue eyes. If a person carries two different alleles for a given trait, he is *heterozygous* for that trait. For example, a person may carry a blue-eye gene in addition to a brown-eye gene, or he may be homozygous, having two brown-eye genes.

In heredity in general, certain alleles may be stronger than, or may mask the presence of, other alleles. For example, in the case of eye color, brown-eye genes will mask the presence of blue-eye genes. In other words, brown-eye genes are *dominant* over blue-eye genes. If a person carries both one brown-eye and one blue-eye gene, his eyes will appear brown. Blue-eye genes are then said to be *recessive* in relation to brown-eye genes. In order for a person's eyes to appear blue, he must have two blue-eye genes. However, in blood banking, the various alleles for a given blood group system are equally dominant, or codominant. If the gene is present (and there is a suitable testing solution available), the gene will be seen or detected.

Two other terms which are often used in blood banking which relate to genetics are *phenotype* and *genotype*. The *phenotype* is the blood type that results from tests which are made directly on the person's blood even though other factors may be present. The *genotype* refers to the actual and total genetic pattern for any system. It is usually impossible to determine the complete genotype in the laboratory. Genotyping usually requires additional studies, especially family studies, to determine the total genetic pattern.

ANTIBODIES AND ANTIGENS

All blood banking is based upon a knowledge of antigens and antibodies. Unfortunately they cannot be defined simply. They have been discussed in terms of factor and anti-factor. In general, an antigen may be thought of as a foreign substance, foreign in the sense that if it is introduced into the body of a person who does not already have the antigen, an anti-substance called an antibody will be produced. The antibody will be found in the plasma and other body fluids. In other words, introduction of foreign antigen stimulates the production of antibodies. The antibody which is produced will react with the foreign antigen in some observable manner. In addition, the antibody is specific for the antigen against which it is formed. This means that the antibody will react with only its corresponding antigen and with no other antigen.

The significance of antigens and antibodies is not limited to blood banking. They are the basis of immunity. Various bacteria have antigenic properties. Therefore, when introduced into a host, they will elicit antibody formation. The antibody formed in response to the foreign antigen (in this case bacteria) protects the person from subsequent infections by that particular bacterium. For example, a person who has had chickenpox is immune to the disease in the future. The immunity is a function of antibody production by the host. However, immunity is not immediate, as can be seen from the fact that upon first infection the person is ill or incapacitated by the disease. This is because antibodies require about 2 weeks to develop sufficiently. After this time subsequent exposure to the antigen will elicit an effective antigen-antibody reaction and therefore protective immunity.

In blood banking, antibody formation does not result in protective immunity. The blood antigens are present on the red blood cells, and the antibody is found in the plasma or serum. The antigen-antibody reaction results in the destruction of the antigen-carrying red blood cell by antibody in the serum of the foreign host. Clinically, the result of this red cell destruction is the hemolytic transfusion reaction. The reaction will vary from patient to patient. Generally the immediate reaction is characterized by chills, high temperature, pain in the lower back, nausea, vomiting, and shock as indicated by decreased blood pressure and rapid pulse. These first effects of the reaction are rarely fatal; however, the by-products of red blood cell destruction pose many problems, primarily severe renal involvement. The patient may eventually die from kidney failure.

Chemically, antigens are usually proteins, although polysaccharides, polypeptides, or polynucleotides may also be antigenic. They are usually large molecules with a molecular weight of 10,000 or more. As mentioned, antigens are highly specific substances and react only with their corresponding antibody. The cause of specificity is not actually known. It may be the shape or spatial configuration of the molecule or the presence and arrangement of amino acids and carbohydrates or other chemical properties.[3] However, not all antigens are equally antigenic. Some are extremely effective in their ability to cause antibody production, while others are relatively weak and not as likely to result in antibodies. If this were not true, blood could never be transfused.

The blood antigens are found not only on the red blood cells but also in other body fluids such as urine, saliva, plasma, and gastric juice.

Antibodies are produced in response to foreign antigenic stimulus. For example, persons whose red blood cells contain group A antigen are unable to form anti-A antibody. However, there are several factors that will influence the amount of antibody that will be formed by foreign antigen stimulation. First, some antigens are stronger, or more antigenic, than others. The stronger the antigen, the greater the antibody response. In blood banking the ABO and D antigens are very strongly antigenic, whereas such antigens as Lutheran and Kidd are relatively weak. The number of foreign antigens which are introduced at a given time will also influence the amount of antibody production. In general, exposure to only one antigen will elicit a stronger antibody response than simultaneous exposure to more than one antigen. The number of exposures to foreign antigen also plays a role in antibody response. Here, repeated exposures will result in greater antibody formation.

The interval between exposure to foreign antigen also has a role in antibody formation. It seems that rapid repeated exposure is less likely to result in antibody formation than the same number of exposures spaced over a longer period of time. The quantity of antigen introduced has some effect; however, the number of exposures and interval between is more effective in terms of antibody production.

It seems that there is a threshold amount of antigen related to antibody production. If more than this threshold amount of antigen is introduced, the amount of antibody produced is relatively small in proportion to the quantity of antigen. In addition it appears that a large excess of antigen may completely inhibit an antibody response. This is important in blood banking, for a relatively small amount of incompatible blood will produce as much antibody as a relatively large amount. In other words, the transfusion of any incompatible blood will result in serious sensitization of the patient.

Finally there are also individual and age differences in antibody formation. Some persons are more prone to form antibodies than others. Newborn infants do not form antibodies but receive them passively from the mother across the placenta. They begin forming gamma globulin and therefore antibody at about three months and normally have a normal gamma globulin level by six months. This fact is important when antibody-typing newborn infants in the ABO blood group system.

It is believed that antibodies are synthesized by lymphocytes or plasma cells from gamma globulin. When foreign antigen is first introduced, antibody cannot be detected immediately in the serum or plasma. Antibody cannot be detected until about 10 to 14 days after antigenic stimulation, and the titer (or concentration) is greatest after about 20 days. After this the titer gradually decreases.

A second exposure to the same antigen, however, will rapidly result in detectable amounts of antibody in the plasma or serum. It seems that some sort of memory phenomenon results in immediate antibody response, or formation, on second or subsequent exposure. This secondary antibody response also produces a higher and longer-lasting titer of antibody. In addition, the secondary antibody formation results in an antibody which is more effective in its reaction with antigen or has better combining properties.

Chemically, antibodies are protein. More specifically they are formed from the gamma globulin portion of the plasma protein. They result from specific antigenic stimulation.

Antibodies have also been classified in terms of physical types.[4] The major classes are slightly different forms of gamma globulin and are called IgG (γ-G), IgM (γ-M), and IgA (γ-A). There are also IgD (γ-D) and IgE (γ-E), about which relatively little is known. Of the first three, IgG is the smallest molecule, with a molecular weight of about 150,000, whereas IgM is the largest, about 900,000. IgA ranges in size from about 150,000 to 350,000 mol. wt. IgG and IgM are probably the most important types. IgM is the type of antibody that results from primary exposure to foreign antigen. Secondary exposure results in IgG formation. Repeated stimulation will result in IgG antibody.

IgM is the first antibody type that the newborn infant is able to form and is effectively synthesized at about nine months. IgG is effectively synthesized at about three to four years of age, whereas IgA is not produced until adolescence.

IgG is the only type of antibody which is able to cross the placenta. Both IgM and IgA lack this ability. This is important in respect to hemolytic disease of the newborn.

A different antibody classification defines *natural* and *immune* antibodies. The natural antibody appears to exist without apparent antigenic stimulus, whereas the immune antibody is the result of specific antigenic stimulation. The only natural antibodies in blood are the anti-A and anti-B antibodies found in the ABO blood group system. In this system if the red cell lacks the A antigen, anti-A antibody will be found in the serum. If the red cell lacks the B antigen, anti-B antibody will be found in the serum. Hence the name natural antibody. The origin of these antibodies is not really known, but there are two theories: one hypothesizes that the natural anti-A and anti-B antibodies are the result of some sort of gene interaction, while the other theory says that there are substances so widely distributed in nature that the antibody will develop in any person if the antigen is not present. The second theory is more popular. There is some evidence that certain bacteria may have A- or B-like antigens. Further, even certain foods may have a similar antigen. At any rate, so-called natural anti-A and anti-B antibodies do exist and are routinely used in testing for a person's ABO blood group. (They are saline solution–active and of the IgM type.) *Primary exposure, largest*

All other antibodies which are encountered in blood banking are of the immune type. These are also referred to as *irregular antibodies*. Immune antibodies are the result of specific antigenic stimulation. They result from immunization by way of *pregnancy, transfusion, injection of red cells,* or *unknown antigenic stimulus.* Once immunization exists, it is permanent. Immune or irregular antibodies are of the IgG, IgA, or IgM type.

MEANS OF DETECTING ANTIGEN-ANTIBODY REACTIONS IN BLOOD BANKING

Two terms which are used in discussing biologic reactions are *in vivo* and *in vitro*. In vivo means in the living body, while in vitro means in glass. A biologic reaction that normally occurs in the body (in vivo) may be demonstrated in vitro, or under laboratory conditions. Blood-banking reactions that are used in determining blood groups and compatibility are in vitro reactions.

In order to demonstrate or determine a person's blood type, some sort of substance must be available to show what antigens are present on the red blood cell. The substance used for this purpose is referred to as an *antiserum*. An antiserum is merely a prepared and highly purified solution of antibody. The antiserum is named on the basis of what antibody it contains. For example, a solution of pure anti-A antibodies is called *anti-A antiserum.*

Most of the antisera that are used in blood banking are prepared commercially and purchased by the blood bank. In general, antiserum is prepared in one of two ways: animals may be deliberately inoculated with antigen and the resulting serum containing antibody purified and standardized for use as an antiserum, or serum may be collected from human beings who have been sensitized to an antigen through transfusion, pregnancy, or intramuscular injection. Antiserum must meet certain requirements to be acceptable for use. It must be specific for the antigen to be detected. It must have a sufficient titer, or concentration, to detect antigen. It must have a certain avidity for, or strength of reaction with, corresponding red cells. It must also be sterile, clear, provided in a good container with a dropper, and stable. It should be marked with an expiration date and must never be used after this date has passed. In addition, it must be stored at 4°C when not in use. Exact requirements for each antiserum are defined by the U.S. Public Health Service. When commercial antiserum is used, the manufacturer's directions should be followed carefully.

When antiserum is mixed with red blood cells, an antigen-antibody reaction may or may not occur. If a reaction does occur, the corresponding antigen must be present on the red cell, and the result is a positive reaction. If a reaction does not occur, the antigen is absent, and the result is negative. A positive reaction with anti-A antiserum demonstrates the presence of A antigen on the red blood cell, and so on.

In the original definition of antibody, it was stated that antibody resulting from antigenic stimulation will react with the antigen in an observable manner. In blood banking there are two types of observable reactions which may occur: *agglutination* and *hemolysis*.

Agglutination is a clumping, or close association, of red blood cells caused by a specific antibody for antigen present on the cell. A positive antigen-antibody reaction results in an immediate combination of antibody and antigen on the red cell followed by the visible agglutination, which takes longer to form. The antibody is thought to be a somewhat cylindrical structure with a reactive site at each end. Each reactive site is capable of combining with corresponding antigen. Agglutination is thought to be the result of a bridging together of red cells by antibody reacting with antigen sites on adjacent red cells. This bridging causes the red cells to stick together. Several such bridges result in visible clumping, or agglutination. The degree of agglutination varies. Very strong agglutination forms a large mass of cells which can be easily seen macroscopically as one large clump of cells. This size ranges down to smaller clumps of cells which can also be seen macroscopically and finally to small clumps of cells which can be seen only microscopically. The ability to observe all degrees of agglutination requires great care and experience. It is not a simple task, yet it is imperative that any degree of agglutination be detected.

Hemolysis is the result of an actual lysis, or destruction, of the red cell by a specific antibody. It is probably the third stage in an antigen-antibody reaction and does not occur in all cases. The antibody causes rupture of the cell membrane with release of hemoglobin. The result is a crystal-clear solution with no cloudiness, since no cells are present. Whenever hemolysis occurs, it is a positive antigen-antibody reaction. However, it is often overlooked and reported as negative, since agglutination is much more common and hemolysis looks much like a negative reaction with no agglutination. In the case of a negative reaction, however, the cells remain in a smooth, cloudy suspension, whereas hemolysis results in a clear red solution. Misinterpretation of hemolysis remains a common cause of false-negative results in the blood bank and may end in disaster for the patient.

In order for hemolysis to occur, a substance called *complement* must be present in the serum. Complement is a complex substance of at least nine components. It is important in blood banking because some antibodies require the presence of complement in order to be demonstrated in vitro and although almost all normal serums contain complement when fresh, complement is destroyed by heat. Therefore, to have complement activity, serums must be either fresh or stored correctly. Complement activity will remain if stored for 24 to 48 hours at 4°C or for 2 months at −50°C. If an antibody is to be detected that requires complement, it must be provided in the test medium.

In summary, the detection of antigen upon red cells requires the demonstration of a positive reaction of that cell with a specific solution of antibodies referred to as an antiserum. The technique by which the red cell and antiserum are brought together varies widely, depending upon numerous factors. The most outstanding factor is the manner of action of the particular antigen-antibody system being tested for; in other words, knowledge of the antibodies of the blood group system involved is necessary.

In general, blood group tests are performed either on microscope slides or within test tubes. When test tubes are used, they are size 10 by 75 or 12 by 75 mm. Other factors are the use of adequate serum, storage of red cells, and concentration of cell suspensions, the testing medium (isotonic saline solution, albumin, or enzymes), the temperature of incubation, the incubation period, centrifugation, reading and interpretation of agglutination reactions, the use of reagents, and the glassware used. The correct conditions are essential to reliable tests. Development of correct techniques requires thorough knowledge of all these considerations as well as of the blood groups themselves. The particular technique will also depend on the brand of antiserum that is being used and the manufacturer's directions, which, as already mentioned, must be followed for accurate results.

THE ABO BLOOD GROUP SYSTEM

The ABO blood group system was first discovered and described in 1900 and 1901 by Karl Landsteiner. By taking the blood of six of his colleagues, separating serum and cells, and mixing each cell suspension with each serum, Landsteiner was able to divide the blood into three groups: group A, group B, and group O. In 1902 the fourth group, group AB, was discovered by von Decastello and Struli, two of Landsteiner's pupils.[5]

The ABO system is now thought to consist of these four groups, or phenotypes, of blood: groups A, B, AB, and O. These four groups of blood may be explained by the presence of two antigens (or factors) present on the red blood cell surface, the A antigen and the B antigen. If the person belongs to blood group A, then A antigen is present on the red cell. Group B persons have B antigen on their red cells. Group AB individuals have both A antigen and B antigen, while group O people have neither A nor B antigen.

The antigen present on the red cell is determined by the presence of determining genes on the person's chromosomes. There are three allelic genes which can be inherited in the ABO blood group system. These are the A gene, B gene, and O gene. Since each person has two genes for any trait, one from each parent, the following combinations of alleles are possible in the ABO system; AA, AO, AB, BB, BO, and OO. These combinations represent the possible genotypes in the ABO system.

If the A gene is present on the chromosome, A antigen will be present on the red blood cell. The presence of B gene results in B antigen on the red blood cell. The presence of O gene results in neither antigen on the red cell.

In actually testing blood for the ABO group, a suspension of red cells in saline solution is prepared. This red cell suspension is then tested by mixing one portion with a solution of known anti-A antiserum, or, in other words, anti-A antibodies. A second portion of red cells is mixed with known anti-B antiserum (anti-B antibodies). The mixtures are then observed for a reaction. A positive reaction is the occurrence of agglutination or hemolysis. A negative reaction is the absence of agglutination or hemolysis. Results may be grouped as follows:

Group A blood—a positive reaction of cells with anti-A antiserum
Group B blood—a positive reaction of cells with anti-B antiserum
Group O blood—a negative reaction of cells with both anti-A and anti-B antiserum
Group AB blood—a positive reaction of cells with both anti-A and anti-B antiserum

In these typing reactions, the blood is merely tested for the presence or absence of A and B antigens. No direct test is made for the presence or absence of the O gene. This is merely phenotyping, or typing by means of tests which are made directly on the person's blood. Since blood is tested only for the presence or absence of A and B antigens, genotypes AA and AO will both type as blood group A. The genotypes BB and BO both contain B antigen and will type as blood group B. Genotype AB will type as group AB, since both antigens are present to react with the appropriate antiserum. All blood that types as group O must belong to the genotype OO, since the blood will not react with either anti-A or anti-B antiserum.

As is the case with any blood group system, corresponding antigens and antibodies cannot coexist in the same person's blood. In other words, persons who are blood group A cannot form anti-A antibodies and will not have anti-A antibodies in their serum. However, unlike other blood group systems, in the ABO system, if the A or B antigen is lacking from the red blood cell, the corresponding antibody will be found in the serum. These are the so-called natural antibodies discussed previously. An adult lacking group A antigen will be found to have anti-A antibody in his serum. The serum of adults with red cells lacking B antigen have anti-B antibody in the serum.

These naturally occurring anti-A and anti-B antibodies are important for several reasons, and the occurrence of natural anti-A and anti-B antibodies is especially important in the actual ABO blood-grouping procedure used in the laboratory. When transfusing blood, it is essential to avoid giving blood to a person whose serum contains an antibody for an antigen present on the transfused red cells. If this did occur, there would be an immediate and severe hemolytic transfusion reaction. It is absolutely essential that the correct ABO blood type be transfused, or a severe reaction and death might result. For these reasons, the occurrence of natural anti-A and anti-B antibodies are made use of in the ABO typing procedure. In addition to testing red blood cells with known antibody, as has been described, in the ABO system serum is tested with known group A_1* and group B red cells to determine what antibodies are present. In these tests, serum from the undetermined blood is separated from the cells. One portion of the serum is mixed with red cells known to contain group A_1 antigen. A second portion of serum is mixed with cells known to contain group B antigen. The mixtures are then observed for a positive or negative reaction as evidenced by agglutination or hemolysis.

If there is a positive reaction of serum with known group A_1 cells, the serum contains anti-A antibodies. If there is a positive reaction of serum with known group B cells, the serum contains anti-B antibodies. If the serum reacts with both group A_1 and group B cells, both anti-A and anti-B antibodies are present. If no reaction occurs with either cell type, both antibodies are lacking. Remembering that in the ABO system the serum contains the corresponding antibody for the A or B antigen lacking from the red blood cell, results may be grouped as follows:

Group A blood—a positive reaction of serum with group B cells
Group B blood—a positive reaction of serum with group A cells
Group O blood—a positive reaction of serum with both group A and B cells
Group AB blood—no reaction with either group A or B cells

Typing reactions which employ undetermined red cells and known antibody or antiserum are referred to as *antigen, cell, direct,* or *front typing reactions*. Typing reactions which employ undetermined serum and known red cells are referred to as *antibody, serum, indirect,* or *back typing reactions*. All these reactions are summarized in Table 5-1.

When the ABO group is to be determined, both the cells and serum should be typed as has been described. The antigen- and antibody-typing

* A_1 is a subgroup of A antigen which will be defined later. For the present it may be considered synonymous with A antigen.

Table 5-1. ABO Typing Reactions

Blood Group	Antigen on Red Cells	Antibody in Serum	Antigen, Front, or Direct Typing		Antibody, Back, or Indirect Typing		Possible Genotype
			Reaction of undetermined cells with anti-A antiserum	Reaction of undetermined cells with anti-B antiserum	Reaction of undetermined serum with A₁ cells	Reaction of undetermined serum with B cells	
A	A	Anti-B	+	−	−	+	AA AO
B	B	Anti-A	−	+	+	−	BB BO
AB	A and B	Neither	+	+	−	−	AB
O	Neither	Anti-A and anti-B	−	−	+	+	OO

275

results should then be compared to be sure that mistakes have not occurred and the results are consistent. This is an excellent way to guard against mistakes in ABO grouping. However, there are certain instances where the antigen and antibody-typing results show discrepancies.

One cause of cell and serum discrepancies involves the occurrence of the natural antibodies. These natural antibodies are expected to occur in most adults. However, they cannot be expected to exist in newborn infants, since infants do not normally begin to produce antibodies until they are three to six months of age. The titer, or concentration, of natural antibodies normally increases gradually through adolescence and then gradually decreases. For this reason, serum-grouping results may also show discrepancies in very elderly patients.

It should also be mentioned that there is a variation of titer, or concentration, of antibody in the random population. In general, the anti-A titer seems to be higher than the anti-B titer. In the laboratory it should also be remembered that the antibody titer of serum will only rarely approach the titer of antibody in commercially prepared antiserum. For this reason, reactions with cell-grouping tests are generally stronger and easier to read than serum-grouping reactions.

The occurrence of subgroups of group A or B antigen might also result in discrepancies between cell- and serum-grouping reactions. The classification of blood in the ABO system into groups A, B, AB, and O is an oversimplification. Both group A and group B may be further classified in units referred to as *subgroups*. The most important subdivision is the division of group A into A_1 and A_2. Practically, these subgroups are of little clinical importance. They are not tested for routinely but should be kept in mind when there is difficulty in ABO grouping or compatibility testing. The concept of an "H substance" as a precursor material from which A and B antigens are produced is involved in the various subgroups. These subjects will not be discussed further. The student should consult a more detailed text such as "Blood Groups in Man" by Race and Sanger[6] or "Technical Methods and Procedures of the American Association of Blood Banks."[7] It is because of the existence of subgroups that A_1 test cells must be used in ABO serum grouping. Subgrouping tests will involve the use, for example, of anti-AB serum, absorbed anti-A serum, and lectins.

It must be stressed that if discrepancies between cell and serum grouping reactions do occur, they must be resolved. These problems should be referred to a person with sufficient training and experience in the area of blood banking.

Thus far, only natural anti-A and anti-B antibodies have been discussed. However, anti-A and anti-B antibodies may also be of the immune type. Serum may contain immune antibodies in addition to the natural anti-A and/or anti-B. As has been mentioned, natural antibodies are normally found in the serum of adults if the red cell lacks the corresponding antigen. They probably arise from the inevitable stimulation by ABH substances widely distributed in nature. Immune anti-A or anti-B antibodies result from specific antigenic stimulation. This stimulation may be by way of incompatible transfusion, through pregnancy, or by injection of ABH substances, or substances having ABH activity.

Immune and natural types of antibodies differ in physical and chemical properties and in their serologic behavior in the laboratory. In addition to other differences, the natural ABO antibodies react best if the red cells are suspended in saline solution and the test is carried out at room temperature, or 4°C. For this reason, ABO blood group reactions are routinely carried out with saline suspensions of cells and incubated at room temperature. Immune antibodies differ in that they react better if cells are suspended in albumin or serum and incubated at 37°C. There are other differences in mode of reaction in the laboratory. These differences must be taken into account in situations in which the occurrence of an immune-type anti-A or anti-B antibody is suspected or possible, for example, in cases of hemolytic disease of the newborn with ABO incompatibility and in screening blood for low titers of anti-A and anti-B.

As to physical and chemical differences between natural and immune anti-A and anti-B, it has already been mentioned that the natural antibody is a larger molecule of a molecular weight of about 900,000 whereas the immune antibody is of about 150,000. Probably, because of this size difference, natural antibodies are unable to cross the placental barrier, whereas immune antibodies may cross. As noted above, this is important in hemolytic disease of the newborn. Natural antibodies are of the IgM (γ-M) type, whereas immune antibodies are of the IgG (γ-G) type.

One concept that must be discussed in conjunction with the ABO system is the idea of so-called "universal donors" and "universal recipients." These are terms familiar to most people, yet to the blood banker the concept is somewhat oversimplified. The idea is used only in cases of extreme emergency.

When blood is to be transfused, there are two questions that must be kept in mind: (1) does the patient's serum contain an antibody against an antigen on the transfused red blood cell, and (2) does the serum to be transfused contain an antibody against an antigen on the patient's red cells? The first situation, in which the patient's serum contains antibody against transfused antigen, is most serious. This situation is said to result in a major reaction and can result in death of the patient. This is because all the transfused blood will be destroyed by antibody in the patient's circulatory system. Besides the transfusion's doing no good, destruction of the transfused blood will result in accumulation of toxic waste products which will probably result in severe renal failure and death.

The second situation, in which the donor (or transfused) serum contains antibody against the patient's red cells, is not as serious. This situation is termed a minor reaction. It is not as serious because only a small amount of blood in proportion to the patient's total blood volume is infused. As a result, only a small proportion of the patient's red cells are actually destroyed by donor serum, and this is offset by the benefits of the donor red cells which remain intact and viable.

These transfusion situations are made use of in the concepts of universal donor and recipient. So-called universal donor blood is group O blood. It is felt that group O blood can safely be transfused into any ABO blood type, because patient serum cannot possibly contain an antibody to group O cells. In other words, a major reaction cannot possibly occur. However, it must be remembered that group O blood does contain anti-A and anti-B antibodies. Therefore, if given to group A persons, a minor reaction can occur with anti-A antibodies. In case of a group B person, there can be a minor reaction with anti-B antibodies, while the AB person can have a minor reaction with both anti-A and anti-B.

Because these minor reactions can occur, any group O blood that is to be used as universal donor blood must be screened with certain additional tests. It is known that the titer, or concentration, of anti-A and anti-B varies from person to person. In selecting blood as universal donor blood, only that blood is chosen which has a "low titer" (or small concentration) of anti-A and anti-B antibodies. There is no universally accepted method of screening for "safe" blood for such use. An additional problem is the possible presence of immune anti-A or anti-B antibodies in addition to the natural forms. For some of the more frequently used techniques see "Technical Methods and Procedures of the American Association of Blood Banks."[7]

In the case of the group AB patient, it is even more dangerous to transfuse group O blood, since both anti-A and anti-B antibodies are present to react with the patient's red cells. For this reason, if group AB blood cannot be secured for transfusion it is preferable to use either group A or group B blood, rather than group O. If group A blood is to be used, the anti-B titer should be determined. If group B blood, the anti-A titer. It should now be obvious that the so-called universal recipient is the person with group AB blood, since these persons may be infused with group A, B, or O blood in emergency situations.

In summary, it should be stressed that ABO type-specific blood should be used whenever possible. Whenever group O blood is used for the A, B, or AB patient and A or B blood for the AB patient, a certain risk does exist. Although screening methods are available to test the titer of anti-A and/or anti-B, these methods are not perfect, and a severe transfusion reaction may still take place. However, a blood bank should always have some tested low-titer blood on hand for use in case of emergency, since a sufficient number of emergencies do present themselves.

These include situations where group-specific blood is not available and blood must be transfused or where there may not be enought time to type and crossmatch the patient. There may be an emergency situation where the patient's blood group cannot be accurately determined. In cases of ABO hemolytic disease of the newborn, group O blood may be necessary. Finally, there may be such unusual circumstances as disasters or military situations where blood cannot be typed for use.[8] Group O blood was routinely used on the battlefield in Korea and is being used in Vietnam.

THE Rh-Hr BLOOD GROUP SYSTEM

DEFINITION OF Rh FACTORS AND INHERITANCE

The Rh blood group system is considerably more complex than the ABO system. Basically, the Rh system consists of six related blood group factors, on antigens, C, D, E, $\underline{c}$, $\underline{d}$, and $\underline{e}$, and the corresponding antibodies anti-C, anti-D, anti-E, anti-$\underline{c}$, and anti-$\underline{e}$. "Anti-$\underline{d}$" antibody has been omitted because it does not exist. Because of the lack of an anti-$\underline{d}$ antibody, the existence of $\underline{d}$ as an antigen is disputed. For this reason, the so-called "presence" of $\underline{d}$ should actually be thought of as the absence of D antigen.

There is more than one system of nomenclature used to define the various antigens of the Rh-Hr system. Basically there is the Rh system of Wiener,[9] the CDE system of Fisher and Race,[10] and the numerical system of Rosenfield et al.[11] These systems are compared in Table 5-2. Because neither the CDE nor the Rh system is universally accepted, all commercial antiserum labels and direction sheets are required by the National Institutes of Health, Division of Biologics Standards, to include both the Rh and the CDE terms. The Rh term is given first and is followed by the CDE term in parentheses. For example, anti-Rh$_o$ (anti-D).

The six antigens which have been defined are not the only antigens in the Rh system, for variants have been described. To date there are at least 28 related factors in the system.[12] However, C, D, E, $\underline{c}$, $\underline{d}$, and $\underline{e}$ are the most important factors of the system.

Table 5-2. Comparative Nomenclature of the Rh-Hr Antigens

CDE System (Fisher-Race)		Rh System (Wiener)		Numerical System (Rosenfield et al.)	
D	$\underline{d}$	Rh$_o$	Hr$_o$	Rh1	
C	$\underline{c}$	rh'	hr'	Rh2	Rh4
E	$\underline{e}$	rh''	hr''	Rh3	Rh5

The various Rh factors, or antigens, which have been discovered on red cells are inherited traits, as are the antigens of the ABO system. However, in the ABO system there were only three allelic genes which could be inherited. In the case of the Rh system, the antigens D, C, E, d, c, and e are not all alleles for the same position. Rather, the antigens C and c are alleles for the same trait, while D and d are alleles for another chromosome position, as are E and e. The various factors are inherited in groups of three, so that a given chromosome will have one position for the Dd allele, a second position for the Cc allele, and a third position for the Ee allele. In other words, each chromosome carrying the Rh determinants has three "closely linked" loci for the three related Rh alleles. Since each person has a pair of chromosomes for any inherited trait, everyone has loci for six Rh genes.

In other words, there are three pairs of Rh-Hr factors which are genetically related. Every person must have on his cells at least one of or both the paired antigens Cc, Dd, and Ee. Since D and d are alleles for the same trait, if D is absent, d must be present. Conversely, if d is absent, D must be present; i.e., if one member of the pair is lacking, the other member must be present.[10] This means that there are three possible combinations of genes for the Dd alleles. A person may possess two D genes, noted as DD, and be homozygous for D. Or a person may possess a D gene and a d gene, noted as Dd, and be heterozygous for D. Finally, the person may possess two d genes, noted as dd, and be homozygous for d. This is also true of the Cc and the Ee alleles. Persons may be homozygous or heterozygous for Ee and for Cc.

Once again the various Rh alleles are inherited in groups of three paired factors. That is, a person has two chromosomes for the Rh factors. One chromosome will carry loci for the D or d, the C or c and the E or e alleles, as will the second chromosome, making a total of six Rh factors for each person. This means that there are eight possible combinations of three factors that can be carried on a given chromosome. These possible combinations of factors in CDE notation, the corresponding Rh notation as devised by Wiener, and approximate frequency are given in Table 5-3.

One of the eight possible Rh-Hr gene combinations is inherited from each parent, so that the total Rh-Hr genotype for a given person would be noted as CDE/cde or CDe/cDe, and so on. In Wiener's Rh-Hr notation corresponding to the CDE system, the capital letter R refers to the presence of D (Rh_0) antigen, while r refers to the presence of d (Hr_0). The superscript in Wiener's notation refers to the antigens C, c, E, and e.

Thus far, only one theory of Rh-Hr inheritance has been presented. This is the theory of Fisher and Race as presented in "Blood Groups in Man," by Race and Sanger.[6] The theory of Fisher and Race views loci for three genes on each chromosome carrying the Rh-Hr determinants.

Table 5-3. Rh Chromosomes and Approximate Frequency

CDE Notation (Fisher-Race)	Rh-Hr Notation (Wiener)	Approximate Frequency in White Population*
CDe	R¹	Common
cDE	R²	Common
CDE	Rᶻ	Rare
cDe	Rº	2%
Cde	r′	1%
cdE	r″	1%
CdE	rʸ	Very rare
cde	r	Common

*F. Stratton and P. H. Renton, "Practical Blood Grouping," p. 154, Charles C Thomas, Publisher, Springfield, Ill., 1958.

However, these genes are felt to be so closely linked that in effect they are inherited as a unit. In other words, the unit of inheritance is considered the chromosome rather than the gene in this particular case. This theory recognizes the existence of six genes, each gene controlling the identical factor in the blood. There is no difference between the gene and the factor.

The other theory of Rh-Hr inheritance is that proposed by Wiener.[9] Wiener differs from Fisher and Race in that he makes a differentiation between genes and factors which are found in the blood. Wiener feels that there is a single gene on each Rh-Hr chromosome which determines the presence of three factors in the blood. Since there are eight possible combinations of Rh-Hr factors, this theory recognizes eight possible genes. In other words, the inheritance of the R^1 gene will result in the presence of C (rh′), D (Rh₀), and e (hr″) antigens on the red blood cells. A person inheriting an R^1 gene from one parent and an R^z gene from the other would be of genotype R^1/R^z (or CDe/CDE), and his red cells will contain C (rh′), D (Rh₀), E (rh″), and e (hr″) antigens. Wiener supports his theory of inheritance with the fact that examples of crossovers (or mutations resulting from paired chromosomes breaking and recombining with the other member of the pair) have not been found. In virtually every other case of closely linked inherited traits, crossovers have been found to occur. For this reason, Wiener feels that the theory of the existence of three closely linked genes is inaccurate.

In any case, the net effect is the same. One person will always have six Rh-Hr factors in his blood: the C and/or c factors, the D and/or d factors, and the E and/or e factors. The only real difficulty is that the two theories of inheritance have resulted in more than one system of nomenclature which must be learned by the student.

HISTORICAL BACKGROUND

The discovery of the Rh system was based upon work by Landsteiner and Wiener in 1940 in addition to studies by Levine and Stetson published in 1939.[10] A woman who delivered a stillborn fetus was studied by Levine and Stetson. The woman had never received a blood transfusion; however, following delivery, she was transfused with her husband's blood. Both the woman and her husband were blood group O. Following transfusion, the woman experienced a severe hemolytic reaction.

Similar transfusion reactions had previously been known to occur following the first transfusion after childbirth which did not seem to be associated with the ABO system. Levine and Stetson developed an explanation of their patient's transfusion reaction which has been proved to be correct. They explained the reaction by proposing that the woman's red blood cells did not contain a "new" antigen. However, the child inherited this so-called "new" antigen from the father, and the fetus cells which contained the "new" antigen found their way into the mother's circulatory system. This resulted in the formation of antibody (or immunization) to the "new" antigen. Therefore, when the woman was transfused with her husband's blood, her serum contained an antibody to the "new" antigen contained on her husband's red cells. It was also found that the woman's serum agglutinated not only her husband's red cells but the red cells of 80 of 104 ABO-compatible bloods. Levine and Stetson did not name this "new" antigen.

The naming of this new factor eventually resulted from studies by Landsteiner and Wiener in 1940.[10] They were working with the red cells of rhesus monkeys with which they inoculated rabbits and guinea pigs. They found that the resulting rabbit antibody agglutinated the red cells of all rhesus monkeys and, more importantly, the red cells of about 85 percent of samples of the white population of New York City. The 85 percent of the cells which were agglutinated by the anti-rhesus serum were called *Rh-positive,* and the remaining 15 percent not agglutinated were called *Rh-negative.* Later it was shown that an antibody found in the serum of certain patients who had hemolytic reactions after transfusion of ABO-compatible blood was apparently the same as the antibody in the anti-rhesus serum. It was also found that the antibody contained within the serum of the women studied by Levine and Stetson in 1939 was the same as the antibody in the anti-rhesus serum produced in rabbits against rhesus monkey cells.

Rh-POSITIVE AND Rh-NEGATIVE

It is now known that the "new" antigen described by Levine and Stetson is the D (or Rh_o) antigen. Persons whose red cells contain D antigen either as D/D or D/d are now termed Rh-positive. These persons represent approximately 85 percent of the population. In other words, the antibody formed by the woman studied in 1939 and the antibody responsible for several transfusion reactions is the anti-D (anti-Rh_o) antibody. Persons whose red cells lack the D (Rh_o) antigen are termed Rh-negative. Rh-negative persons are then d/d. They represent about 15 percent of the population. (The great majority of Rh-negative persons are cde/cde. This genotype is what is meant by a truly Rh-negative person. Other very rare genotypes which are d/d must be considered Rh-negative as blood recipients but Rh-positive as donors.)

CHARACTERISTICS OF THE Rh-Hr ANTIGENS

The factors C, D, E, c, and e are all antigenic. This means that they are capable of stimulating the production of antibodies if introduced into the body of a person whose red cells are completely lacking the antigen. The Rh antigens are permanent inherited characteristics which remain constant throughout life. However, not all the Rh antigens are equally antigenic. The D (Rh_o) antigen is definitely the strongest of the Rh antigens and will result in immunization if introduced into a foreign host. It is for this reason that the term Rh-positive merely refers to the presence of D antigen without respect to the other Rh factors. The antigenic strength of this antigen also makes it imperative that blood be tested for Rh type before transfusion. An Rh-negative person must never be transfused with Rh-positive (D-positive), blood for he will certainly develop an anti-D antibody. This would not be lethal at the time of the first transfusion; however, subsequent transfusion with D-positive blood would result in a hemolytic reaction. In the case of a woman who has been sensitized by an Rh-positive fetus, transfusion with D-positive blood will result in a hemolytic reaction with the first transfusion.

While D is the most antigenic of the Rh antigens, the other factors (with the exception of d) are also antigenic. If strength is to be considered in terms of antibody frequency, anti-c is most common, followed by anti-E, anti-C, and finally anti-e. Combinations of antibodies in the same blood are also seen.

CHARACTERISTICS OF THE Rh-Hr ANTIBODIES

As are all antibodies, the Rh antibodies are made from the gamma globulin portion of the blood plasma. They are specific for the antigen against which they were formed. In other words, anti-D antibody will react only with D antigen and with no other antigen. Unlike the ABO antibodies, all Rh antibodies are immune or irregular antibodies. There are *no* naturally occurring Rh antibodies. They all result from specific antigenic stimulation, whether it be transfusion, pregnancy, or injection of antigen. The lack of natural antibodies in the Rh system is important for several reasons. Practically, it means that antibody typing is impossible in the Rh system. All typing methods in this system depend upon antigen-typing or cell-typing procedures using unknown antigen and known antiserum.

Rh-TYPING PROCEDURES

In terms of testing for the various Rh factors, commercial antiserum is available for the C, D, E, c, and e factors. There is no way of testing for the d factor, since no anti-d antibody has been found. In testing for the various Rh factors it is important to realize that there are two types of Rh antibodies available commercially. One type of antibody is active in saline solution, while the other is of the so-called "incomplete" type and will not react in saline solution. This is extremely important in the laboratory if results are to be accurate.

Antibody of the saline solution–active type is labeled "for saline tube tests." When this preparation is used, reactions must be carried out on saline suspensions of red cells, and the test must be performed in a test tube. Slide tests cannot be performed. The first Rh antibodies discovered were active in saline solution. However, it was found that transfusion reactions would still occur, yet antibody was not detectable.

It was eventually found that some of the Rh antibodies, although not detectable in saline suspensions of red cells, could be demonstrated if a slightly different technique was used. Rather than suspend cells in saline solution, the cells were suspended in serum or a medium containing sufficient protein. These antibodies which were detectable only when suspended in protein were termed "incomplete," or albumin-active, antibodies as opposed to the "complete," or saline solution–active, antibodies. Later, another class of antibody was found to be demonstrable only by means of anti-human globulin, or Coombs' reagent. This type of antibody was termed "incomplete univalent" type antibody. It is now felt that all antibodies are of the bivalent type, although some are detectable in saline suspension while others require sufficient protein concentration and yet others are demonstrable only by means of the anti-human-globulin test.

It appears that the differences in reactivity are dependent upon the length of the antibody molecule. Those molecules which are reactive in saline suspensions of cells are of the larger IgM (γ-M) type. Their length is sufficient to cause a bridging together of adjacent cells in suspension, i.e., agglutination. However, red cells in suspension are known to carry an electric charge which results in a repulsion of cells due to repulsion of like charges. This charge on red cells is referred to as the *zeta potential*. The large IgM-type antibody molecules are so long that they extend beyond the zeta potential and can react with antigenic sites on adjacent cells. Molecules of the smaller IgG (γ-G) type are so short that they do not extend beyond the zeta potential and cannot react with adjacent cells. In order to demonstrate the existence of IgG molecules by means of agglutination, there must be some way of overcoming the repulsion due to the zeta potential. If cells are suspended in a sufficiently high-protein medium (either by suspending cells in their own serum or by adding commercial protein preparations, or both), the zeta potential is reduced. Reduction of the zeta potential allows cells to come closer together, and the IgG antibodies are able to reach antigenic sites on adjacent red cells; thus agglutination occurs. (Other techniques for demonstration of IgG includes high-speed centrifugation and enzyme techniques.)

Commercial Rh antiserum may be of either the saline solution–active or albumin-active variety. In either case, the type of antiserum preparation is stated on the manufacturer's label. It is essential that if the preparation is of the saline solution–active variety, the cells be suspended in saline solution, since the presence of protein may "block" the reaction, resulting in false-negative results. In other words, the manufacturer's direction must be followed for reliable results. In general, saline solution–active antibodies require a test tube method for detection and incubation at 37°C. Slide methods are not adequate. The proper antiserum is labeled "for saline tube tests."

Commercial antiserum of the albumin-active, or high-protein, variety is also available. In this case the commercial preparation contains IgG-type antibodies, which require sufficient protein in order to be demonstrable. Again, manufacturer's directions must be followed. In general, the albumin-active antisera are more avid preparations. For this reason, many of these antisera may be used with either a slide or the test tube technique. In addition, the reaction will take place in less time than with saline solution–active antibody; therefore, incubation time is shortened. The tube methods with albumin-active antiserum may not even require incubation at 37°C but may produce a reaction at room temperature. In general, Rh antibodies will not react unless the preparation is warmed to (or incubated at) 37°C. Antisera of the incomplete, or albumin-active, variety are labeled "for slide or rapid tube test (or modified tube test)." Again, it is essential to follow the manufacturer's directions.

When blood is to be transfused, the patient must be tested for the presence or absence of the D (Rh_o) antigen. This is because the D factor is so antigenic that any person who is D-negative (Rh_o-negative) or d/d will certainly produce an anti-D antibody if transfused with D-positive blood. For this reason, all persons who are D-negative (d/d) must be transfused with Rh-negative or d/d blood. Conversely, since d (Hr_o) has never been shown to be antigenic, Rh-positive (D-positive) persons may be safely transfused with Rh-negative (d/d) blood.

Since the D (Rh_o) factor is the most antigenic of the Rh factors, many laboratories test only for the presence or absence of this factor and transfuse Rh-positive or Rh-negative blood accordingly. In most cases this is sufficient, since other Rh antibodies are comparatively rare and are tested for indirectly through compatibility testing or antibody screening techniques. However, if only the D factor is to be tested for, the incomplete, or albumin-active, anti-Rh$_o$ (anti-D) antiserum "for slide or rapid tube test (or modified tube test)" must be used. Anti-D antiserum is available commercially in both a saline solution–active, or complete, and albumin-active, or incomplete, form. However, there are certain weaker froms of the D antigen (high- and low-grade D^u) which are not detectable with saline solution–active anti-D antiserum. For this reason, if only one test is to be performed, the incomplete, albumin-active form of anti-D must be used. Bloods which are negative with this test must be further tested for the presence of the D^u variant by means of the anti-human globulin (Coombs) reaction.

Although blood must be tested only for the presence or absence of D antigen and transfused accordingly, tests for other Rh factors are often performed routinely. As mentioned previously, antiserum is available for the C, c, D, E, and e factors. Anti-d does not exist. Often bloods are tested routinely for C, c, D, and E. Although anti-e is available, it is so rare that the antiserum is too expensive to be used routinely. There are several reasons for performing tests for C, c, D, and E routinely: In cases of multiple transfusions over extended periods of time, blood which is specific for all these types must be given, for the patient may have developed another Rh antibody. He is likely to develop an antibody if not given type-specific blood for all Rh factors. Both C and c tests are recommended, since anti-c (anti-hr′) is the second most frequent Rh antibody and persons who are c-negative (or C/C) are very likely to develop anti-c (anti-hr′) antibody if transfused with c-positive (hr′-positive) blood.

By performing additional Rh tests, either the complete Rh genotype may be determined positively, or the most probable genotype may be determined by consulting the various frequency charts which are available from these typing reactions. This is especially important in determining the probability of the occurrence of erythroblastosis foetalis in mothers negative for a factor that the father is positive for. In this case both the mother and father are typed and the most probable genotypes determined in order to predict the possibility of erythroblastosis foetalis in their children. Finally, the results of tests with these other Rh-typing sera may be used to check on the laboratory results by consulting frequency charts. Often the occurrence of a very infrequent typing reaction will point to an error in the typing procedure itself.

In using the various typing sera, the anti-D (anti-Rh$_o$) antiserum is available in both a complete, saline solution–active form and an incomplete, albumin-active form. It is often the case that all bloods are routinely tested with both these antisera. This is done as a means of checking the accuracy of the test for D antigen. Since all Rh antibodies are immune or irregular antibodies, it is impossible to antibody-type, as was the case in the ABO system. Therefore, it is quite useful to have a means of checking results for the extremely antigenic D antigen. The saline and the albumin form of anti-D antiserum should give the same result, be it positive or negative. In addition, the use of incomplete, albumin-active anti-D allows for the detection of D antigen in a shorter period of time than that required with saline solution anti-D. In the case of the D^u variants of the D antigen, only the incomplete form of anti-D antiserum will give positive results. Therefore, a combination of reactions with saline solution and albumin anti-D is used in identifying D antigen and some of its variants.

Anti-C and anti-E antisera (in addition to anti-D) are normally available in a saline solution–active form. Antisera of this type will be labeled "for saline tube tests" and require that the tests be performed within test tubes. In general, equal amounts of antiserum and 2 to 4% suspensions of red cells (one or two drops of each) are mixed in 10- by 75 or 12- by 75-mm test tubes and incubated at 37°C for about 1 hour. After incubation, the tubes may be centrifuged. The results are very carefully read macroscopically by resuspending the cells and tipping the tubes. Negative results must be confirmed by observation under the microscope. The exact technique will vary with different brands of antiserum, and the manufacturer's directions must be followed.

The anti-c (anti-hr′) antiserum is normally available in an incomplete, albumin-active form labeled "for slide or rapid tube test (or modified tube test)." This antiserum may be used with a slide technique where a suspension of cells in their own serum is added to antiserum on a warmed microscope slide and observed for agglutination. Or the cells may be suspended either in serum or saline solution and added to antiserum in a test tube. The tube is usually incubated at 37°C; however, the time is generally only 15 minutes or 30 minutes (less than with saline solution-active antiserum). Again the manufacturer's directions must be followed, and the technique will vary somewhat with various brands of antiserum.

CONCLUSION

In summary, the Rh system is considerably more complex than the ABO blood group system. Any person will always have six blood group factors in his blood but only two ABO blood group factors. The person may be either homozygous or heterozygous for the three paired Rh factors, as he may be homozygous or heterozygous for the A, B, or O factors. The ABO system has both natural and irregular (immune) antibodies, while the Rh system has only irregular antibodies. When transfusing blood, ABO type-specific blood should always be given. With the Rh system, blood may be tested for only the presence or absence of D antigen and transfused accordingly. However, it is sometimes necessary to give blood which is type-specific for the various Rh factors.

Commercial Rh antiserum may be of either the saline solution–active or albumin-active type. It is essential that the procedure used be in accordance with the form of antiserum that is being employed. Techniques will vary with different brands of antiserum.

Finally, the in vitro reactions with the anti-A and anti-B antisera are much more easily seen than the reactions with the various Rh-typing sera. For this reason, experience is invaluable when testing for the Rh factors. Techniques must be mastered and performed with great care. Shortcuts must never be taken, and the methods and reasons for them must be thoroughly understood by the laboratory technician.

THE ANTIGLOBULIN REACTION (COOMBS' TEST)

Under Rh-typing Procedures, mention was made of different types of antibodies and their laboratory reactions. Antibodies were classified as being of the complete or incomplete type depending on their ability to react in saline suspensions of red cells or the necessity for additional techniques such as the addition of protein to the test medium. This was related to the size of the antibody molecule and its ability to overcome like electric charges on red cells in suspension (the zeta potential). In general the IgM antibodies are large enough to extend beyond the zeta potential, with resultant agglutination of red cells in saline suspensions. However, many IgG antibody molecules are unable to bring about agglutination unless the zeta potential is reduced by such means as neutralizing the charge by adding protein to the red cell suspension.

Mention was also made of still other antibody molecules which could not cause agglutination, even in the presence of high protein concentrations. These antibodies which are unable to cause agglutination by any of the laboratory techniques mentioned thus far are detectable by means of the antiglobulin, or Coombs, technique. They have been described in the past as being incomplete antibodies of a univalent form; however, they are now felt to be bivalent in action, although undemonstrable without the antiglobulin technique.

The various antibodies which are detectable by the antiglobulin technique react with red blood cells. However, the reaction is not observable in terms of agglutination. Rather, the antibodies merely coat the red cells by reacting with antigenic sites on the cell surface. The other end of the antibody molecule is not able to react with antigen on a second red cell, with resultant bridging and agglutination. In order to demonstrate the coating of red cells by this incomplete "univalent" antibody, some sort of reagent must be available to show that the cells have reacted with antibody. It must be remembered that these "univalent" antibodies are fully capable of reaction in the body and if present will result in severe transfusion reactions.

In the development of a reagent to demonstrate the coating of incomplete antibody on red cells, use is made of the fact that all antibodies are some form of human globulin. The reagent capable of demonstrating any antibody coating a red cell (regardless of its specificity) need only be an antibody to human globulin. This is the basis of the antiglobulin, or Coombs, test. The reagent is an antibody to human globulin, or antihuman globulin antibody. This antiglobulin antibody will react with any antibody coating a red blood cell. Since the antiglobulin antibody is bivalent (has two reactive sites at opposite ends of the molecule) and is sufficiently long (it is actually an IgM-type antibody), it will react with antibody coating adjacent red blood cells, with bridging or agglutination of the red cells as a result.

Anti-human globulin (Coombs) reagent is produced commercially by the various companies which produce blood group antisera. The anti-human globulin reagent is prepared by inoculating laboratory animals with human serum or the globulin fraction of human serum. The laboratory animals will produce an antibody to the human globulin, or anti-human globulin antibodies. The laboratory animal is bled and the serum collected. This serum is purified by various techniques, leaving a serum specific for human globulin. The anti-human serum is prepared in such a way that it reacts with both gamma globulin and complement. The antiglobulin portion of the serum is actually anti-IgG globulin. However, there are antibodies other than those of the IgG type that must be detected by the antiglobulin (Coombs) test. It has been found that some of these other antibodies require complement in order to react. In other words, they are said to *fix* complement. Therefore, anti-human globulin reagent is prepared and standardized in such a manner that it will react both with IgG-type antibodies and with complement. In this way a so-called *broad-spectrum* antiglobulin reagent is produced which will react with a great variety of antibodies.[13,14]

There are actually two ways in which the antiglobulin test is performed. These are the direct and indirect methods.[13,15]

The direct antiglobulin (Coombs) test is performed on cells which are suspected to have been coated with antibody. The red cells suspected of antibody coating are first washed meticulously with saline solution. The washing procedure is essential for reliability of the test. All traces of serum (hence human globulin) must be removed from the test medium. Any serum remaining will react with the antiglobulin reagent, causing neutralization of the reagent and therefore falsely negative results.

The test is performed in test tubes of the 10- by 75- or 12- by 75-mm size. The cells are washed by completely filling the test tube with a forceful stream of saline solution resulting in a homogeneous suspension of cells in saline solution. The tube is then centrifuged, cells being packed at the bottom of the test tube. After centrifuging, the tube is inverted and all of the saline solution decanted in one motion, shaking the tube to remove all saline solution. The tube is then turned upright and shaken to resuspend the cells. The tube must never be covered with the finger or palm of the hand at any stage of mixing, for protein from the skin can inactivate or neutralize the antiglobulin reagent.

The cells are washed with saline solution in this manner a minimum of three times. More washings may be necessary if periodic evaluation of the washing technique shows that three times is not adequate. After the final washing, the saline solution is decanted as completely as possible. The cells are then shaken to facilitate resuspension and the antiglobulin reagent added. The test tube is then incubated and centrifuged as the manufacturer's directions specify, and the results are read macroscopically and microscopically for the presence or absence of agglutination. The direct antiglobulin (Coombs) test is used in the diagnosis of hemolytic disease of the newborn and autoimmune hemolytic anemia, and in the investigation of transfusion reactions.

The indirect antiglobulin (Coombs) test begins a step before the direct method, although it eventually requires the same washing technique and reaction with antiglobulin reagent. The indirect test begins with a serum suspected of containing antibodies. The suspected serum is mixed with red cells which contain antigens for the suspected antibody in the serum. The test cell is suspended in saline solution, albumin, or serum (depending on the antibody involved), mixed with the suspected serum, and incubated for a sufficient period of time for a reaction to occur. Test cells are usually incubated for 15 to 30 minutes at 37°C, but this varies with the antigen-antibody system involved. If the serum contains an antibody for an antigen on the test cell, there will be a reaction, a coating of antibody on the test cell. In order to demonstrate the coating of antibody on the red cell, the cell must be washed with saline solution and treated exactly as is the coated cell in the direct antiglobulin (Coombs) test.

The indirect antiglobulin (Coombs) test has several uses. It is used in cross-matching blood to detect incompatibility before transfusion. The serum of pregnant women is tested using the indirect antiglobulin test when hemolytic disease of the newborn could occur. Donor serum is tested by means of the indirect antiglobulin test for the detection and identification of irregular antibodies. Certain blood group antigens (such as low-grade D^u antigen) require the indirect antiglobulin technique for their demonstration. Finally, various investigative studies require the use of this technique.

It must be remembered that neither the indirect nor the direct antiglobulin tests are specific for any one antibody. They will give the same reaction with any antibody contained within human serum. In order to determine the identity of the antibody responsible for a positive reaction, the antigens present on the red cell must be known. There are certain red cell preparations available commercially where the antigens are known. In screening blood for irregular antibodies, a cell is used which contains a great variety of antigens. If this cell gives a positive reaction, a series of other cells with combinations of antigens are tested, and the antibody is finally identified by elimination.

The antiglobulin (Coombs) test is by no means a simple test. The reagent itself is a particularly unstable preparation and must be stored with great care. It is inactivated in several different ways. The manual of the American Association of Blood Banks lists 10 causes of false-negative and 9 causes of false-positive results.[16] All these mechanisms must be thoroughly understood before the antiglobulin test can be performed with reliability. It is because of these numerous sources of error that positive and negative controls must be included whenever the antiglobulin test is performed.

HEMOLYTIC DISEASE OF THE NEWBORN (ERYTHROBLASTOSIS FOETALIS)

Hemolytic disease of the newborn, or erythroblastosis foetalis, is a condition which may result if a child inherits an antigen for which his mother is negative. The disease most commonly involves factors of the Rh and ABO blood group systems, although it may result from incompatibilities in virtually any blood group system. In order for this disease to occur, however, the child must be positive for an antigen for which the mother is negative.

Hemolytic disease of the newborn is a condition which develops while the fetus is within the uterus. The mechanism involves sensitization or immunization of the mother to foreign antigen present on her child's red blood cells. Although the circulatory systems of a mother and her child are separate closed systems with passage of only smaller molecules such as nutrients across the placenta, there can be some seepage of fetal red cells into the mother's circulatory system. This is most likely to occur very late in pregnancy or at the time of birth. If any incompatible fetal red cells do find their way into the mother's circulatory system, she will develop an antibody to the antigen on the child's red cells and the same antigen on the red cells of any subsequent children. Once such immunization occurs, it is permanent. The antibody formed by the mother is an IgG-type antibody which is fully capable of crossing the placenta into the circulatory system of the fetus. When such maternal antibody does exist, it will cross the placenta and react with corresponding antigen on the red blood cells of the fetus, with resultant destruction of the cells. Hemolytic disease of the newborn is the condition which exists when maternal antibody crosses the placenta and reacts with antigen on fetal red blood cells. This was the cause of death of the child delivered by the woman studied by Levine and Stetson in 1939 which led to the discovery of the Rh blood group system.

Hemolytic disease of the newborn most commonly involves the Rh blood group system. It most often involves the D antigen, the mother being negative for D. In this case, the father is positive for the D antigen, and the child inherits this factor from the father. In other words, the mother is negative for D (or d/d), and the child is D-positive (or D/d). If any of the D-positive red cells of the fetus cross into the mother's circulatory system, she will develop an immune anti-D antibody. This antibody, of the IgG type, will cross the placenta and react with the red blood cells of the fetus. Fortunately, sensitization usually occurs only very late in pregnancy or at the time of delivery, so that the first child is rarely affected by hemolytic disease of the newborn. Further, any child who is D-negative cannot be affected by anti-D antibody in the mother's circulatory system. For this reason, genotyping parents in possible cases of hemolytic disease of the newborn is very useful in predicting the chance of occurrence of the disease. For example, if the husband happens to be heterozygous for the D antigen (or D/d) and the mother is D-negative (or d/d), the chances are that only half of the children will inherit the D antigen (Table 5-4). On the other hand, if the father is homozygous for D (or D/D), then all children will inherit the D antigen, or there is a 100 percent chance of hemolytic disease of the newborn (Table 5-4). (Only those children who are D-positive can possibly be affected by the disease, since only they are positive for a factor which the mother is negative for.)

It has been mentioned that the first child is rarely affected by hemolytic disease of the newborn. In fact, only about 5 percent of Rh-negative women actually become immunized during pregnancy.[17] Although a woman can usually have one or two children both of whom are Rh-positive and encounter no difficulties, once she is immunized, this immunization

Table 5-4. Chance of Development of Hemolytic Disease of the Newborn (Erythroblastosis Foetalis) Based on Genotypes for the D Factor

Father heterozygous for D (D/d)	Father homozygous for D (D/D)
Mother homozygous for d (d/d)	Mother homozygous for d (d/d)
50% chance of hemolytic disease	100% chance of hemolytic disease

	D	d			D	D
d	D/d	d/d		d	D/d	D/d
d	D/d	d/d		d	D/d	D/d

is permanent. Further, once the disease develops in one child, the chances are that subsequent children positive for the antigen in question will be affected at least as severely or more so. Even more important, if a woman has been sensitized prior to pregnancy as a result of transfusion of incompatible blood or injection of antigenic material, even the first child can be severely affected. This is why type-specific blood is recommended for transfusion of women of childbearing age or younger.

It has been mentioned that the anti-D antibody is the most common cause of hemolytic disease of the newborn. Other antibodies causing this disease include anti-c, anti-K (Kell), anti-E, and even incompatibilities in the ABO system. In the case of hemolytic disease due to anti-c, the mother is of genotype C/C, and the child inherits the c factor from the father. This is the second most common cause of hemolytic disease of the newborn and the reason why many laboratories test all patients and donors for the c (hr') factor. Mothers who are C/C are usually D-positive, since this is the most likely genotype or combination of factors in the Rh system. If a D-positive woman who is also C/C is transfused with blood which is merely tested for the presence or absence of D antigen, the chances are she will be transfused with blood which is positive for the c (hr') factor. In such women an anti-c antibody will then develop which may result in severe hemolytic disease of the newborn even in the firstborn c-positive child. Again, this is the rationale for transfusion of type-specific blood to females of or under childbearing age.

Hemolytic disease of the newborn can also occur as the result of factors in the ABO system. In this case, the mother is usually blood group O, whereas the child inherits the A or B antigen from the father. If this does occur and any of the fetal cells actually find their way into the mother's circulatory system, she will develop an immune IgG antibody in addition to her natural IgM anti-A or anti-B antibody. If an immune IgG antibody is produced, it will cross the placenta and react with corresponding antigen on the red blood cells of the fetus. Fortunately, although ABO sensitization may occur fairly often, it seems that hemolytic disease due to ABO incompatibility is less severe and the child may be only mildly affected and require little or no treatment.[18]

When hemolytic disease of the newborn does occur, it will vary considerably in severity. In its most severe form, the child will be stillborn or even abort early in pregnancy. If the child is alive when born, he may be affected so mildly as to require little treatment, or he may be severely affected by the products of destruction of his red cells and anemia. The cell destruction results in hemolytic anemia accompanied by abnormal levels of serum bilirubin with the clinical appearance of jaundice. The bilirubin will result in irreversible brain damage if present in sufficient concentration. If the child survives and is not treated adequately, this brain damage will result in severe mental retardation.

Treatment in severe cases of hemolytic disease of the newborn includes blood transfusion. This is actually referred to as an *exchange transfusion,* for most of the child's blood volume is replaced with the transfused blood. The exchange transfusion will serve to correct the anemia and remove the abnormal levels of serum bilirubin, thus preventing brain damage.

The type of blood which is used for transfusion will vary with the antibody responsible for the disease. The outstanding consideration is to give the child blood which is negative for the factor against which the antibody has been formed. In other words, the child is given blood which is compatible with the mother. In the case of hemolytic disease of the newborn due to the formation of anti-D antibody in the mother's serum, the child is transfused with blood which is D-negative. This is because not all of the child's blood is replaced at the time of exchange; some maternal antibody is left in his system. Therefore, blood is given which will not react with the remaining antibody yet will not harm the child. In this case, the child would be given blood specific for his own ABO type but negative for the D antigen against which the maternal antibody was formed. In the cases of ABO incompatibility which require exchange, the mother is usually group O and the child group A or B. In these cases the child is transfused with low-titer group O blood of his own Rh type.

There are many laboratory studies which are performed in cases of hemolytic disease of the newborn. These are performed on the parents' (primarily the mother's) blood prior to birth and on the child's blood after birth. The first step is to type the mother and father for ABO and Rh during pregnancy to see if hemolytic disease of the newborn can occur. In other words, is the father positive for any factor which the mother is negative for? Depending on the results from genotyping the mother and father with reference to frequency charts and family studies, the probability of the occurrence of the disease can be predicted. If hemolytic disease of the newborn is possible, the mother's serum is tested by means of the indirect antiglobulin (Coombs) test to see if an antibody does exist. If an antibody is found, it is identified and the titer (or concentration) determined. This titer is rechecked throughout pregnancy as an indication of the severity of the possible disease.

After birth, there are several studies which may be performed on the child's blood, in addition to further studies on the maternal serum. Initially, a sample of umbilical cord blood is tested for ABO group and Rh type, and a direct antiglobulin (Coombs) test is performed. Some other laboratory tests include hemoglobin determinations, blood smear examination and differential, reticulocyte count, and serum bilirubin determinations on the child's blood.

The decision to perform exchange transfusion will depend on a combination of various laboratory results and the clinical condition of the child.

Several laboratory tests are of value in making this decision. Preparation can and should be made before birth, so that the exchange can proceed as soon as possible if necessary.

COMPATIBILITY TESTING, OR CROSSMATCHING

Whenever blood is to be transfused, there are two considerations which must be kept in mind. First, blood must be selected which will not be harmful to the patient or result in a transfusion reaction. Second, blood must be selected which will be of maximum benefit to the patient. For these reasons, whenever blood is to be transfused, the *compatibility test,* or *crossmatching,* must be performed. This is an indispensable procedure without which transfusion would be an extremely hazardous treatment.

When blood is selected for transfusion, the patient and donor are tested for ABO type and for the presence or absence of the D (Rh$_o$) antigen. Blood is then selected for transfusion on the basis of matching the ABO group and Rh type in respect to the D factor. Patients whose cells contain the D antigen are given blood positive for the D factor, or Rh-positive blood, while patients who are negative for the D antigen are always given blood which is negative for the D antigen, or Rh-negative. Of course, there are innumerable other antigens both in the Rh system and other blood group systems which collectively make up a person's complete blood type. These are not matched when blood is to be transfused. However, there exists the potential danger of the patient's cells' containing an antigen corresponding to an antibody in the donor's serum in addition to the possibility that the patient's serum contains an antibody corresponding to an antigen on the donor's red blood cells. In order to guard against these situations, which could result in severe transfusion reactions, compatibility tests must be performed. In addition, the compatibility will serve as a means of checking the correct matching of the ABO type of the donor and recipient.

In general, the crossmatch is used to help detect (1) irregular antibodies in the patient's or donor's serum, (2) ABO incompatibilities, and (3) errors in labeling, recording, or identifying patients or donors.[19] Unfortunately, compatibility testing, although indispensable, is not a perfect or foolproof method which guards against all problems which may arise. The most frequent causes of transfusion of incompatible blood are errors of an organizational, clerical, or technical nature. Although these errors may be detected by means of the crossmatch, this is not always the case. In other words, the laboratory must always work with absolute care to avoid mistakes of this nature. In addition, although ABO incompatibility may be detected in the crossmatch, not all such errors are found by this method. Correct typing remains absolutely necessary.

In addition, incompatibility will be discovered only if the patient's serum actually contains an irregular antibody. Crossmatching will not prevent immunization of the patient if he is transfused with foreign antigen. For example, the Rh-negative person who has never been exposed to Rh-positive antigenic material will not show incompatibility if crossmatched with Rh-positive blood, yet he will develop an anti-D antibody. Errors of Rh typing will be detected only if the recipient's or donor's serum actually contains an Rh antibody. Furthermore, there is no single crossmatching procedure which will detect all irregular antibodies which may be present in either the patient or the donor serum. Finally, even though compatible, the crossmatch will not ensure the normal survival of donor red cells. Blood must be processed and stored correctly.[19]

There are several different ways of performing the compatibility test. No method is perfect or can even be said to be preferable. In general, there are (1) the saline solution or serum, crossmatch, (2) the high-protein crossmatch, (3) the antiglobulin (Coombs) crossmatch, and (4) enzyme crossmatches. Each of these types of crossmatch may be performed as a *major* crossmatch or a *minor* crossmatch.

The division into the major and minor crossmatch relates to the principles involved in considering group O persons as universal donors and group AB persons as universal recipients. The major crossmatch involves testing of the donor's red cells with the patient's serum. This procedure is used to detect any antibody present within the patient's serum which will react with the donor's red cells. The presence of such antibody in the patient's serum would certainly result in a major transfusion reaction, for all the infused donor cells would be destroyed by the patient's antibody. Of course, even if the patient's serum did contain an irregular antibody, it would be detected only if the donor's cells contained the corresponding antigen. For this reason, some workers suggest that all patients' serum be screened with a red cell preparation containing a great variety of antigens in order to detect a greater variety of irregular antibody than may be detected by means of the major crossmatch of prospective donors.[20] At any rate, whether patient serum is screened with cell preparations for antibody or not, all blood for transfusion must be matched with donor blood by means of a major crossmatch procedure.

The minor crossmatch is just the opposite of the major. The minor crossmatch tests the donor's serum with the patient's red cells. This is used to detect the presence of an antibody in the donor's serum which is specific for an antigen on the patient's red blood cells. Again, any antibody in the donor's serum will be detected only if the patient's red cells contain the corresponding antigen. The minor crossmatch will not detect every antibody which may exist in the donor's serum. This test is referred to as the minor crossmatch because even if positive, the existence of donor antibody directed against an antigen on the patient's red cells would result in a minor transfusion reaction, minor in the sense that the donor's antibody would be so diluted by infusion into the patient that only a few of the patient's red cells would be destroyed and this would be overcome by benefit of the donor cells, which would remain intact and viable. This was the rationale of using group O blood as universal donor blood and has all the same disadvantages. Although the major crossmatch is required whenever blood is to be transfused, the minor crossmatch may be optional. If the donor's serum is adequately tested for irregular antibody by means of an antibody-screening technique, the minor crossmatch is not absolutely necessary.[21] However, no one technique is perfect, and many investigators feel that both antibody-screening techniques and minor crossmatches should be performed routinely, since each will detect different problems.[22]

Whether the major and minor crossmatch or merely the major crossmatch is to be performed, there are different techniques which may be used. Again, no single technique will detect all irregular antibodies. Usually a combination of techniques is used, since none is preferable. No matter what method is chosen, however, the antiglobulin phase, or test, should be included.

THE SALINE SOLUTION OR SERUM CROSSMATCH[23]

The various general types of crossmatches will be discussed in the paragraphs that follow, although the exact procedures, will not be given.

The saline solution or serum test involves the mixing of serum and a suspension of cells in serum or saline solution. This may be a major test using patient serum and donor cells or a minor test using donor serum and patient cells. The test tube is first incubated at room temperature, centrifuged, and observed for the presence of agglutination or hemolysis. At this stage ABO incompatibility will be observable as will incompatibility caused by antibodies of the P, MNSs, Lewis, Lutheran, or Wright systems.

If negative to this point, the test tube is further incubated at 37°C for a sufficient period of time and observed once again. At this point, saline solution–reacting antibodies of the Rh-Hr and Lewis system will be detected. In addition, antibodies of the P, MNSs, or Kell systems may sometimes react at this stage.

If the saline solution or serum crossmatch is still negative, it may be further tested by means of the antiglobulin crossmatch.

THE HIGH-PROTEIN CROSSMATCH[23]

The higher-protein crossmatch involves the mixing of serum with a suspension of cells in their own serum plus the addition of a commercial preparation of albumin. This may be a major test using patient serum and donor cells or a minor test using donor serum and patient cells. The preparation is mixed, centrifuged, and observed. It is then incubated at 37°C for a sufficient length of time and observed again. The high-protein crossmatch will detect most Rh-Hr antibodies including some which are not detected by the saline solution method. It may also be further tested by means of the antiglobulin test.

THE ANTIGLOBULIN (COOMBS) CROSSMATCH[23]

The antiglobulin, or Coombs, crossmatch may be an extension of either the saline solution or the albumin crossmatch of the major and minor types. It is the one technique which should be included in any crossmatch procedure, since it is the best way of detecting most of the IgG-type antibodies. After incubation of either the saline solution or high-protein preparation at 37°C, the cells are thoroughly washed with saline solution as was described for the direct and indirect antiglobulin tests. The antiglobulin serum is added and the test carried out as recommended by the particular manufacturer. In other words, this is merely an indirect antiglobulin (Coombs) test between a patient and prospective blood donor. The antiglobulin crossmatch will detect almost all Rh-Hr antibodies. In addition, this may be the only means of detecting some antibodies, especially in the Duffy, Kidd, and Kell blood group systems.

ENZYME CROSSMATCHES[23]

There are also various crossmatching procedures which make use of enzyme preparations such as bromelin, ficin, papain, and trypsin. Although these may be useful as additional methods, they should not be used as the only means of compatibility testing and should not replace the antiglobulin test. They may detect some Rh-Hr antibodies not found by other methods but may not detect some antibodies of the MNSs, Kell, and Duffy systems.

SUMMARY

To summarize, some sort of compatibility testing regimen is required whenever blood is to be transfused. Unfortunately, there is no one ideal crossmatching method and no way of guaranteeing that any and all mistakes or incompatibilities have been discovered. Of course, if incompatibility is discovered at any point, the cause of incompatibility must be determined. This determination is far beyond the scope of this brief outline of the crossmatching procedure. In addition, there are numerous technical problems which may be encountered which have not been discussed. Yet, if typing and crossmatching have been performed with absolute care according to the correct routine as determined by the particular blood bank, the transfusion of blood can be a relatively safe procedure of tremendous benefit to the patient.

CONCLUSION

As mentioned at the outset, this chapter is only a brief introduction to the complex field of blood banking. Actual blood-grouping and cross-matching techniques have been purposely omitted, since adequate information has not been given for their complete performance. Other topics which have not been covered completely in this outline but which must be understood before the student can work in the blood bank include causes of error, the cleaning of glassware, organization of the blood bank, selection of blood donors, processing and storage of blood, various types of blood derivatives for transfusion, labeling of blood, records, and types of transfusion reactions. Excellent discussions of these subjects have been published in standard blood bank texts. In addition, knowledge may be gained from firsthand experience in a licensed blood bank.

In the field of blood banking there are numerous situations which may result in error. In general, these may be errors of organization, clerical errors, or technical errors.[1] Organizational and clerical errors may be made by the blood bank staff or by personnel on other services involved in the actual transfusion of blood. These errors often involve incorrect identification of the patient or of the blood removed from a patient and sent to the laboratory for testing.

Transfusion involves a series of tests which are performed by several different persons. Included are clerical manipulations where even a mistake on the part of a typist in transcribing a laboratory report could result in fatal errors if adequate checks did not exist. Because of the series of persons and tests which must be involved in blood transfusion, a blood bank has elaborate organization procedures which must be followed exactly. The exact procedures are beyond the scope of this discussion; however, the American Association of Blood Banks has definite requirements and recommendations. The established systems were developed for definite reasons and must be followed exactly in order to ensure that the correct blood be transfused into the correct patient. The organizational systems involve such items and procedures as request forms, methods of labeling tubes of blood from the patient, the manner in which technicians record results in the laboratory, labeling and numbering of donor blood, selections of blood donors, and storage of blood, to name a few.

Technical errors are the direct responsibility of the blood banking laboratory and its staff. These may be personal errors, where the technician is directly responsible, or impersonal errors due to various factors which enter into the laboratory technique. In any blood grouping or compatibility testing method, there are various impersonal technical factors which will result in false-positive or false-negative results. Some may happen in all tests, and some are peculiar to a specific method. These sources of error are beyond the scope of this outline yet must be thoroughly understood by the blood bank technician if results are to be reliable and accurate.

It is hoped that this discussion of blood banking will serve as a useful introduction to the student. It is to be regarded, however, as only a brief outline. Work in this area will require much additional knowledge and study on the part of the student.

REFERENCES

1. I. Dunsford and C. C. Bowley, "Techniques in Blood Grouping," Oliver & Boyd Ltd., Edinburgh and London, 1955.
2. "Technical Methods and Procedures of the American Association of Blood Banks," 4th ed., p. 33, American Association of Blood Banks, Chicago, 1966.
3. Lot B. Page and Perry J. Culver, "A Syllabus of Laboratory Examination in Clinical Diagnosis," rev. ed., p. 218, Harvard University Press, Cambridge, Mass., 1960.
4. *Ibid.*, pp. 34–36.
5. R. R. Race and R. Sanger, "Blood Groups in Man," 4th ed., p. 17, F. A. Davis Company, Philadelphia, 1955.
6. *Ibid.*
7. "Technical Methods and Procedures of the American Association of Blood Banks," *op. cit.*
8. *Ibid.*, p. 60.
9. A. S. Wiener and I. B. Wexler, "Heredity of the Blood Groups," chap. V, Grune & Stratton, Inc., New York, 1958.
10. Race and Sanger, *op. cit.*, chap. VI.
11. R. E. Rosenfield, F. H. Aleen, Jr., S. N. Swisher, and S. Kochwa, "A Review of the Rh Serology and Presentation of a New Terminology," *Transfusion*, 2:287, 1962.
12. "Technical Methods and Procedures of the American Association of Blood Banks," *op. cit.*, p. 67.
13. "Blood Group Antigens and Antibodies as Applied to Blood Transfusion," pp. 37–41, Diagnostic Division, Ortho Pharmaceutical Corporation, Raritan, N.J., 1960.
14. I. Dunsford and J. Grant, "The Antiglobulin (Coombs) Test in Laboratory Practice," Oliver & Boyd Ltd., Edinburgh and London, 1960.
15. "Technical Methods and Procedures of the American Association of Blood Banks," *op. cit.*, pp. 45–47.
16. *Ibid.*, pp. 48–49.
17. "The Merck Manual of Diagnosis and Therapy," 10th ed., p. 59, Merck Sharp and Dohme Research Laboratories, Division of Merck and Co., Inc., Rahway, N.J., 1961.
18. "Blood Group Antigens and Antibodies as Applied to Blood Transfusion," pp. 59–60, Diagnostic Division, Ortho Pharmaceutical Corporation, Raritan, N.J., 1960.
19. "Technical Methods and Procedures of the American Association of Blood Banks," *op. cit.*, p. 91.

20. "Blood Group Antigens and Antibodies as Applied to Compatibility Testing," pp. 10–11, Diagnostic Division, Ortho Pharmaceutical Corporation, Raritan, N.J., 1967.
21. "Technical Methods and Procedures of the American Association of Blood Banks," *op. cit.*, chap. IX.
22. "Blood Group Antigens and Antibodies as Applied to Compatibility Testing," pp. 12–13, Diagnostic Division, Ortho Pharmaceutical Corporation, Raritan, N.J., 1967.
23. "Technical Methods and Procedures of the American Association of Blood Banks," *op. cit.*, chap. VIII.

6

Microbiology

Microbiology involves the study of organisms so small they cannot be seen with the naked eye. Rather they require the use of a high-power microscope in order to be observable. For most routine studies the bright-field microscope is used where the organism appears dark against a bright background. Other optical systems which are sometimes used in the field of microbiology are the dark-field, phase, ultraviolet, fluorescent, and electron microscopes.

Microorganisms are distributed throughout nature and interact with man and all forms of life. They are present virtually everywhere, and their associations, both intimate and more distant, are essential to all forms of life in a cyclic manner. For example, certain bacteria are normal constituents of man's intestinal tract. These microorganisms benefit from this association, for they derive essential food materials from the host. They also benefit their host, for they synthesize and aid in the digestion of certain vitamins which are essential to the life of man. The life cycle in general involves the bacterial breakdown of dead plants and animals into simpler substances which can be utilized by green plants to make foodstuffs which are further utilized by higher animals. There are microorganisms which inhabit the digestive tract of ruminants such as cows which are essential for the digestion of cellulose by these animals. The major foodstuff of these animals is cellulose, yet animals are unable to digest it. However, the microorganisms which normally inhabit the digestive tract of these animals are plants which are able to digest cellulose into a form utilizable by the larger host, with benefit to the host and its parasite.

Although it must be remembered that mircroorganisms are distributed throughout nature and are generally beneficial and essential to all life, there are certain situations where microorganisms are not beneficial. Rather, some are harmful to their respective hosts. These are disease-producing, or *pathogenic,* microorganisms. This discussion will be concerned with the less numerous, pathogenic microorganisms rather than the more numerous, beneficial microbes.

The pathogenic microorganisms which may cause disease in man include living organisms of both the plant and animal kingdom. The only true microbes of the animal kindom are the *protozoa,* or single-celled animals. Again, most of the protozoa are harmless forms of life, but some may be pathogenic. The protozoa are further subdivided into the amebas, the ciliates, the flagellates, and the sporozoa. An example of disease due to protozoa is amebic dysentery, which is caused by a specific protozoic ameba.

Certain pathogenic worms are often included in the field of microbiology, although they are not microorganisms. Examples of worms which cause disease are the tapeworms such as *Taenia solium;* the fluke *Fasciolopsis buski;* and the roundworm *Strongyloides stercoralis.* An even higher class of animals, the arthropods, are also included in the field of microbiology in some instances. These organisms in themselves rarely cause disease; however, they do serve as vectors in certain microbial infections. Certain insects are essential to one stage of the life cycle of true microorganisms which cause the disease malaria. In addition, there are certain ticks which are bloodsucking parasites in themselves.

The majority of pathogenic microorganisms belong to the plant kingdom, including the fungi and simpler organisms. The systematic classification of these organisms is quite complex. Fungi are simple colorless plants which are further subdivided into the molds, yeasts, and bacteria. Microorganisms simpler than the bacteria include the pleuropneumonia and pleuropneumonia-like organisms, the rickettsiae, and the viruses.

Although the study of microbiology involves more than just bacteriology, this chapter will consist of information and various techniques involved in the growth, or culture, and identification of various pathogenic bacteria.

TYPES AND COLLECTION OF MATERIAL FOR MICROBIOLOGIC EXAMINATION

When a patient exhibits certain disease symptoms, the physician will often want to identify the causative agent if a microbiologic infection is suspected. The positive identification of the causative agent is important in the correct treatment of the patient. Therefore, the physician will send appropriate specimens to the laboratory in order to identify the cause of infection. In the case of a possible kidney or urinary tract infection, a urine specimen will be collected for bacterial analysis. If the patient exhibits a sore throat, the throat will be swabbed with a cotton-tipped applicator, and this will be submitted for analysis. Possible dysentery will require the examination of stool specimens, while examination of infected wounds will require swabs or appropriate material from the area of infection. Other sites of infection from which swabs or material are submitted to the laboratory for culture and identification include the blood; various body fluids; cervix; urethra; vagina; ear; endometrium; eye; spinal, ventricular, or subdural fluid; bronchi or trachea (sputum material); and various tissues.

For each area from which material may be submitted for examination there are certain possible sources of infection. Therefore, the microbiologist must be aware of the possible types of infective agents that may be responsible for the disease and test for these accordingly. Accordingly, for each source of infected material there is a certain set of tests which must be performed in order to discover the cause of infection.

When material is submitted to the microbiology laboratory for culture and identification, certain considerations must be kept in mind that are the responsibility of the people actually collecting the specimen. This is rarely done by the actual laboratory personnel; however, it is the ultimate responsibility of the laboratory to inform the hospital staff of correct procedures for collecting microbiologic specimens and for providing suitable containers for this purpose. The following are general considerations for the collection of specimens.

The treatment of disease or infection often involves the use of antibiotics or other agents which destroy various pathogens. The antibiotics are often administered before the causative agent is identified by the microbiology department, since such identification takes 1 day or more while the patient requires immediate treatment. However, culture of the causative agent will often be impossible once antibiotics have been administered. Therefore, the appropriate specimen should be obtained before antibiotics are administered.

The correct identification of a causative agent requires isolation and growth of a *pure culture* of that organism in the laboratory. The isolation of a pure culture in the laboratory requires that the original specimen be collected in a sterile container and not contaminated at any stage of its subsequent transfer to the laboratory or isolation in the laboratory. In order to ensure sterile collections, the microbiology laboratory should provide sterile containers to the nursing station or physician with specific information as to what type of container should be used for various types of specimens in addition to the actual manner of collection. It is also important for the protection of both the laboratory personnel and anyone handling the specimen that the specimen be placed within the appropriate container and that none of the material be allowed to contaminate the outside. These specimens often contain dangerous pathogens which could infect anyone coming in contact with the infected material.

Once the specimen has been placed in the appropriate container, it should be delivered to the laboratory immediately and not allowed to stand at the nursing station. Although many organisms remain viable (or alive) for long periods of time after collection, certain organisms are extremely fastidious outside the host and require rapid inoculation into a suitable culture medium in order to be detected. In fact, some organisms are so viable that they require special arrangements with the laboratory so that a special culture medium is taken to the patient and the material placed directly on it. Some pathogens will be obscured by the rapid and overwhelming growth of other organisms that are normally present in the material to be cultured. For example, fecal samples normally contain several types of bacteria which will obscure the detection of such pathogens as *Shigella* if not delivered to the laboratory and plated onto a suitable medium soon after collection.

When the specimen reaches the laboratory, it is not always possible to inoculate the correct culture medium immediately. Most specimens may be stored under refrigeration at 4 to 6°C until the culture medium can be inoculated. With certain microorganisms, however, the medium must be inoculated immediately, and it is the responsibility of the laboratory personnel to be aware of which organisms require immediate inoculation.

Finally, the physician should inform the laboratory of the source of the material to be examined and his tentative diagnosis. This information will help the laboratory ensure that the correct medium is inoculated with the specimen and will aid in the correct identification of the pathogen.

PROTECTION OF LABORATORY PERSONNEL AND STERILIZATION OF MATERIALS

Since the material to be examined in the microbiology laboratory contains dangerous pathogens, it is necessary that the laboratory technician or microbiologist protect himself. For this reason, any microbiology laboratory, whether a teaching laboratory or a clinical laboratory, will have certain rules which must be followed for the protection of the worker.

First, nothing should ever be put into the mouth in the laboratory except for a sterile pipet. Smoking, eating, or drinking in the laboratory is absolutely prohibited, as these are ideal modes of infection. In addition, personal objects such as handbags or eyeglasses should not be placed on the work area, as they may become contaminated with pathogens.

The work area should be cleaned with an agent such as Pheneen or 5% phenol before and after use each day. A mild disinfectant such as

Pheneen is used primarily for cleaning. However, it is important to keep the laboratory free from dust, for this can be the cause of infection by dangerous pathogens. If the work area is actually contaminated, a potent disinfectant such as 5% phenol must be used. For example, if a culture is dropped or spilled, 5% phenol should be poured over the contaminated area and covered with paper towels. This should stand at least 15 minutes. Then the contaminated material must be removed and placed in an appropriate container to be autoclaved.

Hands should be washed thoroughly with soap before leaving the microbiology laboratory. Hands must also be washed in case of contamination. In addition, the technician should not work with uncovered open cuts or broken skin. These should be covered with a bandage or some suitable material.

Since open flames are routinely used in the laboratory in order to sterilize the inoculating "loops" and needles in addition to flaming the lips of test tubes before inoculation, there is a constant fire hazard in the microbiology laboratory. This may be minimized by turning off burners whenever they are not in use. In addition, burners should be kept away from lamps and cotton plugs or other material which is flammable.

These are only a few general considerations that must be kept in mind when working in the microbiology laboratory if the personnel is to remain uninfected by the material with which they are working. Specific laboratories will, no doubt, have additional rules which are established for the safety of the personnel.

Reference has been made to the necessity of collecting specimens for microbiologic analysis in sterile containers because the identification of microorganisms generally requires the isolation and growth of a pure culture of the bacteria. If bacteria are placed on suitable culture media, each bacterium will multiply to a fantastic number, which will grow until an isolated colony of bacteria is formed. It is assumed that each colony of bacteria originates from a single bacterium (or single cell). In culturing bacteria in the laboratory, the infected material is treated in such a way that single bacterial cells are separated on the culture medium and allowed to grow into isolated colonies. Material from a single isolated colony is then further inoculated onto additional media so that several colonies will appear, all arising from a single bacterium. The growth of several colonies originating from a single colony, hence a single cell, is what is meant by a pure culture.

Since various microorganisms are so widely distributed in nature, it is essential that sterile media be used for the cultivation of pure cultures of bacteria. In general, all equipment and/or glassware used in the microbiology laboratory plus all media must be absolutely sterile to ensure the preparation of pure cultures of microorganisms. In addition, any equipment in which microorganisms have been cultured or anything contaminated by infected material must be sterilized. Such material must also be sterilized before it is discarded in order to prevent infection of people responsible for its removal. If equipment is to be reused, it must be sterilized before a new microorganism can be isolated and identified.

Sterilization refers to the killing or destruction of all forms of life. There are various ways in which sterilization may be achieved. In general, they involve physical means such as heat or filtration and chemical means such as oxidation.

The effect of heat on organisms is generally known and is the most widely used and efficient method of sterilization by physical means. Actually, heat may be employed in the form of *dry heat* or *moist heat*. Dry heat destroys bacteria by means of oxidation, while moist heat works through the coagulation of protein.[1] Except for actual burning or incineration, sterilization by moist heat is generally more rapid. However, the type of sterilization method which is used will depend on the nature of the material being sterilized, since many materials are destroyed by burning and many are harmed by the application of moist heat. The use of dry heat in sterilization includes burning and sterilization by means of hot air. Sterilization by means of moist heat includes the use of boiling water; "live" steam, which is steam at atmospheric pressure; and steam under pressure.

Sterilization by means of burning is especially useful in the microbiology laboratory in the various steps in the culture and identification of microorganisms. Infected material from the original specimen, material from isolated colonies, or materials from liquid cultures are usually transferred or manipulated by means of a transfer needle or inoculating loop. These needles and loops are made of very inert metals such as platinum or a suitable alloy such as Nichrome. These materials are unharmed when held in a bunsen or alcohol flame and are sterilized in this manner. Therefore, when material is to be transferred, the inoculating, loop, or wire, is flamed to glowing in a bunsen or alcohol flame, cooled to room temperature by waiting approximately 30 seconds, and then reflamed after use to achieve sterilization. The bunsen or alcohol flame is also used to flame the lip of test tubes containing culture media before and after microorganisms are introduced. The top of certain culture media in Petri plates is also flamed when the plates are "poured," or the medium is prepared.

Another form of sterilization by dry heat is the use of *dry air*. This is achieved by means of a dry-air chamber of a type similar to an oven. Sterilization by dry air requires that the material be kept at a temperature between 150 and 160°C for at least an hour.[1] In addition, the material to be sterilized by this method must be a good heat conductor, or it will not be sterilized in this time. This method is most useful for materials which will be destroyed by moist heat. Sterilization by dry heat is often used for pipets in the microbiology laboratory in addition to other glassware.

Moist-heat sterilization by means of *boiling water* is useful in that it requires little special equipment. Boiling in water for 5 minutes is sufficient to kill all vegetative forms of bacteria. Unfortunately, certain species of bacteria of the genus *Bacillus* have the ability to form spores. Spores are highly resistant forms of the bacteria which form during unfavorable conditions but return to the normal vegetative cell once favorable conditions return. Since spores are highly resistant forms of bacteria, they pose a great problem in sterilization. In order to kill spores by means of boiling in water, 1 to 2 hours of boiling is generally required, although certain spores have been known to survive 16 hours of boiling. For this reason, certain chemicals may be added to the water to achieve more rapid sterilization by boiling. For example, 1% sodium carbonate makes the destruction of spores more rapid in addition to preventing rusting of certain metals sterilized in this manner. Also 2 to 5% carbolic acid may be used to achieve more rapid sterilization. This will usually kill anthrax spores in 10 to 15 minutes.[1]

The method of sterilization by means of moist heat that makes use of *live steam,* or steam at atmospheric pressure, usually employes the Arnold sterilizer, although makeshift apparatus may be devised from kitchen equipment. A modification of sterilization with live steam is sometimes required in the microbiology laboratory when a certain medium is to be sterilized. This involves the use of live steam by means of fractional sterilization, or Tyndallization. This method is required for materials or media which cannot tolerate high temperature and pressure. However, live steam will not kill spores, since the temperature of 100°C or slightly higher is not sufficient. In order to achieve the destruction of spores, the material to be sterilized is exposed to live steam for 15 to 30 minutes on 3 successive days. Vegetative cells will be killed by exposure to steam for 15 to 30 minutes. With fractional sterilization, the exposed material is incubated until the next day. During this time, spores will develop into vegetative cells which will be killed during the next period of exposure to steam for 15 to 30 minutes. The third exposure will ensure sterility. This method, however, can be used only if the material to be sterilized is conducive to bacterial growth. For this reason, fractional sterilization is especially useful for sterilizing culture media but will not be effective for such material as glassware.

The most effective means of sterilization with moist heat is the use of *steam under pressure.* This method uses a special device called an *autoclave.* It is the method of choice for any material of a size which can be placed within the apparatus and which is not injured by moisture or high temperature and pressure. Most media prepared in the microbiology laboratory are sterilized in the autoclave before use. Most equipment is sterilized in this manner, as are infected materials which are to be subsequently discarded. There are several types of autoclaves available. All are basically a heavy metal chamber with a door or lid which can be fastened to withstand the internal steam pressure and must have a pressure gauge, safety valve, and temperature gauge. The steam may be supplied by means of boiling water in the chamber or from heating pipes. No matter what type of autoclave is used, it is essential that *all* air be displaced from the autoclave with steam before the system is sealed. If this is not done, the chamber will contain unsaturated steam. This is a mixture of dry heat and moist heat, and is significantly less efficient in achieving complete sterilization.

Exact details in operation of the autoclave may be found in several standard microbiology texts or with the operating instructions provided with the autoclave. In any case, the material is exposed to pure steam in the autoclave at 121°C for 15 to 20 minutes. This temperature is achieved by applying pressure. Generally 15 lb above atmospheric pressure is required to reach 121°C. This time and temperature will kill all forms of bacterial life including spores. The temperature of steam in an autoclave at 15 lb gauge pressure at sea level is 121.3°C.[2]

In the preparation of certain media which are used in microbiology, none of the preceding means of sterilization is applicable, since they result in deterioration of the media. In these cases, some other means such as filtration through sintered Pyrex (unglazed porcelain, infusorial earth, compressed asbestos, or membranes may be necessary. Or, in some cases, chemical methods of sterilization such as the addition of thymol may be employed.

Not all methods of either complete or partial sterilization or disinfection have by any means been covered in this section. Sterilization or disinfection by chemical means has been omitted from this discussion although it is routinely employed in microbiology. In addition, there are other physical means available such as radiation. A complete discussion of sterilization and/or disinfection is beyond the scope of this text.

MICROBIOLOGIC STUDIES

In order for the microbiologist to identify correctly the causative agent of an infection, there are several tests which must be carried out. These tests involve a general knowledge of microorganisms and their mode of action. Several very good microbiology texts are available. The study of microbiology is an extensive field, far beyond the scope of this text. Many of the students using this text will already have taken a general microbiology course. Others will be given more information by means of lecture material or additional texts. Therefore, this section will deal only with the laboratory aspects of the subject.

MORPHOLOGY OF BACTERIA

Something must be said of the morphology and nature of bacteria in general. Bacteria are a form of fungus. Fungi are the colorless plants, that is, plants which do not contain chlorophyll. More specifically, bacteria are one-celled fungi belonging to the class Schizomycetes, which includes bacteria and related forms of the group Protophyta, the primitive plants.

Each specific bacterium has a shape characteristic of that species. Yet all species of bacteria have one of three basic shapes: If the bacterium is spherical or round, it is a *coccus. Bacilli* are straight, rod-shaped bacteria. If the bacterium is a spiral rod, it is a *spirillum.* Most bacteria are either cocci or bacilli, the bacilli being the most numerous.

There are certain variations of the three basic shapes such as club-shaped bacilli and bacilli with square ends. The particular species of bacterium may be further classified according to whether the cells normally occur singularly; in diploids, or pairs; in chains; or in clusters.

Although bacteria can be seen with the ordinary compound light microscope, they are extremely small structures. They are normally observed under oil immersion using a $97\times$ objective giving a magnification of $970\times$ when the $10\times$ ocular is used. Bacteria are measured in terms of microns. One micron (μ) is one one-thousandth of a millimeter, or about one twenty-five-thousandth of an inch. There is a good deal of variation in the size of different bacteria. Cocci may range from 0.15 to 2 μ in diameter, although most pathogens are from 0.8 to 1.2 μ. The bacilli show an even greater size variation. *Hemophilus influenzae* is a very small rod, about 0.5 μ in length by 0.2 μ in width. *Bacillus anthracis* is a relatively large rod which is 5 to 10 μ in length and 1 to 3 μ in width.[3] A typical red blood cell measures approximately 7 μ in diameter. Bacteria, obviously, are quite small structures.

If bacteria are merely placed on a glass slide and observed under the microscope, they appear as transparent, colorless structures which may be homogeneous or granular. The refractive index of the bacteria is nearly that of water; therefore, they should be stained in order to be more visible. Various staining procedures may be used depending on what information is desired. If only gross morphologic features are to be observed, a simple stain such as with crystal violet, fuchsin, methylene blue, or safranin may be used. However, the most widely used stain in the bacteriology laboratory is the Gram stain, which differentiates bacteria as being gram-positive or gram-negative, besides observing gross morphologic features. There are various other stains such as the acid-fast stain, capsule stains, flagella stains, stains for metachromatic granules, spore stains, relief stains, in addition to stains for spirochetes, rickettsiae, yeast, and fungi. Some specific staining procedures and preparation of slides will be described later in this section.

Each bacterium has four distinct morphologic parts: the protoplasm, cytoplasmic membrane, cell wall, and capsule. Various stains may be used which will accentuate certain of these parts. Other morphologic structures have also been discovered by means of the electron microscope.

CULTURAL REQUIREMENTS OF BACTERIA

In the ultimate discovery of the identity of a particular bacterium, its morphologic character is a useful tool. Determinations should be made concerning the general shape of the bacteria (cocci, bacilli, or spirilla), Gram-staining reaction, and association with other bacterial cells—whether single, in chains, or in clusters—in addition to other determinations that may be required. However, these and other morphologic characteristics will only rarely lead to the final identification of the bacteria under examination. Another essential tool for this final identification of the particular species of bacterium concerns its cultural characteristics. Many (but not all) microorganisms may be grown in the laboratory away from their natural habitat. The artificial growth of microorganisms, however, does require that the proper nutrients and growth conditions be provided. The growth of microorganisms on such artificial material is referred to as a *culture* of the microorganism. The particular mixture of nutrients upon which the microorganism is grown is the *culture medium*) plural, *media*).

In order to culture any microorganism, certain factors must be taken into account, as described in the "Difco Manual of Dehydrated Culture Media and Reagents."[4] First, the *proper food elements* must be available. Different microorganisms will differ in their particular food requirements. Some will grow on media containing simple mixtures of inorganic salts, since they are able to synthesize their own organic compounds. Others, especially many pathogens, or disease-causing organisms, are very fastidious, or particular in their food requirements. These may require complex mixtures of nutrients which include many of the B-complex vitamins, certain amino acids, and other requirements. In general, the culture media must supply an available source of carbon, nitrogen, and inorganic salts. Peptone is used in a variety of culture media to supply a form of nitrogen which can be used by microorganisms. Most organisms are able to use the amino acids and simpler nitrogen compounds present in peptone. Certain bacteria require media to which serum, blood, or ascites have been added. In some media, it is advantageous to add carbohydrates. In some instances, salts such as salts of calcium, manganese, magnesium, sodium, and potassium are required by the microorganism for growth.

In addition to growth requirements, certain dyes, or indicators, may be added to the culture media. These substances may serve as indicators of metabolic activity by the microorganism or as means of selecting the growth of only certain microorganisms by inhibiting the growth of others.

Finally, certain microorganisms either require or will be enhanced by the presence of growth-promoting vitaminlike substances in the media.

Another factor that must be considered in the culture of microorganisms is the requirement for the presence or absence of *oxygen*. Certain microorganisms require the presence of oxygen for growth and will multiply and grow under ordinary conditions of oxygen tension. These oxygen-requiring organisms are called *aerobes,* or *aerobic organisms.* However, certain microorganisms are able to derive oxygen from their food substances. These organisms are actually inhibited by the presence of atmospheric oxygen, and culture requires that atmospheric oxygen be excluded. The organisms which require the exclusion of atmospheric oxygen for growth are called *anaerobes,* or *anaerobic organisms.* There are also organisms with oxygen requirements between the obligate aerobes and obligate anaerobes. The *facultative anaerobes* are able to grow under either aerobic or anaerobic conditions. The *microaerophilic* organisms grow best under conditions of low oxygen tension, and high oxygen tension is inhibitory.

There are various ways in which anaerobic conditions may be obtained in the laboratory. These include such methods as displacement of air by carbon dioxide, the use of special media such as thioglycolate broth, inoculation into the deeper layers of solid media, and addition of small amounts of agar to liquid media.

All microorganisms require a certain amount of *moisture* for growth, since water is a universally required nutrient of all microorganisms. Bacteria in general require a high concentration of water in their environment for growth and multiplication. The formation of highly resistant spores by those bacteria which are spore formers is stimulated by drying, or lack of water. Water is required for the various metabolic reactions which take place within the bacterial cell in addition to being the means through which nutrients are supplied and waste products removed from the cell. Water forms an integral part of the organism's protoplasm and accounts for much of the weight of the bacterial cell.

The actual degree of moisture in various culture media will vary with the type of media used. Media may be used as a liquid, solid, liquefiable solid, or semisolid. Liquid media are frequently referred to as *broths*. They may be converted into solid media by adding whole eggs, egg white, or blood serum and heating until the mixture coagulates. Alternatively, potatoes may be used as a solid medium.

Liquefiable solid media are prepared by adding gelatin, which is a low-melting-point protein, or agar-agar, which is a complex carbohydrate prepared by adding certain seaweeds to a liquid medium such as nutrient broth. Agar-agar is superior to gelatin in a liquefiable solid type of medium. Agar-agar melts just before boiling, solidifies just above body temperature, and is digested by only a few bacteria; it is therefore an ideal additive. Gelatin has a lower melting point than agar-agar, and many organisms will not develop satisfactorily at temperatures below its melting point. In addition, many organisms liquefy gelatin. When gelatin is added to a broth, the medium too is referred to as a *gelatin*. For example, gelatin added to nutrient broth is termed *nutrient gelatin*. When agar-agar is added to a liquid medium, the medium is referred to as an *agar*. In this case, agar-agar added to nutrient broth would be called *nutrient agar*.

Semisolid media are prepared in much the same way as the liquefiable solid media. However, a much smaller amount of agar-agar is added than is used for a true agar, or liquefiable solid media.

Another factor affecting the growth or culture of microorganisms is the *pH* of the medium. Not only must a culture medium contain the proper nutrients in the correct concentration, but the medium must have the correct degree of acidity or alkalinity, or hydrogen ion concentration. Most microorganisms prefer culture media which are approximately neutral, although some require a medium which is distinctly acid. Most microorganisms grow within a pH range of 3.0 to 9.0. Although changes in pH may not actually prevent growth of a particular bacteria, the normal metabolic activities may not exist if the pH is not optimum for the organism. Therefore, most media will be controlled as to their actual pH. This is done by means of buffers, substances which resist changes in hydrogen ion concentration. Buffers are especially useful in the growth of microorganisms which produce acid as part of their metabolic process. These acid producers would kill themselves as a result of their own acid production if a suitable buffer were not present. Conversely, some bacteria produce alkaline products such as ammonia which must also be buffered, or the culture will destroy itself. Blood, milk, and sea water are all solutions which are naturally buffered and therefore useful as culture media. Synthetic media are often buffered by means of phosphate buffer systems.

All organisms have a minimum *temperature* below which development ceases, an optimum temperature at which growth is maximum or luxuriant, and a maximum temperature above which death occurs. The majority of bacteria will grow within a temperature range of 15 to 43°C. However, in general the pathogens have a narrow temperature range with optimum growth at 35°C, and for this reason most cultures in the medical microbiology laboratory are incubated at 35°C. Besides heat, sufficient moisture should also be provided. Since the heat of an incubator would promote drying, the incubator should always be equipped with containers of water or some other suitable source of humidity. In addition, most microorganisms grow in the absence of light, and sunlight should be avoided.

In order to obtain a pure culture of a microorganism, the culture media must be *sterile*. Not only is sterilization necessary for the separation of the inoculated organism, but also contamination by other forms may influence or prevent the growth of the desired microorganism. Most culture media are sterilized by means of the autoclave. Quantities of medium up to 1 liter should be autoclaved for 15 minutes at 121°C. Larger volumes may require a longer period for sterilization. The culture media should be prepared according to directions and then placed in test tubes or erlenmeyer flasks. These are plugged with nonabsorbent cotton, or loosely capped, and placed in the autoclave. Test tubes should be placed in the autoclave in racks or loosely placed in baskets, while flasks should not be filled more than two-thirds full. Oversterilization or prolonged heating must be avoided, as they will change the composition of the medium. This may cause agar media to show a precipitate and may result in an increase in acidity. Some culture media may be harmed by autoclaving. These may require methods such as tyndallization or filtration for sterilization.

Finally, culture media must be protected from *external contamination*. This is achieved by plugging test tubes or flasks with cotton before sterilization. The plug must not be too tight or too loose, and it must protect the lip of the container from contamination by dust. Media and cultures within Petri dishes are protected from such external contamination by the design of the dish. Tubes and flasks may also be covered with screw caps or loosely fitting metal covers. Screw caps must be used with care, for they may result in anaerobic or partially anaerobic conditions. Cotton plugs are useful for preventing the entrance of foreign microorganisms and debris while allowing the entrance of sterile filtered air, which is necessary for the growth of aerobic microorganisms. Loosely fitting metal caps are becoming more popular, for they decrease the fire hazard of cotton plugs and do not tend to fall out of test tubes which have been entered repeatedly, as do cotton plugs.

Although media should not be stored for prolonged periods of time, they are generally prepared in reasonably large batches. Usually these should be stored under refrigeration until they are to be used. This is done to prevent deterioration and dehydration of the media. Certain media require special storage, but such information will be provided with directions for preparation of the specific medium. In general, a medium should be allowed to warm to room temperature before it is inoculated, or microorganisms may be destroyed.

COLONIAL CHARACTERISTICS OF BACTERIA

When inoculated onto suitable semisolid nutrient media with proper temperature and moisture, bacteria will rapidly multiply and form macroscopic colonies. Bacteria multiply by means of binary fission, or division into two equal parts. Macroscopic bacterial colonies will form in 24 to 48 hours. The bacterial colonies originate from an individual cell, although the colony is a mass of individual cells, each one of which functions independently. Different species of bacteria form colonies of different appearance; therefore, colony appearance is useful in identifying a particular species of bacterium. Colony characteristics which are observed in such identification include the following:

1. Bacteria without slime capsules will produce colonies which appear dry and rough.

2. Bacteria with slime capsules appear smooth and shiny.

3. Bacteria may possess a pigment which gives a characteristic color (e.g., white, red, yellow, orange) to the colony.

4. Bacteria may spread from the original colony, motility thus being indicated, while nonmotile bacteria remain in discrete colonies.

Therefore, bacterial colonies should be observed for their relative size, shape, elevation, texture, marginal appearance, and color. This information in addition to morphologic appearance under the microscope and various staining reactions such as the Gram stain reaction will help in the eventual identification of a particular species of bacterium.

SELECTIVE, DIFFERENTIAL, AND ENRICHMENT MEDIA

Although cultural characteristics in addition to morphologic features are invaluable in the identification of bacteria, additional determinations are often necessary. Besides supplying essential nutrients and enabling observation of characteristic colony appearance, culture media may be employed to give additional information. In this sense, the medium may be a selective, differential, or enrichment medium.

Selective media are prepared by adding various dyes, antibotics, or other chemical compounds to certain media. These substances selectively inhibit the growth of certain microorganisms yet permit the growth of others. In other words, they select certain microorganisms for culture.

Enrichment media are usually liquid. These media are used because they permit one organism to grow rapidly while inhibiting the growth of other organisms. Enrichment media are especially useful in the isolation of *Salmonella* or *Shigella* from stool cultures. Such material normally contains several bacteria which are referred to as the *normal intestinal flora.* Yet these organisms are so numerous that they will obscure the growth of the pathogenic *Salmonella* and *Shigella* which must be identified. Therefore, the culture of stool specimens for pathogens normally includes an enrichment medium which will inhibit the normal intestinal flora yet promote the growth of the pathogens which must be identified.

Differential media are especially useful in the microbiology laboratory. These are media which contain certain dyes, indicators, or other constituents which give colonies of a particular organism distinctive and easily recognizable characteristics. The final identification of an organism often requires isolation on a suitable culture medium and then characteristic reaction or growth on a differential medium. Use of such media constitutes a confirmatory test for the microorganism.

SPECIAL EQUIPMENT AND TECHNIQUES FOR
MICROBIOLOGIC STUDIES

Microbiologists have developed special techniques and equipment in order to isolate and grow pure cultures of microorganisms free from the contamination of other microorganisms which are present everywhere. Such techniques and equipment include use of the inoculating needle and bunsen burner, tube cultures, the Petri dish, and preparation of artificial media.

USE OF THE INOCULATING NEEDLE AND LOOP

Probably the most often used and most important tool of the microbiologist is the inoculating needle or loop. This implement may be either a straight wire or wire with a loop at the end inserted into a suitable holder. The wire is usually platinum or an alloy such as Nichrome which can be heated to glowing without being harmed and returned to room temperature fairly rapidly. An object which can be safely heated to red heat will be sterilized almost instantaneously. Therefore, the inoculating needle is extremely useful as the means of transferring microorganisms from one medium to another or from a culture to a microsope slide. Because it can be sterilized in an instant over the flame of a bunsen burner, it can be used quickly and repeatedly for this purpose. Whenever a transfer is to be made, the inoculatiing needle is sterilized in a flame, used to perform the actual transfer, then resterilized before setting the needle aside. The actual procedure for sterilizing the inoculating needle by flaming is as follows (Fig. 6-1):

1. Hold the inoculating needle by the handle as you would a pencil. This leaves the three outer fingers free to remove cotton plugs or tops from test tubes, etc.

2. Push the loop into the upper flame of the bunsen burner at an angle of about 45 to 60 degrees. (Observe special technique for use of a wet needle.) Continue heating until the entire needle is red hot. Then briefly flame the hub of the needle holder.

3. Allow the needle to cool to room temperature before using. If used hot, it will kill the organism under study.

A flame normally consists of two portions: the outer portion of the flame is referred to as the *outer cone,* and within this extending down to the base or origin of the flame is the *inner cone.* It must be remembered that the hottest part of the flame is the upper portion, above the top of the inner cone. The inner part at the base of the flame (inner cone) is cool. If an inoculating needle or loop filled with bacteria is inserted into the hottest part of the flame, a small amount of steam will form. This will result in an explosive sputtering of the material from the loop to the desk top, hands, and clothing of the worker. This is extremely

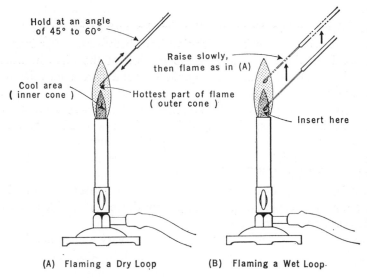

Hold at an angle
of 45° to 60°

Raise slowly,
then flame as in (A)

Cool area
(inner cone)

Hottest part of flame
(outer cone)

Insert here

(A) Flaming a Dry Loop   (B) Flaming a Wet Loop

Fig. 6-1. Flaming of wet and dry inoculating loops.

dangerous, as the bacteria are often still alive when this sputtering of material occurs and can result in accidental infection. In order to prevent this, an alternative method of flaming must be followed: If the needle is wet, it must be first inserted into the cool inner cone at the base of the flame. The needle is then slowly raised through the inner cone and then flamed in the hottest part of the flame. The needle must always be flamed before it is set aside.

TUBE CULTURES AND TUBE CULTURE TRANSFERS

Microorganisms are commonly grown and maintained in test tubes containing liquid or liquefiable solid medium which have been plugged with cotton or covered with loose fitting metal caps or screw caps and sterilized before use. The actual technique used in the introduction and transfer of material from these tubes should be demonstrated by an instructor. In general, the closure is removed by, and held in the outer three fingers of, the hand holding the inoculating needle. The lip of the tube is flamed before and after entry to prevent contamination of the culture. The actual transfer is performed with a sterilized inoculating needle.

PLATE CULTURES AND TRANSFERS

If culture medium is not contained within test tubes, Petri dishes are often used. Petri dishes are shallow glass or plastic plates with loose fitting covers of the same material, shape, and depth as the dish but slightly larger in diameter. The deep cover prevents contamination of the dish. Petri dishes are used for liquefiable solid media. The medium is poured into the dish, allowed to harden, covered, and stored in an inverted position in order to prevent condensation on the surface of the medium. The plates are stored in an inverted position both before and after inoculation. Plates are labeled on the back of the portion of the plate in which the medium is contained. Plates of liquefiable solid media may be used as *streak plates* or as *pour plates*.

Streak plates are prepared by streaking material across the surface of the desired hardened medium contained within a Petri dish. Streaking is especially useful as a means of isolating individual colonies originating from a single bacterial cell. These isolated colonies may then be transferred to another medium. Thus pure cultures may be prepared from mixtures of bacteria. Colony characteristics may also be observed from isolated colonies on streak plates, which leads to the eventual identification of the microorganism under question.

The exact technique of streaking a plate will vary and should be demonstrated. Techniques differ from laboratory to laboratory and even within a given laboratory, depending on the source of material and particular characteristics of the microorganism under investigation. It should be remembered that the streak plate is used primarily as a means of obtaining isolated colonies of microorganisms. In general, a small and sometimes measured amount of the desired material is streaked onto the periphery at one side of the plate. Streaking is achieved by drawing the inoculating loop across the surface of the medium in a zigzag motion. The first streaking is continued across approximately half of the plate. The plate is then turned at right angles and streaked again, beginning at the periphery, overlapping both the previously inoculated area one or two times and the previously uninoculated area. The second streak is continued across half the plate. Finally, the plate is turned at right angles once again and streaked a third time, beginning at the periphery, drawing the loop through the second streaking once, and continuing across the remaining quarter of the plate (Fig. 6-2). The isolated colonies will generally be found in this third area of streaking.

Sometimes the needle must be flamed between each streaking operation besides the essential sterilization before and after inoculation. Sheep blood agar plates are often cut one or more times with the inoculating loop at the conclusion of streaking in the third and/or first area of streaking in order to observe hemolysis reactions of certain bacteria. Some of these techniques will be described under Media Used in Medical Bacteriology.

Pour plates represent another manner of inoculation of culture media within Petri dishes. Although streak plates are far more common in the medical microbiology laboratory, pour plates are sometimes used. Pour plates are generally used as a means of determining the number of viable organisms in a liquid. This method is especially useful in testing such liquids as milk and water for bacterial contamination. In the medical micro-

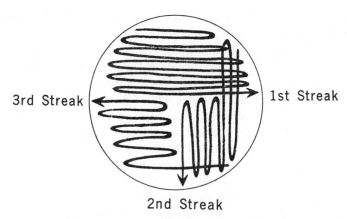

Fig. 6-2. Preparation of a streak plate.

biology laboratory, the pour plate may be used in cultures of blood in addition to other types of specimens.

In general, the pour plate is prepared by first diluting the specimen serially in order to achieve isolation of colonies. The diluted specimen is then inoculated into a liquefiable solid medium which is in the liquid state. The medium and inoculum may be mixed in a test tube or within the plate itself, depending on the particular technique being used. Thorough mixing must be achieved in any case. When the medium has been inoculated at the appropriate temperature for the desired length of time, it is allowed to harden. Plates are then observed for growth and the colonies counted, giving an approximation of the concentration of microorganisms in the original specimen. The use of pour plates rather than streak plates results in at least partially anaerobic conditions in the deeper layers of the plate, facilitating the culture of anaerobic microorganisms. As with streak plates, colonies may be observed on the pour plate itself or introduced into additional media for purposes of obtaining pure cultures or growth on differential media.

PREPARATION OF ARTIFICIAL CULTURE MEDIA[5]

The preparation of artificial culture media for the growth of microorganisms in the laboratory used to be a difficult task. The microbiologist needed to be something of a chef, for he had to concoct a medium suitable for growth of the microorganism under question. He had to be acutely aware of the various growth requirements (nutrients, oxygen, moisture, pH, temperature, and sterility), for he had to be certain that they were all correctly accounted for in his medium.

Today, with the advent of new techniques, the microbiologist is certainly better off, even though he cannot be the creative concoctionist of the past. Although microorganisms have the same requirements for growth as before, the microbiologist no longer needs to assemble his media completely and cook them. The "home" preparation of artificial culture media has been replaced by the availability of commercially prepared dehydrated culture media. The advent of dehydrated culture media has made the preparation of culture media much like the preparation of any reagent in the laboratory. The medium is supplied in a dry form. Basically, all that is necessary is rehydration. Of course, certain precautions must be observed which take into account microbial requirements. The medium is generally supplied in a labeled bottle which gives its exact chemical composition. In addition, the label contains instructions for preparation, in terms of quantity of dehydrated culture medium necessary per liter of reconstituted medium. The person preparing the culture medium must accurately weigh the necessary amount of dehydrated medium, dissolve it in freshly distilled water or freshly boiled distilled water which has been cooled to room temperature, and sterilize the reconstituted medium.

It is important to use distilled water, which should be either freshly distilled or distilled water that has been boiled and cooled to room temperature. If distilled water has been stored, it will have absorbed gases from the atmosphere which alter the composition and pH of the medium. Of course, it is necessary to avoid contamination of the medium while it is being prepared, even though it is to be sterilized before it is ready for use. It is absolutely essential that only chemically clean, sterile glass-

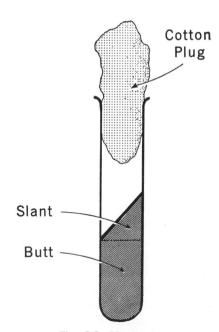

Fig. 6-3. Slant tube.

ware be used for medium preparation. It is extremely important that all traces of detergent be removed from the glassware, as residual detergent will inhibit the growth of bacteria which are to be cultured.

If the medium is to be used in test tubes, it is usually dispensed and autoclaved in the tubes. If liquefiable solid media is to be used in "slant" tubes, the media is dispensed in the liquid state into test tubes, autoclaved, and allowed to harden while set at an angle (Fig. 6-3). If the media is to be used in plates, it is generally autoclaved in erlenmeyer flasks and dispensed into sterile plates under aseptic conditions. The exact techniques will require demonstration by an instructor.

The work of the microbiologist has been made even easier since the advent of dehydrated artificial culture media. It is also possible to purchase a culture medium which has been rehydrated, dispensed in sealed plates or tubes, and sterilized. In other words, the medium is completely ready for use. Although this is more expensive per unit, purchasing such prepared media may be very useful in certain situations such as very small laboratories or physicians' offices with limited storage and preparation facilities.

STAINING TECHNIQUES

One step necessary in the eventual identification of a particular species of bacterium involves morphologic observation under the microscope. Since bacteria are such small structures having a refractive index approximately equal to glass, an observation of bacterial structure requires the use of a stain in order to accentuate the microorganism.

In order to stain bacteria, the material to be examined is thinly spread on a glass microscope slide and allowed to dry. The film should be thin enough to see individual bacteria. If the material to be examined is a liquid, such as a broth culture, the material may be transferred by means of a sterile, cooled inoculating loop and spread directly on the dry slide. If the material is taken from an isolated colony on a Petri plate or other dry material, a drop of sterile water must first be placed on the slide and the desired material added and mixed with the sterile, cooled inoculating loop.

After the material has air-dried, it must be fixed to the slide. To *fix* in a microbiologic sense means to kill, harden, and preserve for microbiologic study. The fixing process prevents many of the bacterial cells from washing off the slide in subsequent operations. Fixing is achieved by merely passing the back of the microscope slide through the burner flame two or three times. The film side of the slide must not be exposed to heat. In addition, the bottom of the slide must not be so hot that it cannot be held against the back of the hand. This heating coagulates the bacterial protein, causing cells to adhere to the slide. However, the air drying and fixing do not necessarily kill all bacterial cells on the slide. Since bacteria encountered in medical microbiology are generally danger- ous pathogens, in order to prevent accidental infection slides must be handled carefully and placed in containers to be autoclaved before being discarded.

SIMPLE STAINING PROCEDURES

Simple staining procedures employing such stains as crystal violet, fuchsin, methylene blue, or safranin have only limited use in the micro- biologic laboratory. They are termed *simple* stains, for they involve the use of only one stain and all structures present are stained the same color. In other words, they accentuate the otherwise colorless bacterial cell, but that is about all. When a simple stain is used, organisms should be observed for size, shape, and uniformity of staining. The staining pro- cedure for one such simple stain used in microbiology, the methylene blue stain, may be performed as follows:

1. Prepare the slide by spreading a thin film of material on the clean microscope slide, air-dry it, and heat-fix it. Place the slide on the staining rack.

2. Flood the surface of the slide with methylene blue staining solution. Allow the stain to remain on the slide for 2 minutes.

3. Wash the slide gently with running water to remove excess methylene blue stain.

4. Allow the slide to dry naturally.

5. Examine the smear with the oil-immersion microscope lens, noticing the size, shape, and uniformity of stain of the microorganisms present.

DIFFERENTIAL STAINING METHODS

Differential staining methods are very useful in the microbiology labora- tory, for, in addition to showing gross morphologic features, they serve to differentiate bacteria or divide them into useful groups. Two of the most widely used differential stains are the Gram stain and various acid- fast stains such as the acid-fast method of Ziehl and Neelsen.

The Gram Stain

Gram's stain is a particularly useful stain in bacteriologic studies. There are several modifications of the method itself, but the stain generally in- volves the primary stain crystal violet; the addition of iodine, which serves as a mordant; decolorization with alcohol-acetone solution, and counter- staining with a secondary stain such as safranin. By using this staining method, bacteria may be divided into two broad groups: Bacteria which stain *purple* as a result of retention of the crystal violet–iodine complex are termed *gram-positive*. Bacteria which stain red by the counterstain are termed *gram-negative*. Differentiation into gram-positive and gram-negative categories is very useful to the microbiologist. Such a differentiation is particularly helpful in determining subsequent tests and means of culture for eventual identification of the particular bacteria. It is also useful in treatment of the patient, for certain antibiotics are generally effective against gram-positive bacteria, while gram-negative bacteria are not as susceptible to their action.

One manner of performing the Gram stain procedure (basically the Hucker modification) is as follows:[6]

Reagents

1. Crystal violet stain.
   a. Stock crystal violet. Dissolve 20 g of crystal violet 85% dye in 100 ml of 95% ethanol.
   b. Stock oxalate solution. Dissolve 1 g of ammonium oxalate in 100 ml of distilled water.
   c. Working solution. Dilute the stock crystal violet solution 1:10 with distilled water. Mix this with 4 vol of stock oxalate solution. Store in a glass-stoppered bottle.
2. Gram iodine solution. Dissolve 1 g of iodine crystals and 2 g of potassium iodide in 5 ml of distilled water. Add to this 240 ml of distilled water and 60 ml of a 5% aqueous solution of sodium bicarbonate. Mix well and store in an amber glass bottle.
3. Alcohol-acetone decolorizer. Mix 250 ml of 95% ethanol and 250 ml of acetone. Store in a glass-stoppered bottle.
4. Safranin counterstain.
   a. Stock safranin. Dissolve 2.5 g of safranin stain in 100 ml of 95% ethanol.
   b. Working safranin. Dilute stock safranin 1:5 or 1:10 with distilled water. Store in a glass-stoppered bottle.

Technique

Step 1:
   a. Flood the heat-fixed slide with crystal violet stain and wait 30 to 60 seconds.
   b. Pour off the stain and rinse with iodine solution.
Step 2:
   a. Cover with iodine solution and wait 1 to 2 minutes.
   b. Rinse with running water shaking off the excess.
Step 3: Decolorize quickly with the alcohol-acetone solution or with 95% alcohol if the alcohol-acetone decolorization proves to be too rapid. Decolorize until no more color is extracted by the

solvent. This usually takes from 20 seconds to 1 minute, but take care not to over decolorize the film.

Step 4:

    a. Flood with safranin for 30 to 60 seconds.

    b. Rinse with water, then allow to air-dry.

To review the steps of the staining procedure:

In the first step, all organisms present are stained violet by the primary stain, crystal violet. The addition of the mordant iodine in the second step results in a violet-iodine complex which is fixed or retained within gram-positive organisms. (A mordant is a substance used in dyeing in general. It combines with the particular dyestuff, forming an insoluble complex, or "lake," which results in a fixed color in the substance to be dyed.) Although it seems that a violet-iodine complex is formed within both gram-positive and gram-negative organisms, this complex is retained within only the gram-positive organisms, and the gram-negative organisms are unaffected by this stain, or dye complex. The exact mechanism involved in retention of this complex within gram-positive and not gram-negative organisms has not been completely defined, although it reflects significant differences between the two groups.

The third step involves decolorization with a mixture of acetone and alcohol. This step removes all color from gram-negative organisms but does not affect the gram-positive organisms, which remain purple because of retention of the violet-iodine complex within the cell. Since the gram-negative organisms are colorless after the third step, they require counterstaining in order to be visible under the microscope. Therefore, the fourth step involves staining of the colorless gram-negative organisms with the red secondary stain safranin.

If a slide were observed under the microscope after each step of the Gram staining process, the following results would be noted. After Step 1, all organisms would be colored purple, as they would be after Step 2. After Step 3, gram-positive organisms would appear purple, while gram-negative organisms would be colorless. After Step 4, the final step, all gram-positive organisms would appear purple and all gram-negative organisms red.

Acid-fast Stain

Another differential stain which is widely used in the microbiology laboratory is the acid-fast stain. This staining technique is used mainly to detect organisms which cause tuberculosis and leprosy. These organisms are extremely difficult to stain by ordinary methods because of their highly resistant fatty (or lipid) cell membranes. Once stained, they retain the dye color, and decolorization is difficult, even with acid-alcohol. Since these organisms resist decolorization by the acid alcohol reagent, they are known as acid-fast bacteria. Other bacteria are easily decolorized by the acid alcohol reagent.

The Ziehl-Neelsen acid-fast method uses carbolfuchsin as the primary stain, heat as the mordant, a mixture of hydrochloric acid and alcohol as the decolorizer, and methylene blue as the counterstain. The Kinyoun acid-fast method uses a slightly different carbolfuchsin preparation and Tergitol number 7 rather than heat as the mordant. After the first step, all bacteria present on the slide appear red. Following decolorization with acid-alcohol reagent, the acid-fast bacteria appear red, while all other bacteria are colorless. After counterstaining with methylene blue, the acid-fast bacteria appear red, while all other cells appear blue.

The acid-fast stain, Kinyoun carbolfuchsin method, may be performed as follows:[7]

Reagents

1. Kinyoun carbolfuchsin stain. Dissolve 4 g of basic fuchsin in 20 ml of 95% alcohol. Add 100 ml of distilled water slowly while shaking the preparation. Melt phenol in a 56°C water bath. Add 8 ml of melted phenol to the stain using a pipet with mechanical suction. (Do not pipet by mouth.) In order to accelerate the staining procedure add 1 drop of Tergitol number 7 to every 30 to 40 ml of the Kinyoun carbolfuchsin stain.

2. Acid-alcohol. Add 3 ml of concentrated hydrochloric acid 97 ml of 95% ethanol.

3. Counterstain. Dissolve 0.3 g of methylene blue in 100 ml of distilled water.

Method

Step 1: Flood the heat-fixed smear with Kinyoun's carbolfuchsin stain with Tergitol number 7 for 1 minute.

Step 2: Wash with water.

Step 3: Decolorize with the acid-alcohol reagent added drop by drop with continual agitation until more carbolfuchsin fails to wash off. This requires approximately 2 minutes for smears of average thickness.

Step 4: Wash with water.

Step 5: Counterstain with methylene blue for 20 to 30 seconds.

Step 6: Wash with water and air-dry.

MEDIA USED IN MEDICAL BACTERIOLOGY[8-12]

Since the eventual identification of a particular species of bacteria requires the culture of that organism on various media (selective, enrichment. and differential), it is important that the student have some knowledge of the more commonly used media in the medical bacteriology laboratory. The media discussed in the remainder of this chapter do not include all media employed in the medical bacteriology laboratory. Some of the more commonly used media have been included, but since there is no one system that is universally employed in the identification of pathogens, some routinely used media have no doubt been omitted. It is hoped that the student will be able to make certain generalizations from the information given and apply it to other situations.

The student should keep in mind certain objectives in terms of what sort of information he should have in his immediate grasp after this study of media. He should be able to recognize the commonly used media by their appearance. He should recognize what change in the appearance of a medium constitutes a positive reaction. He should be able to correlate a characteristic change in the medium with the ability of organisms to carry on certain chemical reactions. In other words, he should be able (1) to recognize the reactions of various indicators at different pH levels, (2) to associate the ingredients of the medium with the stated purpose for using the medium, and (3) to interpret a change in the indicator in relation to the metabolic product which caused the change. Since most media have rather cumbersome names, they are commonly known by certain abbreviations with which the student should be familiar.

Since most commonly used media are contained within either test tubes or Petri dishes, the following material will be divided in two sections, namely, media in test tubes and media in Petri dishes.

MEDIA IN TEST TUBES

Trypticase Soy Broth (Tryp Broth)

Contains: Trypticase soy
Yeast extract
PABA
Agar (0.15% to provide anaerobic conditions)

Tryp broth is a very good general purpose media. Almost everything grows well in it. There are many similar broths with slightly different names. All contain dextrose, some type of peptone, inorganic salts, and water. Most cultures are inoculated into trypticase soy broth to maintain the growth of *all* organisms in the specimen. A small amount of agar is added to the medium to make it thicker, but not enough to solidify it. This permits the growth of some anaerobic organisms, since oxygen does not diffuse to the bottom of the medium if agar is added.

Thioglycolate Broth (Thio Broth)

Contains: Trypticase
    Cystine
    Dextrose
    Sodium chloride
    Sodium thioglycolate
    Resazurin (an oxidation-reduction indicator)
    Small amount of agar

Thio broth is used particularly for the cultivation of anaerobic organisms. It contains thioglycolic acid and agar to encourage anaerobic growth. The medium is in a reduced state, and contains the indicator resazurin, which turns pink if the medium becomes oxidized. If more than one-third of the medium is pink, it contains too much oxygen for anaerobic growth. The oxygen can be driven off by heating the tube of medium. All cultures in which an anaerobic organism is suspected are inoculated into thio broth.

Sugars

Contains: Beef extract
    Peptone
    Sodium chloride
    Bromcresol purple
    One percent sugar solution

Different bacteria ferment different sugars with the production of either lactic acid or lactic acid and gas. The ability of microorganisms to ferment certain sugars often serves to identify them. Sugar tubes contain peptone broth in addition to a 1% solution of the sugar in question. The medium also contains a pH indicator, bromcresol purple, which is purple in alkaline solutions, and yellow in acid solutions. The tube of medium contains a smaller tube which is inverted into the larger tube. This smaller tube indicates the production of gas by the inoculum if it becomes filled with the gas carbon dioxide. If a microorganism ferments the sugar into which it has been inoculated, it will produce lactic acid from the sugar. As a result, the pH of the medium will be lowered. This change of pH is indicated by a color change of the bromcresol purple indicator from purple to yellow. Hence, the presence of a yellow color indicates fermentation of the particular sugar, or a positive reaction. If gas is also produced by the inoculum, the smaller inverted tube will become filled with carbon dioxide. Growth may occur in the various sugar tubes without the production of lactic acid (i.e., without actual fermentation). However, there will be no color change in this case. The three most important sugars used in the identification of bacteria are dextrose, sucrose, and lactose.

Maltose and mannitol fermentation studies are also occasionally desired. The sugar contained within the culture tubes must be indicated by the color of the cotton plug (or other suitable system), since all sugar tubes look exactly alike.

Agar Slants

Agar slants are liquefiable solid media made by heating nutrient agar, placing it in a sterile tube, and cooling the tube at a slant. An agar slant is usually used to preserve a pure culture of a microorganism, either for maintenance of the culture or so that further chemical tests may be conducted on the organism. Slants are inoculated by streaking the desired inoculum on the slant in a zigzag movement from bottom to top.

Simmons Citrate Agar

Contains: Magnesium sulfate
Monoammonium phosphate
Dipotassium phosphate
Sodium citrate
Sodium chloride
Agar
Bromthymol blue

Simmons citrate is also an agar slant. Rather than being nutrient agar, Simmons citrate contains simple inorganic salts. The medium tests the ability of the organism to utilize sodium citrate as its sole source of carbon, and monoammonium phosphate as its sole source of nitrogen. The medium also contains an indicator, bromthymol blue, to indicate growth. Bromthymol blue remains green (the color of the uninoculated medium) when the organism is not growing and turns blue to indicate growth. Therefore, a positive reaction is seen as a change of color of the medium from green to blue. This medium is important in separating different types of gram-negative rods.

Peptone Water with Tryptophan (Indole Medium)

This is the culture medium used for the *indole test*. Tryptophan is an amino acid. The ability of bacteria to split indole from the tryptophan molecule is highly diagnostic. If a microorganism growing in peptone water with tryptophan has produced indole, the addition of Kovac's reagent to the culture results in a red color. Therefore, a positive test for indole production is the production of a red color after addition of Kovac's reagent. The indole test is useful in the identification of the gram-negative rods.

Clark-Lubs Broth (Voges-Proskauer Medium and Methyl Red Medium)

Contains: Peptone water
Two percent dextrose

The Clark-Lubs medium is important as the culture medium for two differential tests: the methyl red test and the Voges-Proskauer test.

The Methyl Red Test

This is merely a test of hydronium ion concentration, or pH. The organism is inoculated into Clark-Lubs broth and incubated at 35°C for 48 hours. After incubation, four to five drops of methyl red indicator is added to the broth. The appearance of a reddish color indicates a pH below 4.4. A yellow color indicates a pH above 4.4.

Voges-Proskauer Test

This tests the ability of the inoculum to produce acetylmethylcarbinol from glucose. The addition of potassium hydroxide to the culture produces a red color if the test is positive (i.e., if acetylmethylcarbinol is formed).

The methyl red and Voges-Proskauer tests are both important in the identification of various gram-negative rods.

Triple Sugar Iron Agar (TSI Slants)

Contains: Nutrients.
One percent lactose.
One percent sucrose.
0.1% dextrose.
Phenol red indicator. Shows yellow in acid pH and red in alkaline pH.
Ferrous sulfate. Becomes black in the presence of hydrogen sulfide.

TSI slants are slant tubes having a lump, or butt, of medium at the bottom and a slant above (Fig. 6-3). It is essential that these slants be inoculated with a pure culture. Therefore, a single, well-isolated colony should be used for the inoculum. The medium is inoculated by streaking the slant and then stabbing the butt with a straight inoculating needle.

The medium is especially useful as a first step in the identification of gram-negative rods. The medium tests the ability of gram-negative rods to ferment dextrose, sucrose, and lactose, and to produce hydrogen sulfide (H_2S). The fermentation of sugars is accompanied by acid production and indicated by a change in color of the phenol red indicator from red to yellow. Production of hydrogen sulfide is indicated by the formation of a black color resulting from combination of hydrogen sulfide with ferrous sulfate. Splitting of the agar in the butt indicates gas production.

Since there are a variety of reactions which occur in the TSI slants, there must be a scheme for reading and recording these reactions. These are noted by recording reactions in the slant and butt as acid (A) or alkaline (Alk) and indicating the production of hydrogen sulfide (H_2S) and/or gas (G). An acid (A) reaction refers to the presence of a yellow color, while an alkaline (Alk) reaction refers to a red color. Various reactions are noted as follows:

Notation	Color Change	Metabolic Change
A/A	Yellow slant, yellow butt	Dextrose fermented, lactose *or* sucrose *or* both fermented.
Alk/A	Red slant, yellow butt	Dextrose fermented, lactose and sucrose not fermented.
Alk/Alk or NR	Red slant, red butt	None of the three sugars fermented, or no reaction.
H_2S	Black in butt	H_2S production
G	Splitting of agar in butt	Indicates gas production.

As indicated, failure of the organism to ferment any of the three sugars results in an Alk/Alk reaction (or no reaction) indicated by a red slant and butt. An Alk/A reaction (red slant and yellow butt) results when only dextrose is fermented. Organisms fermenting dextrose only will originally give an A/A reaction, or yellow slant and butt. However, because of the small amount of dextrose present, the dextrose is used up as the incubation continues. The slant is under aerobic conditions and reverts to alkaline (or red) in 18 to 24 hours. In the butt, however, anaerobic conditions exist. Because of these conditions, there is no reversion to alkaline pH, and the acid (or yellow) reaction remains in the butt.

An A/A reaction (yellow slant and butt) results when dextrose and lactose or sucrose or both are fermented. There is ten times more lactose and sucrose present in the medium than dextrose. Therefore, organisms fermenting lactose or sucrose or both do not use up the sugars except after very prolonged incubation. Therefore, such fermentation of sucrose and/or lactose is indicated by acid (yellow) conditions in both the slant and the butt. However, with prolonged incubation of 48 to 72 hours, lactose and sucrose may also be used up, and formerly acid reactions may revert to alkaline. Therefore, the time of incubation is critical. The time recommended to obtain typical reactions is 18 hours.

There are other media available similar to TSI slants. One such medium is Kligler's iron agar. This medium differs in that it tests fermentation of only dextrose and lactose. Sucrose is not included.

Christianson's Urea Slant (with 1-in. Butt)

Contains: Peptone
　　　　　Urea
　　　　　0.1% glucose
　　　　　Phenol red indicator
　　　　　Buffer

This is an enrichment agar slant which tests the ability of a microorganism to utilize urea as its only source of nitrogen. In order to utilize urea, the organism must produce the enzyme urease. Breakdown of urea by the action of urease results in ammonia production. Ammonia raises the pH of the medium, as indicated by a color change of the phenol red indicator to red. The organism is streaked onto the slant only. The butt is *not* stabbed. Some organisms will result in red color in only the slant, while others will color both the butt and the slant.

Tests for urease production may also be done on urea broth which contains a buffered urea solution and phenol red indicator.

Selenite Broth

Contains: 0.4% sodium selenite

This is an enrichment medium used for stool cultures. The medium inhibits the growth of gram-positive organisms and the coliforms (i.e., gram-negative organisms which are part of the normal intestinal bacterial flora) while favoring and therefore isolating *Shigella* and *Salmonella,* the causative agents of dysentery and typhoid fever, respectively. The medium suppresses growth of organisms other than *Shigella* and *Salmonella* for 12 to 18 hours. After this time coliforms and enterococci grow rapidly. Therefore, subcultures of growth in selenite broth after 18 hours of incubation must be made onto a MacConkey plate or other suitable differential medium. Selenite broth is most effective under reduced oxygen tension. Therefore, it is dispensed into tubes to a depth of 2 in. The broth should be inoculated heavily with fecal material, an amount about the size of a pea.

Motility Test Medium

This is a semisolid medium used to test bacteria for motility. The sterile medium is inoculated by stabbing through the center of the medium with a straight wire to no more than one-fourth the depth of the tube. Motility is indicated by growth of the organism away from the stab.

Loeffler's Slant

Contains: One part dextrose
Three parts coagulated beef serum

This medium is used for detection of *Corynebacterium diphtheriae,* the causative agent of diphtheria. The medium is inoculated with swabs of material taken from the throat. After 24 hours' incubation the growth is smeared and stained with Loeffler's methylene blue and examined for typical morphologic features of the diphtheria bacteria.

Litmus Milk

Contains: Skim milk
Litmus

This medium is used to determine the action of bacteria on milk. Bacteria may ferment, coagulate, peptonize (that is, convert to a clear fluid), or reduce milk. The litmus indicates acid (pink) and alkaline (blue) changes. It also indicates reduction, by turning colorless.

MEDIA IN PETRI DISHES

Sheep Blood Agar (SB, or BA)

Contains: Trypticase soy
Yeast extract
Sodium chloride
Agar
PABA
Five percent fresh sterile sheep blood

This medium is a 5% concentration of sterile sheep blood added to nutrient agar. The medium supports the growth of most ordinary bacteria. It is therefore used for primary plating and for subculturing. It is a good general medium for the growth of pathogens, since the blood adds many of the accessory substances which pathogens require. Most pathogens can be recognized on sheep blood. It is also useful in distinguishing different types of streptococci by their ability to hemolyze the red blood cells present in the medium. They are differentiated as follows:

Alpha streptococci—green hemolysis
Beta streptococci—clear hemolysis
Gamma streptococci—no hemolysis

Human blood can also be used in nutrient agar; however, false hemolysis is often observed. Horse blood works well. SB may inhibit the growth of *H. influenzae,* a common respiratory pathogen in children. Rabbit blood, however, promotes the growth of this organism.

Rabbit Blood Agar (RB)

This medium is a 5% concentration of fresh sterile rabbit blood in nutrient agar. RB is used as the primary culture medium for nose and throat cultures of material taken from pediatric patients or when *Hemophilus* infection is suspected. It is used for the isolation of *H. influenzae,* since it contains the X and V growth factors required by this organism. RB is rarely used for other cultures, because it produces too diffuse hemolysis.

Chocolate Agar

Contains: GC base medium (Difco). This nutrient base medium has a low concentration of agar (1%) which provides the higher moisture content required by some fastidious organisms.

Supplement B (Difco) or Isovitalex (BBL). These supply glutamine, X factor, V factor, cocarboxylase, and other growth factors.

Hemoglobin.

Chocolate agar is prepared by adding blood to the base medium at a temperature of 75 to 80°C. The heat denatures proteins in the blood, causing the blood to coagulate and turn brown. This gives a richer medium than ordinary blood agar and is used in the cultivation of the pathogenic *Neisseria* species. These organisms cause gonorrhea and meningitis, and are difficult to grow. They require an atmosphere of 10% carbon dioxide in addition to the special medium. The medium also supplies the special growth requirements for *H. influenzae*.

Phenylethyl Alcohol Agar (PEA)

Contains: Trypticase
Peptone
Sodium chloride
Agar
0.25% phenylethyl alcohol
Five percent fresh sterile sheep blood

This is essentially SB (sheep blood agar) with phenylethyl alcohol added. The medium inhibits the growth of gram-negative organisms except *Pseudomonas aeruginosa*. PEA allows growth of gram-positive organisms and permits their identification and separation even when they are mixed with gram-negative organisms. If *P. aeruginosa* is present in a mixed culture and isolation of gram-positive organisms is desired, the culture is mixed with ether and then streaked onto the PEA plate, since ether destroys *Pseudomonas*. Hemolysis cannot be read on the PEA plate.

Bordet-Gengou Agar (BG)

Contains: Potato agar base
Fifteen percent fresh sterile rabbit or sheep blood
One percent glycerol (to conserve moisture)

This is a special plate used in the diagnosis of whooping cough, caused by *Bordetella pertussis*. Colonies of the organism have a special diagnostic appearance on this medium. Penicillin may also be added to the medium to inhibit growth of the normal bacterial flora. However, certain strains of *B. pertussis* are also inhibited by penicillin. Therefore, two BG plates should be inoculated, one with and one without penicillin.

Levine's Eosin Methylene Blue Agar (EMB)

Contains: 0.20% eosin. Gives metallic sheen to *Escherichia coli*.
0.005% methylene blue. Inhibits gram-positive organisms.
One percent lactose.

This medium promotes the growth of gram-negative organisms and inhibits gram-positive organisms. In addition, many gram-negative organisms take on a characteristic appearance on EMB. Lactose fermenters produce acid which precipitates the two dyes and give colonies of the lactose-positive organisms a purple center. Urine cultures are inoculated onto EMB plates as well as SB, since many urinary tract infections are caused by gram-negative rods.

MacConkey's Agar (Mac)

Contains: Nutrients.

0.15% bile salts.

One percent lactose.

Neutral red. An acid-base indicator: red indicates acid reaction; yellow, alkaline reaction.

Crystal violet. Inhibits gram-positive organisms.

Mac is a differential medium used in the primary plating of routine stool cultures. The medium should be lightly inoculated. Crystal violet in the medium inhibits growth of gram-positive organisms. Bile salts are included to inhibit growth of nonpathogenic gram-negative organisms. The medium is used in the diagnosis of dysentery, typhoid, and paratyphoid bacteria. These organisms do not ferment lactose. Colonies of organisms which do ferment lactose are red in this medium because of the action of acids resulting from fermentation on the bile salts and subsequent absorption of neutral red. Therefore, the nonlactose fermenters (of which isolation is desired) are yellow or colorless colonies on this medium.

Mac medium is sometimes used in place of EMB, since it tends to inhibit the spread of *Proteus* species more than EMB.

Salmonella-Shigella Agar (SS)

Contains: Nutrients

One percent lactose.

0.85% bile salts (higher concentration than Mac).

Sodium citrate. Inhibits coliforms.

Sodium thiosulfate. Inhibits coliforms.

Ferric citrate. H_2S indicator.

Neutral red. Acid-base indicator.

Brilliant green. Inhibits gram-positive organisms.

SS is a highly selective medium very inhibitory to coliforms and gram-positive organisms. It is used along with Mac in routine stool cultures. The medium should be heavily inoculated. It is designed to isolate the *Salmonella* and *Shigella* species in the presence of other gram-negative organisms. Colonies of lactose fermenters are red and nonfermenters yellowish or colorless on this medium. Organisms which produce hydrogen sulfide colonies show black centers on this medium.

Sabourands Agar

This medium is used to promote the growth of fungi while inhibiting bacterial growth. The medium has a low pH and high osmotic pressure. It should always be incubated at room temperature. Chloramphenicol may be included to inhibit gram-positive and gram-negative organisms. Actinodine may be included in the medium to inhibit nonpathogenic fungi.

CONCLUSION

In determining the cause of a bacterial infection (or disease), it is necessary to separate the various bacteria present in the specimen submitted to the laboratory in order to isolate and identify the causative agent. Specimens will be submitted to the laboratory which are derived from various types of material and different locations in the body. For example, if the patient is suffering from a urinary tract infection, a urine specimen will be submitted for analysis. Respiratory infections will require tests on swabs of material taken from the nose and/or throat. The existence of possible typhoid fever or dysentery will require tests on fecal material. Infections of wounds or presence of abscesses will require examination of material from the site of infection.

In each type of infection or disease, there are certain bacteria which are most likely to be the organism (or pathogen) responsible for the infection. For this reason, each type of specimen that is submitted to the laboratory (be it urine, feces, throat swab, material from wounds, or any other material) will require culture on a certain combination of media which have been found to facilitate identification of the most common pathogens of that area of the body. Each area will have a certain set of media which are used for the primary culture of the organism. After this initial growth and isolation, individual colonies will be subcultured onto various media and undergo various chemical tests in order to confirm the identity of the organism.

It should be understood that there is no one set of tests or culture media which is used in every microbiology laboratory for identification of pathogens from a given source. In fact, numerous schemes for identification may be used. However, certain considerations and generalities will be true of all systems, because of characteristics of the microorganism responsible for infection.

REFERENCES

1. David T. Smith, Norman F. Conant, et al., "Zinsser Microbiology," 12th ed., p. 102, Appleton-Century-Crofts, Inc., New York, 1960.
2. *Ibid.,* p. 104.
3. *Ibid.,* pp. 13–14.
4. "Difco Manual of Dehydrated Culture Media and Reagents for Micro-

biological and Clinical Laboratory Procedures," 9th ed., pp. 16–20, Difco Laboratories Inc., Detroit, 1953, reprinted 1960.

5. *Ibid.,* pp. 21–22.
6. W. R. Bailey and Elvyn G. Scott, "Diagnostic Microbiology," 2d ed., pp. 320–321, The C. V. Mosby Company, St. Louis, 1966.
7. *Ibid.,* pp. 318–319.
8. "Diagnostic Procedures and Reagents," 4th ed., American Public Health Association, Inc., New York, 1963.
9. "Difco Manual of Dehydrated Culture Media and Reagents for Microbiological and Clinical Laboratory Procedures," 9th ed, Difco Laboratories Inc., Detroit, 1953, reprinted 1960.
10. "Difco Supplementary Literature," Difco Laboratories Inc., Detroit, 1962.
11. P. R. Edwards and W. H. Ewing, "Identification of Enterobacteriaceae," Burgess Publishing Company, Minneapolis, 1962.
12. "Products for the Microbiological Laboratory," 4th ed., Baltimore Biological Laboratory, Inc., A Division of Becton, Dickinson and Company, Baltimore, 1959.

7

Electrocardiography and Basal Metabolic Rate Tests

There are two tests performed in most laboratories which require the use of special machines and, in addition, require direct patient contact. Learning to operate these machines is a basic part of many teaching programs for the laboratory technician. One of these tests employs a machine called the electrocardiograph; the other test uses a machine for detecting the patient's basal metabolic rate (BMR). Upon the results of the BMR test and electrocardiography may depend the physician's diagnosis of certain disorders and eventual treatment of the patient. Tests for BMR and electrocardiography are done routinely in most laboratories. In some instances, these tests are run by other departments in the hospital. For example, in some hospitals the x-ray department is in charge of running the electrocardiography tests ordered. Both the BMR tests and electrocardiography are tests which can adequately be performed by a laboratory technician. The ability to approach a patient comfortably and to perform these tests properly are important assets of a competent laboratory technician.

ELECTROCARDIOGRAPHY

Electrocardiography is the graphic recording of the action potentials, or voltages, given off by the heart muscle as it beats. Any muscular activity is accompanied by electrical activity within that muscle. The heart muscle is unique among the muscles of the body in that it possesses the quality of automatic rhythmic contraction. The impulses which precede the actual contraction begin in the conduction system of the heart. Once the impulses are given off, muscle fibers throughout the entire myocardium (heart muscle) are excited. These impulses and their conduction produce weak electric currents which spread through the entire body.

As the heart muscle beats, it gives off a characteristic electrical pattern. This electrical pattern can be recorded by connecting the patient to a machine which receives the voltage from the patient, amplifies it, and produces a tracing of it on tape. This machine is called an *electrocardiograph*. The tape produced by the machine and the information recorded on it are called an *electrocardiogram*, which is abbreviated to ECG (or EKG). By applying a series of electrodes to various positions on the body and by connecting these electrodes to an electrocardiograph machine, the electrocardiogram is made.

THE ELECTROCARDIOGRAPH MACHINE

The history of electrocardiography goes back as far as 1903, when a Dutch physiologist devised the first string galvanometer. The heart currents deflected a quartz fiber, called the "string," and this was magnified and recorded on photographic paper. Since that time, many changes have been made.

There are several types of machines available for making the electrocardiogram. The two types used in the modern laboratory are the string galvanometer type and the electronic amplifier type. Of these two, the electronic amplifier type is the more commonly used machine. Several companies manufacture electrocardiograph machines, most of which are very similar to one another in operation.

The minute voltages which the heart generates as it beats are directed to radio tubes in the machine by means of electrical connections attached to the patient. These connections will be discussed under Leads and Placement of Electrodes and under Patient Preparation. The radio tubes magnify the voltages and also simplify them (Fig. 7-1). From the radio tubes the amplified impulses are directed to a galvanometer. The galvanometer is an extremely sensitive device for measuring electric current. Within the galvanometer is a coil which moves when it receives an electric impulse. The movement, or deflection, is proportional to the strength of the voltage of the electric impulse received. The coil in the galvanometer moves under the slightest influences of the amplified heart voltages. Attached to the coil is a writing arm, or stylus. As the coil moves up and down, so does the stylus. At the end of the writing arm is an electronically heated ribbon of metal called the *stylus ribbon*. The stylus ribbon is placed so that it just slightly touches the moving paper, or tape.

The paper used in the electrocardiograph machine is heat-sensitive. It consists of two layers of plastic, a white coating covering a black layer. When this heat-sensitive paper unrolls beneath the stylus ribbon, the heated ribbon melts away the top white plastic coating, and the black

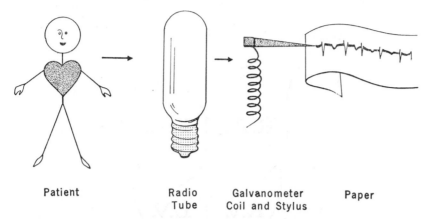

| Patient | Radio
Tube | Galvanometer
Coil and Stylus | Paper |

Fig. 7-1. Pathway of the electric impulse for an electrocardiogram.

layer shows through. As the heated stylus ribbon is deflected by the impulses from the heart, the impulses are recorded permanently on the moving tape, the resulting tape and record being the electrocardiogram.

Each manufacturer of electrocardiograph machines supplies a complete manual with directions for the operation and care of that particular machine. Anyone using such a machine for the first time should read the manual accompanying it. The procedure for the operation of one type of electrocardiograph machine will be described under Operation of the Electrocardiograph Machine.

THE HEART AND THE CIRCULATION OF THE BLOOD

Since the electrocardiograph is a machine used to measure the electric potentials originating from the heart muscle, it is necessary to understand something about the structure of the heart itself. The heart is a hollow, muscular organ which pumps blood through the body's circulatory system. The heart can also be considered a generator of electric energy submerged in a conducting mechanism, the body. There are thousands of individual muscle fibers which produce this electrical activity.

The basic anatomy of the heart includes the four chambers (the right atrium, the left atrium, the right ventricle, and the left ventricle) and e four vessels serving these chambers (Fig. 7-2). The right atrium receives blood from the vena cava. This blood has circulated through the body and has picked up carbon dioxide and other waste materials. When the right atrium contracts, it sends the blood into the right ventricle. After the right ventricle receives the blood from the right atrium, it contracts and sends the blood through the pulmonary artery to the lungs. In the lungs, the carbon dioxide and other waste materials are removed from the blood, and oxygen is added. The blood returns to the heart

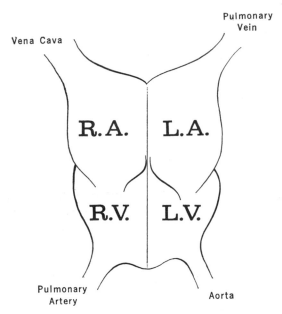

Fig. 7-2. The heart.

by way of the pulmonary vein. The left atrium receives the purified blood from the lungs through the pulmonary vein. When this chamber contracts, it sends the purified blood to the left ventricle. After the left ventricle receives the blood, it contracts and sends the oxygen-containing blood into the aorta. The aorta is the main vessel leaving the heart. It eventually subdivides, sending oxygenated blood to all parts of the body.

The two atria contract at the same time, followed by the contraction of the two ventricles. When the two atria are emptying, the ventricles are filling. Likewise, when the ventricles are emptying, the atria are filling. The contraction of the atira is instigated by a special tissue within the heart called the sinoatrial node, or the "pacemaker." The sinoatrial (S-A) node excites the atria at regular intervals and causes them to contract. When they contract, they send their contents to the ventricles. As the blood flows into the ventricles, another node, the atrioventricular (A-V) node is stimulated. This stimulation causes the contraction of the ventricles, thereby sending the blood out into the body or to the lungs.

CARDIAC WAVES

As mentioned previously, the heart is made up of thousands of tiny muscle fibers. The electric impulses from a normal heart contraction cause definite deflections of the stylus writing arm in the electrocardiograph machine. These deflections follow a definite pattern. Originally, the cause of each of the deflections was not known, so the man who did much of the early work in this field (a man named Einthoven) used letters to label the deflections. The deflections which occur each time the heart beats are known as the *cardiac waves*. These waves are repeated each time the heart beats, and each set of waves is identical with all other sets. The letters P, Q, R, S, T, and sometimes U are used to identify the normal cardiac waves in each set (Fig. 7-3).

The P wave is the first wave of the electrocardiogram. This wave is due to the contraction of the atria, after they have been stimulated by the sinoatrial node. The P wave is usually upright and is short in duration and in height. The Q, R, and S waves are actually a complex wave, referred to as the QRS complex. This group of three waves occurs after the excitation and contraction of the ventricles takes place. The contraction of the ventricles is stimulated by the atrioventricular node. The atria are relaxed during this time. The Q wave is a downward wave. The R wave is upright. The S wave is a downward deflection. The T wave is the last of the normal cardiac cycle waves. It is due to the relaxation of the ventricles. It is an upright wave, a little larger and longer in duration than the P wave. Sometimes the Q and S waves are so small that they do not appear on the electrocardiogram.

In between the P and QRS waves an interval of little or no electric potential exists. This is often referred to as the P-Q interval. Likewise, there is an interval of little electric potential in between the S wave and T wave, called the S-T interval. There is also an interval before the P wave begins again to form another cardiac wave series. There is another cardiac wave, known as the U wave, which is sometimes seen following the T wave and preceding the next P wave. Little is known about the cause for the presence of this wave in the cardiac cycle.

INTERPRETATION OF THE ELECTROCARDIOGRAM

As mentioned previously, a normal heart produces a characteristic electrical pattern. Many heart abnormalities will produce a pattern which deviates from the normal in a diagnostic electrocardiogram. Interpretation of the electrocardiogram can be attempted only by a physician experienced at reading these tracings. Since a normal electrocardiogram has a characteristic pattern, the physician will notice several features before deciding

Fig. 7-3. Normal cardiac wave.

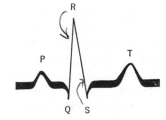

whether a tracing is normal or abnormal. Some of the features noted by the physician are the absence or presence of each of the waves, the shape of the waves (rounded, peaked, smooth, or notched), the direction of the waves (upright, inverted, or diphasic), the time duration of the waves (how long they last), the height or depth of the waves in millimeters, the rate at which they occur (how many heart beats per minute), the rhythm (regular or irregular), and the electrical axis.

All these factors are taken into consideration when the electrocardiogram is judged to be normal or abnormal in appearance. At this point it is pertinent to note that the electrocardiogram is a laboratory test only and is not the only tool available to the physician in diagnosing the presence of heart disease. The electrocardiogram should always be interpreted in conjunction with the other clinical findings available to the physician.

LEADS AND PLACEMENT OF ELECTRODES

For each routine electrocardiogram, a number of sections, or leads, are used each of which measures the electric potential from a different angle. With the most commonly run electrocardiogram there are 12 different leads, or sections. The body serves as the conductor of the electric impulses from the heart. In general, the 12 leads are divided into two main categories, the 6 limb leads and the 6 chest leads. For the limb leads, the connections, or electrodes, are placed on the arms and legs of the patient. For the chest leads, the electrodes are placed at various positions on the chest of the patient.

The first three limb leads are called *bipolar leads,* because they measure the electric potential from one limb to another. These are called leads I, II, and III and are the original leads selected by Einthoven to record the electric potentials in the frontal plane of the body. Lead I measures the potential from the right arm to the left arm. Lead II measures the potential from the right arm to the left leg, and lead III measures the potential from the left arm to the left leg (Fig. 7-4). The bipolar leads actually represent a difference of electric potential between two selected sites as expressed algebraically by Einthoven's equation: lead II = lead I + lead III. It is not necessary for the person running an electrocardiograph machine to comprehend this equation and its use, but the physician reading the resulting electrocardiogram should understand it thoroughly.

With most modern electrocardiographs the right leg is also connected to the machine by means of an electrode. Leads I, II, and III require the use of only the two arms and the left leg. The right leg, when connected to the machine, serves to ground the patient but does not serve as an active electrode in any lead. It may be necessary to extend a grounding wire from the machine to a metal object, such as a water pipe, to eliminate any possible electrical interference.

Electrodes are attached to the patient's arms and legs by means of

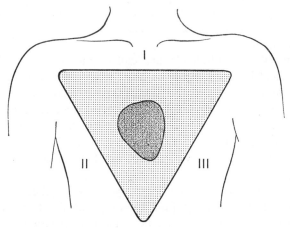

Fig. 7-4. Inverted triangle formed by limb leads I, II, and III.

a strap connection (see also Patient Preparation). Electrode paste or jelly is used to assure good contact between the skin and the metal electrode. The electrodes are made of silver, which is a good conductor of electricity. The paste or jelly which is used in the application of the electrodes to the patient is harmless and noncorrosive. It contains a jellylike base to moisten the skin, salt to promote conductivity, and quartz, an abrasive which slightly reddens the skin and dilates the capillaries to promote better contact. The electrodes should be kept clean and free from tarnish. Any tarnish which occurs may be removed with cleansing powder. Steel wool should not be used on the electrodes. If the electrodes are properly cleaned after each use, corrosion and tarnish will be eliminated.

The three active electrodes placed on the left and right arm and on the left leg, leads I, II, and III, form an inverted triangle around the heart (Fig. 7-4). The electric potential being measured will be the same no matter where the electrode is placed on the extremity. It is therefore not necessary to place the electrodes at a particular place on either the arms or the legs. The formation of the inverted triangle around the heart is of primary importance. The electrodes on the arms may be placed at any point between the wrists and the shoulders. The leg electrodes may be placed at any point between the ankles and the thighs. However, the electrodes are usually placed just above the elbows and ankles. If an extremity has been amputated, the electrode may be placed on the stump remaining. It is also possible to place both electrodes on the same leg, if one leg has been amputated, since only one point of the inverted triangle is formed by the leg. In the case of amputation, it does not matter on which leg the electrode is placed, as long as the electrodes are at least 6 in. apart. In such an instance there must not be any electrode jelly between the electrodes. Since both the arms form a point in the inverted triangle, each arm must have an electrode attached to it. If a patient has an uncontrollable tremor, it is advisable to apply the electrodes on the upper part of the limbs.

The second three limb leads are called *unipolar leads,* because they measure the electric potential of the heart from one particular place. These leads are also called augmented vector (AV) leads. The three unipolar limb leads are designated AVR (augmented vector, right arm), AVL (augmented vector, left arm), and AVF (augmented vector, left foot or leg). Together with the three bipolar limb leads (I, II, and III), the leads AVR, AVL, and AVF make up half of the routine 12-lead electocardiogram.

The last six leads of an electrocardiogram are called the *chest leads.* These leads are obtained by placing an electrode at various positions on the chest. The electrodes must be accurately positioned on the chest. There are specific places at which each electrode must be placed in order to obtain a satisfactory electrocardiogram. The six chest leads are also unipolar, since they each measure the potential at one particular place on the chest. The six chest leads are designated as V1, V2, V3, V4, V5, and V6. The standard positions (as recommended by the American Heart Association) for these six chest leads are listed below (Fig. 7-5):

Lead V1—in the fourth intercostal space at the right sternal border.
Lead V2—in the fourth intercostal space at the left sternal border.
Lead V3—equidistant between V2 and V4.
Lead V4—in the fifth intercostal space in the left midclavicular line,

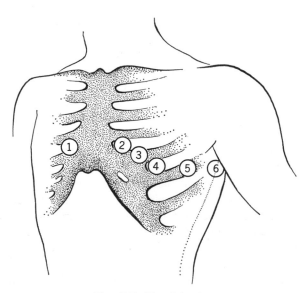

Fig. 7-5. Chest leads.

or at the outer border of the apex beat area. All subsequent leads are taken in the same horizontal plane as lead V4.

Lead V5—in the same plane as V4, in the anterior axillary line.

Lead V6—in the same plane as V4, in the midaxillary line.

There are additional chest lead positions, if more than the usual 12 leads are desired. A seventh chest lead, V4R, is used for all children under sixteen years of age. The position for the V4R lead is in the midclavicular line in the fifth intercostal space to the right of the sternum (the same position as lead V4, except on the right side of the sternum).

Each lead of the electrocardiogram is marked according to a code. This marking system identifies each lead for the physician. The marking pen is heated, like the stylus ribbon, and when the marking button is pressed, it burns the code into the plastic tape. One code which can be used is given below:

Lead I	▬	Lead V1	▬▬ ▬
Lead II	▬ ▬	Lead V2	▬▬ ▬ ▬
Lead III	▬ ▬ ▬	Lead V3	▬▬ ▬ ▬ ▬
Lead AVR	▬ ▬▬ ▬	Lead V4	▬▬ ▬ ▬ ▬ ▬
Lead AVL	▬ ▬▬ ▬ ▬	Lead V5	▬▬ ▬ ▬ ▬ ▬ ▬
Lead AVF	▬ ▬▬ ▬ ▬ ▬	Lead V6	▬▬ ▬ ▬ ▬ ▬ ▬ ▬

STANDARDIZATION

Since not only the shape of the recorded waves but also their height and length can indicate abnormalities, it is necessary for the physician who reads the tracing to know how much voltage a deflection represents. He must also know how long this particular voltage lasted in the heart. For this reason, all electrocardiograms are standardized to make certain that a certain amount of voltage will produce the same deflection in every electrocardiogram. It is necessary to standardize both voltage and time with respect to the ruled tape, in order to determine the time element and voltage strength of an electrocardiogram.

The electrocardiograph paper, or tape, is a graph which is made up of horizontal and vertical lines at 1-mm intervals. There is a darker, heavier line every 5 mm. Time is measured along the horizontal lines: 1 mm represents 0.04 second, and 5 mm represents 0.20 second. Voltage is measured along the vertical lines and is expressed in millimeters. The routine electrocardiographic recording speed is usually 25 mm/second.

An electrocardiogram reads from left to right and measures the passage of time horizontally. Time standardization is not done routinely with every electrocardiogram, but the speed at which the paper moves should be checked occasionally. This can be done simply by running the paper for exactly 1 minute and then checking to see if the proper amount of paper has moved out of the machine. Each of the smallest squares of the paper is 1 mm long and is equal to 0.04, or $\frac{1}{25}$, second. In other words, the paper moves the length of one square, or 1 mm, in $\frac{1}{25}$ second. Each of the large squares is 5 mm long. Each of these large squares is equal to 0.2, or $\frac{1}{5}$, second.

The height of the electrocardiographic waves is measured in millivolts (mv). The vertical lines of the paper are spaced 1 mm apart. A voltage standardization must be done routinely with each and every electrocardiogram that is run. The International Standard is the accepted standard used when measuring an electrocardiogram. Every physician reading an electrocardiogram knows that 1 cm of deflection represents 1 mv of current (Fig. 7-6). If an electrocardiograph is understandardized or overstandardized, that is, if 1 mv of current produces less or more than 1 cm of deflection, the measurements of the entire electrocardiogram will be inaccurate. One millivolt is equal to 0.0001 volts, or 1/10,000 volt. To standardize an electrocardiograph, a potential of 1 mv is applied, causing the writing arm to deflect 1 cm. The sensitivity of the machine must be adjusted until this amount of electricity produces a deflection of 1 cm (or 10 mm). The height of the deflection is always measured from the bottom edge of the baseline to the bottom edge of the deflection. (In this way, the width of the line is not being measured as part of the voltage deflection.) A standardization must accompany each electrocardiogram.

Occasionally, the patient's voltage output will be so great that his deflections will exceed the width of the paper. When this happens, it is necessary to make the standardization smaller by adjusting the sensitivity of the machine so that 1 mv of current produces only 0.5 cm (or 5 mm) of deflection. The machine should be run with this smaller standardization only for those leads which show the great voltage output. As soon as possible, the machine should be returned to its normal standardization. This should be indicated by running a new standardization at 1 cm.

TECHNICAL DIFFICULTIES

Because obtaining an accurate and readable electrocardiogram is so important and because the inherent difficulties of mechanical devices are numerous, it is necessary to consider carefully the many technical factors which can affect the end result of this test.

Tenseness on the part of the patient will show up on the tracing as something called *somatic tremor*. The result of somatic tremor is irregular

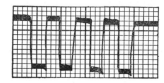

Fig. 7-6. Correct standardization.

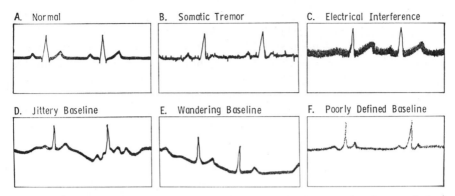

Fig. 7-7. Examples of electrocardiograms—normal and showing technical difficulties.

peaks, uneven in space and unequal in height (Fig. 7-7). The baseline appears fuzzy, and the stylus quivers. There are several remedies for eliminating somatic tremor. The patient should be made comfortable, and his arms should be completely supported. A cot or bed on which the patient can really relax is preferable to a chair. The patient should also be made free from apprehension and should be as quiet as possible. All conversation should be avoided during the running of the test. Sometimes somatic tremor is impossible to eliminate completely. When the patient is very old, nervous, or extremely ill, somatic tremor can be difficult to eliminate. At times, allowing the patient to relax for 10 to 15 minutes can reduce the presence of the tremor. In cases of tremor due to diseases of the thyroid gland or nervous system, the electrodes should be fastened to the patient at a site where the movement is at a minimum—where the limb joins the trunk of the body.

Electrical interference is another common difficulty encountered. In alternating-current (ac) interference, there is a regular "sawtooth" notching of the baseline (Fig. 7-7). Alternating-current interference is usually caused by leakage of alternating electric current from neighboring appliances or wiring. This current is picked up by the patient and enters the machine through the patient cable cord. This type of interference can be distinguished from other types of interference by noting that there are 12 notches or peaks for each $\frac{1}{5}$ second (for each large square on the paper) and 60 peaks for each full second. This shows that the interference is produced by the conventional 60-cycle current. The source of the alternating-current interference must be remedied in order to produce a readable tracing for the physician. No x-ray or diathermy equipment should be in operation near the patient. If no other cause can be found for this interference and the patient is in an oxygen tent, ask a nurse to turn off the tent for a short while. As soon as the electrocardiogram has been run, the nurse must be told to turn on the oxygen tent again. The laboratory technician should never assume the responsibility of turning off an oxygen tent—this should be done by a nurse or doctor. If the patient is on a cooling blanket, ask if it can be turned off for the duration of the test. If a patient is on a litter, a cloth sheet should be placed over the leather in order to avoid any possible interference. The patient must not be touching anything metal. Electrical interference will be seen if this is the case. If a limb is too close to a wall, and hidden wiring is present in that wall, electrical interference will result. If the remedies just discussed fail or do not apply and electrical interference is still seen, an additional grounding wire may be needed. Connect the grounding wire from the machine to something which is metal.

A *wandering baseline,* in which the baseline of the electrocardiogram "drifts" slowly up and down during the tracing, is usually caused by movement of the patient (Fig. 7-7). A wandering baseline is usually a temporary difficulty. To remedy this problem, make certain that the patient is comfortable and fully relaxed at the beginning of the test and during the test. All conversation should be avoided. Wandering may also be caused by a strain, or "drag," on one or more lead wires in the patient cable cord. This difficulty can be remedied by moving the machine and the patient closer together and by resting the crotch of the cable on the patient's body. Poor contact between the electrode and the patient and between the electrode and the cable cord can also cause a wandering baseline to appear. Re-rub the electrodes and check to see that the connections are tight between the cable cord and the electrodes.

A *jittery baseline* is one which moves up and down erratically with quick, jerky movements (Fig. 7-7). This type of difficulty may be caused by poor electrical contact. It may also be caused by having the electrode straps too loose or too tight, or there may not have been enough electrode jelly applied in the initial preparation of the patient. All points of contact should be rechecked. Contaminated electrode jelly may cause a jittery baseline, particularly if it is contaminated with metallic particles. If contamination of the jelly is suspected, the only remedy is to throw away the tube of jelly and use a new one. If the patient's skin has any metallic particles on it, thorough cleaning of the skin at the sites of electrode attachment will eliminate this type of interference. A less likely cause of a jittery baseline is a broken patient cable cord.

A *poorly defined baseline* is another technical difficulty. This occurs when the contact between the paper and the stylus is unsatisfactory. A poorly defined baseline appears thin and gray, and the record is difficult to read (Fig. 7-7). The poorly defined baseline may be due to insufficient heat in the stylus. This may be easily remedied by adjusting the stylus heat with the temperature control button. An accumulation of plastic on the stylus ribbon can also cause a poorly defined baseline. This plastic can be burned off the stylus ribbon with its own heat. If there is insufficient pressure, caused by a slightly bent stylus, for example, a poorly defined baseline may result. If this is the case, it would be wise to let someone with more detailed knowledge of the machine do the adjusting and repair.

PATIENT PREPARATION

Since the attitude, comfort, and general state of mind of the patient can affect the tracing so critically, it is important that the person operating the electrocardiograph machine use the best possible patient approach. The patient should be in a warm, quiet room where complete relaxation is possible. During the test, the patient should be lying down on a comfortable bed, and he should not be touching any metal objects which are grounded. It is not necessary for the patient to remove jewelry or a wrist watch, however, as these will not interfere with the test.

To obtain the best electrocardiogram, as already noted, the patient should be made to feel free from apprehension about the test. The person running the test should assure the patient that the test is a simple one, that it causes no discomfort, and that the best result will be obtained if he lies quietly and is as relaxed as possible. The patient must also be told to avoid any talking during the test and to avoid any movement.

In order that the electric potential from the patient's heart be carried to the electrocardiograph machine, electrodes are first placed on the limbs and the chest. These electrodes are made of silver and are good conductors of electricity. The electrodes are attached to the patient's body by means of a rubber suction cup or strap. A conducting paste, or electrode jelly, is applied between the skin and the electrodes to give better electric conduction. This paste is harmless and noncorrosive. A small amount of the jelly is squeezed from the container onto the inner curved surface of the electrode. The electrode is then fastened on the side of the arm or leg with the connection screw closest to the middle of the body. One electrode is fastened to each of the four limbs. The rubber strap should be fastened tightly enough to provide firm contact between the skin and the electrode. The patient should feel no discomfort; that is, the straps should not be fastened too tightly. Strap electrodes are usually used for the limb leads.

In the same manner, the chest electrode is applied to the first position on the chest wall, by first applying electrode jelly to the chest and then attaching the suction electrode. Suction electrodes are usually used for the chest leads. No electrode jelly should extend beyond the electrode, for the chest leads are point contacts. An excess of jelly is equivalent to a larger electrode, and it may distort the result.

After every test is taken, the electrode jelly is thoroughly wiped off the electrodes. They are washed in hot water and dried well. Carefully done, this will eliminate corrosion and tarnish of the electrodes.

After the electrodes are in place, the patient cable cords are attached to the proper electrode. By means of the cable cord, the electrode is connected to the electrocardiograph machine. The cable cords are identified as to which electrode they are to be attached to. The initials RA for right arm, LL for left leg, and C for chest, are examples of this identification. The cable cord must be firmly screwed into the electrode in order to have the proper contact. A second check should be made to ensure that the correct lead cord is attached to the correct electrode. Mixing up these lead cords will cause abnormalities in the tracing.

OPERATION OF THE ELECTROCARDIOGRAPH MACHINE

Once the patient has been properly connected to the machine, the actual test can be started. As mentioned previously, there are several different companies producing electrocardiograph machines of a good quality (Sanborn, Hewlett and Packard, Cambridge, and Burdick, for example). Each machine requires specific instructions for its use, but, by and large, they all operate on a similar principle. The procedure to be used will depend on the kind of machine which is available. For the purposes of this textbook, the following generalized procedure has been devised.

Procedure

1. Plug the machine into an electric outlet, and check to make certain that it is properly grounded. The machine will not produce a readable tracing unless it is correctly grounded. Usually the machines ground themselves, but this is possible only if the polarity of the power cord is correct. Grounding eliminates alternating-current interferences.

2. Turn the power switch to "on." Be sure to allow the machine to warm up for at least 1 minute.

3. Check to make certain that the patient is lying comfortably on the bed and that the patient is properly connected to the machine.

4. Turn the lead selector switch to the proper position for the standardization. At the beginning of every electrocardiogram, record a standardization to assure the physician that 1 mv of current will produce a deflection of exactly 1 cm. If the standardization does not check out exactly, adjust the sensitivity of the machine until it does. When the standardization is correct, record the rest of the leads.

5. At the time of the standardization, note the thickness of the baseline. The correct width of the baseline is 1 mm, or the width of one small square. The thickness of the baseline is controlled by the amount of heat in the stylus ribbon. If any adjustment is necessary, manipulate the heat control button. Also, at the time of the standardization, note the position of the deflections on the paper. The deflections should be approximately in the middle of the paper (not touching the upper or bottom edges of the paper). There is a positioning, or centering, button which can be adjusted to change the stylus position, should this be necessary.

6. Record the limb leads in this order: leads I, II, III, AVR, AVL, and AVF. Turn the lead selector dial to the appropriate position (there is a position for each of these limb leads, and the dial is switched from position to position for each reading taken). In order that the deflections be recorded properly, the paper must be moving. The power control knob must be turned to the position whereby the paper will move at the stipulated rate (usually 25 mm/second). During the recording of each of the leads, depress the marking button to code or identify each lead properly. Record 8 to 10 in. of each limb lead.

7. Take the six chest leads last, in numerical order: V1, V2, V3, V4, V5, and V6. To switch from one lead to the next, change the position of the chest electrode, according to the standard positions discussed previously. To record the chest leads, turn the lead selector switch to the V position; the paper must be moving. Between each of these chest leads, move the electrode to the next position on the chest wall by turning the lead selector switch to a neutral point, to avoid damage to the machine. Any time a lead is switched or an electrode is changed, the lead selector should be in a neutral position. Each lead should be marked according to the established code. Record 8 to 10 in. of each chest lead.

8. When the last lead has been taken, turn off the power switch, leaving the lead selector switch in the neutral position.

9. Remove the finished tracing from the machine. Write the patient's name and hospital number directly on the tracing. One convenient spot to record this information is somewhere near the standardization. Also record on the tracing the date of the test, the time it was taken, and the initials of the person running the test. This labeling procedure will help to prevent mix-ups and errors. The tracing is then ready to be given to the physician for reading.

10. At the completion of the test, disconnect the cable cords from the electrodes, and remove the electrodes from the patient. Thoroughly wipe off any jelly left on the patient. Clean the electrodes with hot water, and dry them with a towel. Then unplug the power cord from the wall, and put the machine in order for the next test.

FACTORS IN AN ACCEPTABLE ELECTROCARDIOGRAM

Only if the tracing is technically correct can the physician read it with any degree of accuracy. An accurate electrocardiogram should show good electric contact and conduction; that is, no electrical interference should be seen. There must be no somatic tremor. The correct standardization is a necessary part of the electrocardiogram and must be present. The leads must be marked properly. The baseline should be straight (no wandering baseline should be present). The electrocardiogram should be labeled properly with the patient's name, hospital number, date of the test, etc. (see Step 9, under Procedure).

ISOLATION TECHNIQUE FOR TAKING AN ELECTROCARDIOGRAM

When a patient is in isolation, special precautions are necessary to keep the machine and its parts free from contamination. Two operators are necessary. Both operators must be masked and gowned.

One operator remains "clean." This person is responsible for handling the machine and giving to the other operator (without touching the person) any equipment needed during the test. The "clean" operator must also make certain that the electrocardiogram tracing does not touch the floor. This can be done by folding up the tracing as it leaves the machine. When the test is done, the "clean" operator should immediately tear off the tracing and place it safely in the machine drawer or other convenient spot until the physician can read it. The "clean" operator must not touch the patient, the bed, anything in the patient's room, or the other operator.

The second operator is the "dirty" operator. This operator is responsible for plugging in the power cord, attaching the electrodes and the cable cords to the patient, changing the position of the chest electrode, and cleaning up the patient. Since the hands of the "dirty" operator are contaminated, this person must not touch the machine or the other operator.

The special equipment which is needed for an isolation electrocardiogram is an extra set of electrodes and a container of 70% medicated alcohol. When the test has been completed, the "clean" operator soaks gauze with the alcohol and gives this gauze to the "dirty" operator. With it the "dirty" operator then cleans the cable cords and the power cord thoroughly. The "clean" operator follows, also swabbing the cords with alcohol. As they are cleaned, the cords are wound around the machine. The used electrodes are dropped into the alcohol container by the "dirty" operator. These electrodes should remain immersed in the alcohol for at least 20 minutes. Then they are removed and cleaned in the regular manner.

When the cords have been cleaned and the electrodes placed in the container of alcohol, the "clean" operator wheels the electrocardiograph machine out of the patient's room. After the machine is out of the room, this operator returns to the room to discard the gown. The "dirty" operator also discards the gown inside the patient's room. All contaminated gowns are to be left inside the patient's room. Both operators then leave the room and wash their hands very well at a special isolation sink. After their hands are clean, the operators may remove their masks. Isolation masks should be left in a designated place.

THE MASTER TWO-STEP EXERCISE ELECTROCARDIOGRAM

The Master test is an exercise electrocardiogram. It is used to aid in the diagnosis of coronary artery disease and is used in conjunction with other test results and the patient's history.

To perform the Master two-step test, the patient should be at ease and should have had no medications before the test. Smoking can affect the test results; the patient therefore must not smoke prior to the test. A routine 12-lead resting electrocardiogram is first taken. This must be normal before the test is continued. A physician must be present to read the resting electrocardiogram. Leaving the electrodes and cable cords attached to the patient, the cable cord can be unhooked from the machine. The patient is instructed to travel over the specially constructed steps at an easy pace a number of times. The number of times is dependent on the patient's weight, age, and sex. The steps consist of a two-step platform constructed according to specific dimension specifications. In a single Master test, 1½ minutes is allowed for this exercise. In a double Master test, 3 minutes of exercise is allowed. At the end of the exercise on the step platform, the patient immediately returns to the bed, and the exercise electrocardiogram is taken at once. Only short leads need be taken, omitting V2, V3, and V5. Another electrocardiogram is taken 4 minutes after cessation of the exercise, again omitting V2, V3, and V5.

The test should be stopped if the patient complains of chest pains or if he becomes overfatigued. A physician should be present at the time of the exercise, in the event of any severe chest pains. If the patient is sick, the test should not be done.

In normal subjects the test is usually negative. It is positive in at least 95 percent of patients who suffer from coronary artery disease. An S-T depression or elevation and the contours of the T wave may indicate a positive test. False positives are occasionally found in nervous patients. A negative test can direct the physician's attention to other causes of chest pain, such as arthritis, gallbladder disease, peptic ulcer, and hernia.

BASAL METABOLIC RATE

The human body requires energy to carry on its life processes, such as respiration, the heart beat, digestion, and muscle tone. The fuels used for the release of energy are the various proteins, carbohydrates, and fats which are included in the diet. These fuels undergo chemical changes in the body and release their energy slowly. The chemical changes taking place in the body after food is absorbed is known as *metabolism*. The standard unit used to measure metabolism is the *calorie* (cal). The calorie is a measurement of heat, and heat is the form of energy measured in metabolism rate tests. The basal metabolic rate (BMR) is the measurement of energy, or heat, produced by the body at rest. It is the percentile variation of the observed measurement compared with the normal or predicted heat production for an individual of a given height, weight, age, and sex in the postabsorptive state and in complete mental and physical repose.

FACTORS INFLUENCING THE BMR

One of the several factors which influence the BMR of an individual is age. The BMR is low at birth, shows its first rise at the age of three or four years, drops 20 to 25 percent from five to ten years, shows a second rise at puberty, and then shows a gradual decline. It is, therefore, most important that the age of the patient be noted.

The sex of the patient also influences the BMR. The BMR is 7 to 10 percent lower in females than in males.

The BMR correlates closely with the surface area of the body in square meters. The surface area varies inversely with the BMR. For this reason, the patient must be weighed accurately and the weight recorded properly. The height must also be measured accurately.

For each degree rise in Fahrenheit temperature above 98.6° there is a 7.2 percent increase in the BMR. Therefore the patient's temperature is necessary information.

The patient must be in the postabsorptive state. This term means that the patient has had no food for a minimum of 14 hours. The patient is instructed to eat nothing after 7 P.M. the night before the test and to have no breakfast the following morning. When a person is in the postabsorptive state, he is burning a certain combination of food so that his respiratory quotient is constant. This constant is equal to 0.82. The respiratory quotient equals the carbon dioxide (CO_2) expired divided by the oxygen (O_2) taken in (CO_2 expired/O_2 intake). The entire calculation of the BMR is dependent on this constant respiratory quotient and therefore on the patient's being in the postabsorptive state when the test is run. At standard conditions (760 mm barometric pressure and 0°C, or 273° absolute temperature), the calorific equivalent of 1 liter of oxygen is a constant 4.825 calories/hour. The calculation of the BMR is dependent on this fact also.

The patient must also be in a state of physical repose. The patient is instructed to have a minimum of 8 to 10 hours of sleep the night before the test and to come to the laboratory with the least possible exertion on the morning of the test. If the patient is in the hospital, the factor of physical repose is easier to control. A controlled rest period of ½ hour in a comfortable bed and in a quiet cheerful room that is comfortably warm is essential for maintaining the basal conditions. This rest period is necessary for patients coming into the laboratory on an outpatient basis for the BMR test.

Mental repose is another factor which can greatly affect the BMR. It is essential that the patient be free from fear and apprehension about the test. The laboratory technician plays an important role in allaying any such fear and apprehension. A medical laboratory technician dealing with patients directly, as is the case in performing the BMR test, must use tact and consideration. In a quiet, gentle manner, the patient should be instructed as to what will be required of him during the test. During the course of the test, too, the laboratory technician should show a quiet and efficient manner.

Certain medications can influence the measurement of the BMR. Thyroid extract can affect the BMR if it has been taken by the patient within 1 to 3 weeks of the test, depending on the dose. No caffeine, epinephrine, or sedatives should be taken by the patient for at least 24 hours prior to the BMR test.

METHODS FOR MEASURING THE BMR

A method used mainly for research pertaining to the BMR is a direct method whereby the heat produced is measured in a calorimeter. The carbon dioxide expired and the nitrogen excreted are measured by this direct method also.

There are also indirect methods which can measure the BMR. These methods employ the measurement of the oxygen consumption per unit time. One mechanism which is used to measure the BMR indirectly is called the Tissot apparatus. In using this method, the patient breathes outside air into a cylinder. The volume is measured, and samples of the expired air are taken from the cylinder after 1 unit time and analyzed for oxygen and carbon dioxide content. In using this method, the respiratory quotient (RQ) is also obtained in addition to the oxygen consumption.

By and large, the most commonly used methods for determination of the BMR are modified indirect methods. One such method is known as the Benedict-Roth method. This method employs the Benedict-Roth water machine and measures the time it takes for the patient to consume a unit of oxygen. The unit most commonly used is 1 liter. Another machine, called the Sanborn Waterless, measures the oxygen consumption in 1 unit time. Rubber bellows are used in this machine, and a special scale is provided which allows the results to be obtained directly by placing the scale on the test graph. The record is taken on waxed paper. A third machine, employing a modified indirect measurement of the BMR, is called the McKesson Recording Metaboler. This is a waterless machine measuring the oxygen consumption in 1 unit time (usually 6 minutes). This type of machine is used widely and for this reason will be discussed in more detail than the other types mentioned. Most BMR machines contain the same principal parts and operate in a similar manner. Again, the person using any special machine should always consult the direction manual supplied by the manufacturer.

BASIC PARTS OF THE BMR MACHINE

1. Bellows. The bellows expands and contracts with the patient's respirations and is enclosed in the body of the machine. It is supported on

ball bearings and mounted in such a way that it can open and close like a book. A safety valve on the bellows prevents any possible damage to it from overfilling with oxygen.

2. Oxygen tank. The oxygen tank is connected to the bellows by means of a rubber tubing and a stopcock. The rubber tubing is attached to a yoke which fits all oxygen tanks. The bellows is filled with oxygen from this reserve tank by opening the stopcock and turning the oxygen tank handle. The bellows should be filled slowly. After filling the bellows with oxygen, the stopcock should be closed to prevent any seepage of oxygen into the bellows, which would give lower-than-basal, or invalid, test results. When the oxygen tank no longer contains enough oxygen to fill the bellows completely, a new tank must be attached to the BMR machine.

3. Inhaling valve, inhaling tube, inhaler (two-way valve), exhaling valve, and exhaling tube. The patient is connected to the bellows by means of these valves and breathing tubes. The inhaling and exhaling valves look alike externally but are constructed in such a manner that the passage of air can be in only one direction. By means of the inhaler, or two-way valve, it is possible for the patient to have the mouthpiece and noseclip on and at the same time be breathing air from the outside atmosphere and not oxygen from the bellows. In other words, when the inhaler is closed, the patient is breathing outside air; when it is opened, the patient is breathing air from the bellows. Consequently, the inhaler is opened only when the test is actually being run or when the bellows is being emptied of its oxygen contents for some reason.

4. Chart paper. The special paper for this test is fitted onto a studded roller so that there is no danger of its slipping. One roll of paper contains enough paper for about 200 BMR tests. The completed chart can be removed by a tear-off bar. An electric time drive moves the paper on the roller. The paper is so calibrated and the time drive so synchronized that 1 in. vertically is equivalent to 1 liter of oxygen and 1 in. horizontally is equivalent to 1 minute. Therefore, if each test is run for 6 minutes, the common time interval used, 6 in. of paper will have passed over the studded roller. For each 6-minute test, the oxygen consumption line can be drawn. The oxygen consumption line is a diagonal line which connects as many points as possible on the 6-in. distance recorded. Considering the point where the oxygen line intersects the baseline (a dark horizontal line) as the starting point and measuring over 6 in., the oxygen consumption in liters can be read directly off the chart by reading up from the 6-in. point to where the diagonal line crosses this vertically drawn point (Fig. 7-8). The consumption of oxygen in liters is used in the final calculation of the basal metabolism.

5. Recording pen. The pen is a fine capillary instrument that must be able to move freely on a sliding rod. The pen is filled with red recording ink from a reserve supply kept in a small bottle on the BMR machine.

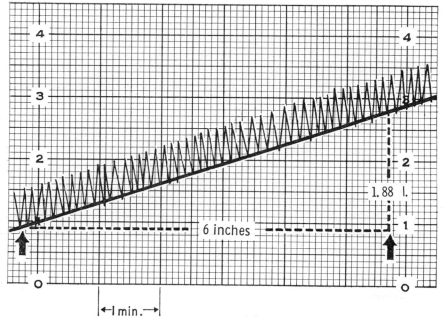

Fig. 7-8. BMR oxygen slope line.

When the pen is not in use, it should be supported by the metal rider and should not be touching the paper. If the sliding rod is not clean, the pen will not move smoothly, and the jerking of the pen and the noise produced can make the patient apprehensive and nervous about the test. The rod can be cleaned by using carbon tetrachloride or zylol.

6. Chemical to remove carbon dioxide from expired air. On the machine is a container with a chemical to remove the carbon dioxide from the expired air. One chemical which is used frequently is called *soda lime*. It consists of sodium hydroxide and calcium oxide. In order to find out the type of chemical which is best for the particular machine being used, contact the manufacturer. The particles of soda lime or other chemical must be of the correct size for maximum efficiency. If the particles are too small, the passage of air can be obstructed; if the particles are too large, there will not be enough surface for absorption purposes. One change of soda lime should suffice for 15 to 20 tests. If the chemical used is not removing all the carbon dioxide and water vapor from the system, the BMR result obtained will be lower than the correct result, because the carbon dioxide goes back into the bellows and is mistaken for unconsumed oxygen. Since carbon dioxide is a respiratory stimulant, it is to be expected that the respirations of the patient will be deeper and more frequent if there is carbon dioxide in the system instead of

the usual oxygen. In this case, a bizarre tracing is usually produced with an irregular oxygen line and exaggerated inspirations and expirations. In some machines there is an indicator crystal which shows the condition of the chemical used to remove the carbon dioxide.

7. Dial thermometer, or spirometer. A dial thermometer, or spirometer, read in degrees centigrade gives the temperature of the oxygen in the bellows. This information, in addition to the barometric pressure, allows the conversion of the consumed oxygen volume to standard conditions. The dial thermometer temperature is taken for each 6-minute test that is run on a patient. This figure is most commonly recorded halfway through the test. As the machine is used, the temperature of the oxygen in the bellows rises. For this reason, the dial thermometer reading must be recorded for each test run.

8. Barometer. Some BMR machines have a barometric unit built into the system. The built-in systems are not usually satisfactory. A separate barometer is more satisfactory, and one must be available, as the barometric pressure of the day is an essential piece of information for the BMR calculation.

9. Oxygen volume viewing scale. This allows the volume of oxygen in the bellows to be approximated.

10. Knob to compress the bellows manually. This knob allows the bellows to be compressed, or emptied of its oxygen contents. It also is used to test the machine for any possible leaks (this is done before any test is run).

11. Mouthpiece and noseclip. The mouthpiece connects the patient to the breathing tubes. The mouthpiece is made of rubber and is curved to fit the mouth. There are usually two sizes, one for adults and most children and one small enough for extremely small-mouthed children. The noseclip has two rubber pads that can be held apart or pinched together. Care must be taken in placing the noseclip in position, so that the passage of air is completely obstructed through the nasal channels. The mouthpieces and noseclips are sterilized after each use. A special mask is available for situations in which the regular mouthpiece and noseclip cannot be used. This is held in place by a strap placed under the patient's head. The mask is placed with the top over the bridge of the nose and the bottom securely over the chin of the patient. In order that leaks do not occur, the mask must be very tightly strapped onto the patient and the edges of the mask properly inflated so that a cushioning effect is produced. When the mask is used, the patient may breathe either through his nose or through his mouth. The mask is attached to the inhaler and breathing tubes of the machine. It should be used only when needed, as in some patients with no teeth or if the patient has a sore nose or one so small that the noseclip may slip off.

PATIENT PREPARATION

The many factors which can influence the BMR have previously been discussed. These factors (age, sex, height, weight, postabsorptive state, mental repose, physical repose, and medications) must all be taken into consideration when preparing the patient for the BMR test. The information regarding these factors must be requested from the patient and recorded on the patient file. A patient should be asked if he has ever had a BMR test before. Often if this test has not been run on a patient before, he can be quite apprehensive about it. Since it is the duty of the laboratory technician to allay the fears and apprehensions of the patient, it is wise to anticipate just what the patient might be worrying about. If the patient is not in the basal condition (if food has been consumed, sleep is inadequate, or the general physical or mental state is not good), the test must be rescheduled. The good judgment of the laboratory technician must be used in these cases, as the answers from some patients, upon questioning, can be quite inadequate.

The patient must be weighed and his height measured. If he is a hospital patient, this information can be taken from the chart. Heights and weights taken from the chart of the patient should be no more than 1 day old. Height can be measured in centimeters, feet, or inches, and weight can be measured in either pounds or kilograms. Using the height and weight for a patient, the surface area may be calculated by using a prepared chart. The surface area is in square meters and is necessary information for the proper calculation of the BMR result.

Mental repose on the part of the patient is essential. The most ideal conditions for taking a BMR would be at the bedside of the patient as soon after he awakens in the morning as possible. This is not usually possible for ordinary laboratory schedules. The patient should come to the laboratory with the least possible exertion and is required to rest for a minimum of ½ hour before the test is taken. There are some exceptions to this rest period. For small children, the rest period is not as long, and the BMR test is taken as soon as they are comfortably settled in the bed. A rest period makes small children even more restless. For extremely nervous persons too the rest period is cut down, since long rest periods tend to make these patients more nervous also. The room should be comfortably warm, and it should be clean, quiet, and restful in atmosphere. The patient should be encouraged to relax as completely as possible.

During the rest period, the patient's temperature is taken. Three minutes is usually a sufficient length of time to leave the thermometer in the patient's mouth. If the patient has lipstick on, it is wise to ask that it be removed with a tissue, as it is difficult to remove lipstick both from the thermometer and from the mouthpiece for the BMR machine. The thermometer should be rinsed in water and wiped off, and the mercury column shaken down below the 97°F mark. The patient should be instructed to hold the thermometer under his tongue for 3 minutes. At the end of 3 minutes, the temperature is read and recorded. After being used, the thermometer is rinsed off with soapy water, wiped with a tissue, and left in a dilution of Zephiran chloride, medicated alcohol, or other suitable solution. The patient should be allowed to rest undisturbed as much as possible.

During the rest period, any information collected concerning the patient is recorded neatly on a permanent record, and any necessary special attention is given to the preparation of the BMR machine.

The patient's pulse rate also is determined during the rest period. The pulse rate is the expansion and contraction of an artery which may be felt with a finger. The pulse is usually felt on the radial artery at the wrist, though it may be felt over the temporal, carotid, ulnar, brachial, or femoral arteries. After the pulse is located, the number of pulsations per minute are counted. Exact timing is necessary for this determination. The regularity of the pulse is also recorded (whether the pulsations are regular or irregular). The pulse is most satisfactorily located by placing the first two fingers of the hand over the radial artery of the patient's wrist; the thumb should not be used to locate the pulsations, as there is a beat in the thumb which can be mistaken for the patient's pulse. The pulse rate should be recorded.

If the patient is coming to the laboratory on an outpatient basis, the blood pressure must also be checked. If the BMR test patient is a patient in the hospital, this information can be obtained from his chart. In order to record the blood pressure for a patient, special equipment must be available, and a certain procedure must be followed.

The blood pressure is the pressure of the blood on the walls of the arteries. It is dependent on the energy of the heart action, the elasticity of the walls of the arteries, the resistance in the capillaries, and the volume and viscosity of the blood in the heart. Two pressures are routinely recorded when taking the blood pressure of a patient. These pressures are called the *systolic pressure* and the *diastolic pressure*. The systolic pressure is the maximum pressure felt at the time of the contraction of the left ventricle of the heart. The diastolic pressure is the minimum pressure felt at the time of the dilatation of the left ventricle of the heart.

To determine the blood pressure accurately, the laboratory technician should have normal acute hearing, since variations in auditory acuity are important. The patient may be either in a reclining position or comfortably seated. The patient should be made to feel at ease, and time should be allowed for recovery from any unusual recent exercise, or apprehension. The arm should be bared, abducted, and perfectly relaxed. If the patient is in a sitting position, the forearm should be supported at the level of the heart, by resting the arm on a smooth surface. The hand may be pronated or supinated later, depending on which position is found to yield the clearest sounds. The deflated blood pressure cuff (called a *sphygmomanometer*) should be applied evenly and snugly around the arm with the lower edge about 1 in. above the antecubital space. If the veins of the forearm are prominently filled or if there is evidence of congestion, the cuff should be applied while the arm is elevated in order to promote venous drainage.

To determine the systolic pressure the mercury level on the sphygmomanometer gauge must be vertical. This applies only when the mercury sphygmomanometer is being used. Many blood pressure cuffs have a sphygmomanometer gauge attached for easier reading. There is no mercury level on this type of sphygmomanometer gauge. A stethoscope receiver should be applied snugly over the artery in the antecubital space, free from contact with the cuff. The pressure in the cuff should then be raised rapidly by vigorous squeezing of the bulb. The air valve on the tubing connecting the bulb to the cuff must be closed before inflating can take place. Once the cuff is properly inflated, the valve is slowly opened, thus decreasing the pressure, a small amount at a time. With the stethoscope still in place over the antecubital space, the first sound of the systolic pressure is listened for intently. When a sound is heard with each heart beat, the reading on the sphygmomanometer is noted as the systolic pressure. With the continued deflation of the cuff below the systolic pressure at a rate of 2 to 3 mm Hg/heart beat, the sounds undergo changes in intensity and quality. As the cuff pressure approaches the diastolic reading, the sounds often quite suddenly become dull and muffled and finally cease altogether. It appears that the point of complete cessation is the best index of the diastolic pressure. This reading is noted as the diastolic blood pressure.

The blood pressure cuff and stethoscope must be in good working condition. Any leaks in the cuff or stethoscope can result in inaccurate readings. Good technique in taking blood pressure is gained, as in so many other laboratory tests, from experience through practice and repetition.

OPERATION OF THE BMR MACHINE

As mentioned previously, there are several companies manufacturing machines for use in determining the BMR. Each manufacturer will supply the purchaser of the machine with a complete manual with directions for operation of that particular machine. Most of the commonly used BMR machines employ the same general parts and involve the same general principles as far as operation is concerned. Again, for the purposes of this textbook, a simplified, general method for the operation of the BMR machine is described.

Procedure

1. Insert the electric plug into the wall outlet.

2. Fill the ink pen with red recording ink from the reserve supply located on the machine.

3. Empty the bellows of oxygen by manually compressing the bellows.

4. Connect the inhaling and exhaling breathing tubes to their respective valves. Close the inhaler.

5. Fill the bellows with oxygen from the supply tank, being certain to open the oxygen stopcock prior to addition of any oxygen. Slowly open the reserve oxygen tank handle, and fill the bellows completely. The bellows is full when the indicator almost reaches "full" on the oxygen volume viewing scale or when the ink pen falls to the 1-in. horizontal line on the chart paper. After filling the bellows with oxygen, close the stopcock so that there will be no further seepage of oxygen from the tank into the bellows. This seepage would give a falsely low BMR.

6. Test the machine for possible leaks by manually compressing the bellows so that the oxygen occupies a smaller volume. The pen will be seen to rise on the movable rod during this compression step. When the pressure is released, the volume of gas (oxygen) should go back to the original volume (the pen goes down on the rod to the same point where it originally rested before the bellows was compressed). The paper may be moved slightly and this procedure repeated several times. If the system is without leaks, the pen returns to its original position each time the bellows is compressed (Fig. 7-9). If, however, there is a leak in the system, each time the volume of oxygen is compressed some gas is forced out through the leak, and the total volume of oxygen decreases slightly. The pen does not come back to its original position. This is shown by a definite "step arrangement" recorded on the chart paper (Fig. 7-9). This method of checking for leaks can be used during the actual test also, when the patient is connected to the machine and breathing into it. In this case, the oxygen slope will change in a "step arrangement" if a leak is present but remain constant with no leak.

7. Connect the patient to the machine by first securely attaching the mouthpiece to the inhaler portion of the machine so that it will be in a parallel position to the mouth of the patient. The inhaler should be

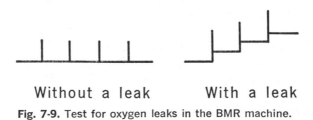

Without a leak   With a leak

Fig. 7-9. Test for oxygen leaks in the BMR machine.

in a closed position, so that the patient can breathe outside air. Do not handle the mouthpiece with bare hands but rather hold it with paper or gauze while positioning it on the machine. Explain to the patient what is expected of him during the test. Show him the mouthpiece, and ask him to hold the rubber prongs between the teeth or gums and the rest of the rubber part between the teeth and the inner lips. The mouthpiece must be held securely in place by the patient. Difficulty can arise at this point when the patient has dentures or no teeth at all. It is important that the arm supporting the breathing tubes be adjusted in such a way as to support the mouthpiece completely. In this way, the patient does not have to strain his neck to support the mouthpiece, and the whole procedure can be made more comfortable for the patient, with better end results.

8. Always adjust the machine to the patient, and be certain that the breathing tubes hang freely and are not distorted. Any distortion produces extra tension on the mouthpiece.

9. Instruct the patient to breathe as naturally as possible through his mouth, as the nose will be closed off with the noseclip. Place the noseclip on the nostrils so that there is complete obstruction of air through the nasal passage. The patient can be told to close his eyes and pretend he is asleep. This often makes him less conscious of his breathing. Also tell the patient that each test is only 6 minutes long.

10. When the patient is comfortably resting, open the inhaler, and turn on the electric timing device. The timing device drives the paper on the rollers at a rate of 1 in./minute. Run each test for 6 in., or 6 minutes. Give every patient a minimum of two 6-minute tests.

11. During each of the 6-minute tests, note and record the following: the temperature of the oxygen in the bellows, read from the spirometer dial; the patient's respirations and any observations regarding his attitude and emotional stability; the regularity of respirations (regular, irregular, natural, deep, shallow, or forced); and physical signs (moistness of skin, tremor, or exophthalmos).

12. At the end of the 6-minute test, turn off the electric timer, and remove the 6-minute test from the chart roller. The mouthpiece and nose-clip are usually not removed between the first and second tests.

13. Before starting the second 6-minute test, refill the bellows with oxygen, if necessary, following the same procedure as previously used.

14. To start the second 6-minute test, turn on the electric timer. Follow the same directions as given for the first test.

15. After the second test, remove the mouthpiece and noseclip from the patient. Draw the oxygen slope line for the tests and calculate the oxygen consumption per 6 minutes. If tests 1 and 2 do not check within 0.06 liter of oxygen, then a third test is started. For a third test, follow the directions for tests 1 and 2.

16. Always begin a fourth test without stopping between tests 3 and 4. However, if test 3 checks out within 0.06 liter of oxygen with either test 1 or test 2, then discontinue the fourth test. If test 3 does not check out, allow the fourth test to run for the usual 6 minutes. In this way, time is not wasted between the tests, and the benefit of a continuous series of tests is obtained without interruption and disturbance to the patient.

17. Use the lowest test, that is, the test showing the least amount of oxygen consumed in 6 minutes, for the calculation. It is assumed that the lowest test is the one closest to the basal state.

18. After use, wash the mouthpiece and noseclip in hot soapy water, rinse them in warm water, and finally boil them for 5 minutes. After boiling, sprinkle the noseclips with talc powder. Wrap the mouthpiece and noseclip in a clean paper towel, and secure them with a rubber band. If the mask is used instead of a mouthpiece and noseclip, wash it thoroughly, but never boil it.

19. Disconnect the breathing tubes from the valves, and rinse them with cold running water several times. Rinse the inhaler during this procedure also. Then place the tubes back on the supporting arm of the machine, and allow them to drain dry.

CALCULATING THE BMR

As already mentioned, the number of liters of oxygen per 6 minutes obtained from the actual breathing test run on the patient is only a part of the information needed for calculating the BMR, other items being the surface area of the patient, the temperature of the oxygen in the BMR machine, and the barometric pressure of the day. In some instances these calculations are made easier by the use of specially prepared reading charts. In order that the laboratory technician student understand thoroughly, however, the steps necessary in the calculation of the BMR, the entire calculation is described as follows:

1. The number of liters of oxygen used by the patient in 6 minutes is obtained by running the breathing test, drawing the oxygen slope line, and calculating this value to the nearest 0.01 liter.

2. The number of liters of oxygen per 6 minutes is multiplied by 10, the result being the number of liters of oxygen consumed in 1 hour.

3. The number of liters of oxygen per hour multiplied by the gas factor equals the calories per hour that the patient used. The gas factor is a mathematical factor which allows correction to standard conditions of barometric pressure (760 mm Hg), temperature (0°C, or 273° absolute), and vapor saturation (80%). In using the gas factor, the calorific equivalent constant (4.825 cal/hour for 1 liter of oxygen) is also employed. Under standard conditions and at a constant respiratory quotient of 0.82 (provided the patient has had no food for a minimum of 14 hours),

the calorific equivalent of 1 liter of oxygen is a constant 4.825 cal/hour. A special conversion table is provided to calculate the gas factor (Table 7-1). To use this table, the information necessary is the barometric pressure of the day and the temperature of the oxygen in the BMR machine.

4. The calories per hour divided by the surface area of the patient in square meters equals the calories per square meter per hour. The surface area of the patient is found by using the Du Bois surface area formula, which involves the height and weight of the patient. The surface area of the patient in square meters is the factor that most closely correlates with the BMR, which varies inversely with the surface area. A special table is provided to find the surface area of a patient (Table 7-2).

5. The calories per square meter per hour compared with the average normal for a person of the same sex, age, and living environment, giving the result in terms of percentile variation of the observed from the normal. The normal standards of the Aub-Du Bois table are used for this discussion. It has been found, however, that the Harris-Benedict standard predictions are the most reliable for average normal subjects. The Du Bois results in normal cases are about 4 percent too high. The Du Bois standards show less deviation than any of the other standards, however, and for this reason they are used commonly. The normal values for comparison purposes are obtained from a table prepared especially for calculation of the basal metabolic rate (Tables 7-3 and 7-4). To use these tables, the age and sex of the patient must be taken into consideration.

6. Once the normal value has been obtained, the observed value is compared with it to obtain the percent BMR by using the following equation:

$$\frac{\text{Normal value } - \text{ observed cal/m}^2\text{/hour (patient)}}{\text{Normal value}} \times 100 = \text{BMR}\%$$

The difference between the normal value and the observed value, divided by the normal value, and multiplied by 100 gives the result in percent. This is the unit desired for reporting the BMR. The BMR is reported as a plus ($+$) or minus ($-$) figure, depending on whether the observed value is greater ($+$) or less ($-$) than the normal value. Plus or minus fifteen (± 15) is considered within the normal range.

7. A temperature correction must be made if the patient's temperature is greater than 99°F. No correction is made if the temperature of the patient is less than 98.6°F (the normal body temperature). For each degree rise in Fahrenheit temperature above 98.6°, there is a 7.2 percent increase in the BMR result. An example of applying the temperature correction factor in the calculation of a BMR result is seen below:

The patient's temperature is 99.8°F. The normal body temperature

Table 7-1. BMR Calculations—Gas Factor

The calorific equivalent of one liter of oxygen (4.825) combined with factors for reduction of volumes to 0°C., 760 M.M. pressure and 80% aqueous vapor saturation.

BAROMETRIC PRESSURE IN M.M.	TEMPERATURE °C																						
	15	16	17	18	19	20	21	22	23	24	25	26	27	28	29	30	31	32	33	34	35	37	38
615	3.65	3.63	3.61	3.59	3.57	3.55	3.53	3.52	3.50	3.48	3.46	3.44	3.42	3.40	3.38	3.36	3.34	3.33	3.31	3.29	3.27	3.23	3.21
620	3.68	3.66	3.64	3.62	3.60	3.58	3.56	3.55	3.53	3.51	3.49	3.47	3.45	3.43	3.41	3.39	3.37	3.36	3.34	3.32	3.30	3.26	3.24
625	3.71	3.69	3.67	3.65	3.63	3.61	3.59	3.58	3.56	3.54	3.52	3.50	3.48	3.46	3.44	3.42	3.40	3.39	3.37	3.35	3.33	3.29	3.27
630	3.74	3.72	3.70	3.68	3.66	3.64	3.62	3.61	3.59	3.57	3.55	3.53	3.51	3.49	3.47	3.45	3.43	3.42	3.40	3.38	3.36	3.32	3.30
635	3.77	3.75	3.73	3.71	3.69	3.67	3.65	3.64	3.62	3.60	3.58	3.56	3.54	3.52	3.50	3.48	3.46	3.44	3.42	3.40	3.38	3.34	3.32
640	3.80	3.78	3.76	3.74	3.72	3.70	3.68	3.67	3.65	3.63	3.61	3.59	3.57	3.55	3.53	3.51	3.49	3.47	3.45	3.43	3.41	3.37	3.35
645	3.83	3.81	3.79	3.77	3.75	3.73	3.71	3.70	3.68	3.66	3.64	3.62	3.60	3.58	3.56	3.54	3.52	3.50	3.48	3.46	3.44	3.40	3.38
650	3.86	3.84	3.82	3.80	3.78	3.76	3.74	3.73	3.71	3.69	3.67	3.65	3.63	3.61	3.59	3.57	3.55	3.53	3.51	3.49	3.47	3.43	3.41
655	3.88	3.86	3.84	3.82	3.80	3.78	3.76	3.75	3.74	3.72	3.70	3.68	3.66	3.64	3.62	3.60	3.58	3.56	3.54	3.52	3.50	3.46	3.44
660	3.91	3.89	3.87	3.85	3.83	3.81	3.79	3.78	3.76	3.74	3.72	3.70	3.68	3.66	3.64	3.62	3.60	3.58	3.56	3.54	3.52	3.48	3.46
665	3.94	3.92	3.90	3.88	3.86	3.84	3.82	3.81	3.79	3.77	3.75	3.73	3.71	3.69	3.67	3.65	3.63	3.61	3.59	3.57	3.55	3.51	3.49
670	3.97	3.95	3.93	3.91	3.89	3.87	3.85	3.84	3.82	3.80	3.78	3.76	3.74	3.72	3.70	3.68	3.66	3.64	3.62	3.60	3.58	3.54	3.52
675	4.00	3.98	3.96	3.94	3.92	3.90	3.88	3.87	3.85	3.83	3.81	3.79	3.77	3.75	3.73	3.71	3.69	3.67	3.65	3.63	3.61	3.57	3.55
680	4.04	4.02	4.00	3.98	3.96	3.94	3.92	3.90	3.88	3.86	3.84	3.82	3.80	3.78	3.76	3.74	3.72	3.70	3.68	3.66	3.64	3.60	3.58
685	4.07	4.05	4.03	4.01	3.99	3.97	3.95	3.93	3.91	3.89	3.87	3.85	3.83	3.81	3.79	3.77	3.75	3.73	3.71	3.69	3.67	3.63	3.61
690	4.10	4.08	4.06	4.04	4.02	4.00	3.98	3.96	3.94	3.92	3.90	3.88	3.86	3.84	3.82	3.80	3.78	3.76	3.74	3.72	3.70	3.66	3.64
695	4.13	4.11	4.09	4.07	4.05	4.03	4.01	3.99	3.97	3.95	3.93	3.91	3.89	3.87	3.85	3.83	3.81	3.79	3.77	3.75	3.73	3.69	3.67
700	4.16	4.14	4.12	4.10	4.08	4.06	4.04	4.02	4.00	3.97	3.95	3.93	3.91	3.89	3.87	3.85	3.83	3.81	3.79	3.77	3.75	3.71	3.69
705	4.19	4.17	4.15	4.13	4.11	4.09	4.07	4.05	4.03	4.01	3.99	3.97	3.94	3.92	3.90	3.88	3.86	3.84	3.82	3.80	3.78	3.74	3.72
710	4.22	4.20	4.18	4.16	4.14	4.12	4.10	4.08	4.06	4.04	4.02	4.00	3.97	3.95	3.93	3.91	3.89	3.87	3.85	3.83	3.81	3.77	3.75
715	4.25	4.23	4.21	4.19	4.17	4.15	4.13	4.11	4.09	4.07	4.05	4.02	4.00	3.98	3.96	3.94	3.92	3.90	3.88	3.86	3.84	3.80	3.78
720	4.28	4.26	4.24	4.22	4.20	4.18	4.16	4.14	4.12	4.10	4.08	4.05	4.03	4.01	3.99	3.97	3.95	3.93	3.91	3.89	3.87	3.83	3.81
725	4.31	4.29	4.27	4.25	4.23	4.21	4.19	4.17	4.15	4.13	4.11	4.08	4.06	4.04	4.02	4.00	3.98	3.96	3.94	3.92	3.90	3.86	3.84
730	4.34	4.32	4.30	4.28	4.26	4.24	4.22	4.20	4.18	4.16	4.14	4.11	4.09	4.07	4.05	4.03	4.01	3.99	3.97	3.95	3.93	3.89	3.87
735	4.36	4.34	4.32	4.30	4.28	4.26	4.25	4.23	4.21	4.19	4.16	4.13	4.11	4.09	4.07	4.05	4.03	4.01	3.99	3.97	3.95	3.91	3.89
740	4.39	4.37	4.35	4.33	4.31	4.29	4.27	4.25	4.23	4.21	4.19	4.16	4.14	4.12	4.10	4.08	4.06	4.04	4.02	4.00	3.98	3.94	3.92
745	4.42	4.40	4.38	4.36	4.34	4.32	4.30	4.28	4.26	4.24	4.22	4.19	4.17	4.15	4.13	4.11	4.09	4.07	4.05	4.03	4.01	3.97	3.95
750	4.45	4.43	4.41	4.39	4.37	4.35	4.33	4.31	4.29	4.27	4.25	4.22	4.20	4.18	4.16	4.14	4.12	4.09	4.07	4.05	4.03	3.99	3.97
755	4.48	4.46	4.44	4.42	4.40	4.38	4.36	4.34	4.32	4.30	4.28	4.25	4.23	4.21	4.19	4.17	4.15	4.12	4.10	4.08	4.06	4.02	4.00
760	4.51	4.49	4.47	4.45	4.43	4.41	4.39	4.37	4.35	4.33	4.31	4.28	4.26	4.24	4.22	4.19	4.17	4.15	4.13	4.11	4.09	4.05	4.03
765	4.54	4.52	4.50	4.48	4.46	4.44	4.42	4.40	4.38	4.36	4.34	4.31	4.29	4.27	4.25	4.23	4.21	4.18	4.16	4.14	4.12	4.08	4.06
770	4.57	4.55	4.53	4.51	4.49	4.47	4.45	4.43	4.41	4.39	4.37	4.34	4.32	4.30	4.28	4.26	4.24	4.21	4.19	4.17	4.15	4.11	4.09
775	4.60	4.58	4.56	4.54	4.52	4.50	4.48	4.46	4.44	4.42	4.40	4.37	4.35	4.33	4.31	4.29	4.27	4.24	4.22	4.20	4.18	4.14	4.12
780	4.63	4.61	4.59	4.57	4.55	4.53	4.51	4.49	4.47	4.45	4.43	4.40	4.38	4.36	4.34	4.32	4.30	4.28	4.25	4.22	4.20	4.16	4.14

is 98.6°F. The normal is subtracted from the observed

$$(99.8 - 98.6 = 1.2°F)$$

to arrive at the difference between the two. A proportion problem is set up as the next step:

$$\frac{7.2\%}{1°F} = \frac{x\%}{1.2°F}$$
$$x = 8.64, \text{ or } 9\%$$

that is, a 9 percent increase in the BMR due to the elevated temperature. This means that the calculated BMR percent minus the temperature correction percent equals the corrected BMR percent. In applying the correction factor it is important to remember the plus and minus signs affixed to the BMR percent. For example, if the result of the BMR calculation is plus 15 percent ($+15\%$) and a temperature correction factor of 9 is to be applied, the corrected BMR result would be plus 6 percent ($+6\%$). If the BMR result is a minus 15% (-15%) and the same temperature correction factor of 9 is to be applied, and the corrected BMR result would be minus 24% (-24%). The corrected result is the one reported to the physician.

If the patient's temperature is more than 2°F above normal, the BMR cannot be accurately determined. In this case, the test is not run, and it is rescheduled for a time when the patient's temperature is lower.

8. The test is considered satisfactory if two tests check within 0.06 of a point and if the oxygen consumption lines were easily drawn and connect most of the points. If the basal requirements are fulfilled but two tests do not check within 0.06 or if they check but the oxygen consumption lines were difficult to draw, then the test is considered fairly satisfactory. If the tests do not check, if the oxygen slope lines were impossible to draw accurately, or if the patient is not under basal conditions, the test is considered unsatisfactory.

9. The chart-paper tracing is usually cut to fit a report sheet for the patient's chart, and the BMR percent is recorded and reported to the physician.

OTHER TESTS

There are other tests which can be determined using the BMR machine or the results of the regular breathing test for BMR previously discussed. One such test is called the *vital capacity* test. The patient is placed almost in a sitting position for this test and the regular noseclip and mouthpiece are attached as for a routine BMR test. The patient is asked to take a deep breath and exhale all the air about five or six times with about ½-minute intervals of normal breathing between. The greatest inhalation

Table 7-2. BMR Calculations—Surface Area

HEIGHT IN CENTIMETERS

WEIGHT IN KILOGRAMS

	100	102	104	106	108	110	112	114	116	118	120	122
18	.692	.702	.712	.721	.731	.741	.751	.761	.770	.780	.789	.799
20	.723	.734	.744	.754	.765	.775	.785	.795	.805	.815	.825	.835
22	.753	.764	.775	.786	.796	.807	.818	.828	.839	.849	.860	.870
24	.782	.793	.804	.815	.826	.837	.848	.859	.870	.881	.892	.903
26	.81	.82	.83	.84	.86	.87	.88	.89	.90	.91	.92	.93
28	.83	.85	.86	.87	.88	.89	.91	.92	.93	.94	.95	.96
30	.86	.87	.88	.90	.91	.92	.93	.94	.96	.97	.98	.99
32	.88	.90	.91	.92	.93	.95	.96	.97	.98	1.00	1.01	1.02
34	.91	.92	.93	.95	.96	.97	.98	1.00	1.01	1.02	1.03	1.05
36	.93	.94	.96	.97	.98	.99	1.01	1.02	1.03	1.05	1.06	1.07
38	.95	.96	.98	.99	1.00	1.02	1.03	1.04	1.06	1.07	1.06	1.10
40	.97	.99	1.00	1.01	1.03	1.04	1.05	1.07	1.08	1.09	1.11	1.12
42	.99	1.01	1.02	1.03	1.05	1.06	1.08	1.09	1.10	1.12	1.13	1.15
44	1.01	1.03	1.04	1.05	1.07	1.08	1.10	1.11	1.13	1.14	1.15	1.17
46	1.03	1.06	1.06	1.07	1.09	1.10	1.12	1.13	1.15	1.16	1.18	1.19
48	1.06	1.06	1.08	1.09	1.11	1.12	1.14	1.15	1.17	1.18	1.20	1.21
50	1.07	1.08	1.10	1.11	1.13	1.14	1.16	1.17	1.19	1.20	1.22	1.23
52	1.09	1.10	1.12	1.13	1.15	1.16	1.18	1.19	1.21	1.22	1.24	1.25
54	1.10	1.12	1.13	1.15	1.17	1.18	1.20	1.21	1.23	1.24	1.26	1.27
56	1.12	1.14	1.15	1.17	1.18	1.20	1.22	1.23	1.25	1.26	1.28	1.29
58	1.14	1.15	1.17	1.19	1.20	1.22	1.23	1.25	1.27	1.28	1.30	1.31
60	1.15	1.17	1.19	1.20	1.22	1.24	1.25	1.27	1.28	1.30	1.32	1.33
62	1.17	1.19	1.20	1.22	1.24	1.25	1.27	1.29	1.30	1.32	1.34	1.35
64	1.19	1.20	1.22	1.24	1.25	1.27	1.29	1.30	1.32	1.34	1.35	1.37
66	1.20	1.22	1.24	1.25	1.27	1.29	1.30	1.32	1.34	1.35	1.37	1.39
68	1.22	1.23	1.25	1.27	1.29	1.30	1.32	1.34	1.35	1.37	1.39	1.41
70	1.23	1.25	1.27	1.28	1.30	1.32	1.34	1.35	1.37	1.39	1.41	1.42
72	1.25	1.27	1.28	1.30	1.32	1.34	1.35	1.37	1.39	1.41	1.42	1.44
74	1.26	1.28	1.30	1.32	1.33	1.35	1.37	1.39	1.40	1.42	1.44	1.46
76	1.28	1.29	1.31	1.33	1.35	1.36	1.38	1.40	1.42	1.44	1.46	1.47
78	1.29	1.31	1.33	1.35	1.36	1.38	1.40	1.42	1.44	1.45	1.47	1.49
80	1.30	1.32	1.34	1.36	1.38	1.40	1.42	1.43	1.45	1.47	1.49	1.51
82	1.32	1.34	1.36	1.37	1.39	1.41	1.43	1.45	1.47	1.49	1.50	1.52
84	1.33	1.35	1.37	1.39	1.41	1.43	1.45	1.46	1.48	1.50	1.52	1.54
86	1.34	1.36	1.38	1.40	1.42	1.44	1.46	1.48	1.50	1.52	1.53	1.55
88	1.36	1.38	1.40	1.42	1.44	1.45	1.47	1.49	1.51	1.53	1.55	1.57
90	1.37	1.39	1.41	1.43	1.45	1.47	1.49	1.51	1.53	1.55	1.56	1.58
92	1.38	1.40	1.42	1.44	1.46	1.48	1.50	1.52	1.54	1.56	1.58	1.60
94	1.40	1.42	1.44	1.46	1.48	1.50	1.52	1.54	1.55	1.57	1.59	1.61
96	1.41	1.43	1.45	1.47	1.49	1.51	1.53	1.55	1.57	1.59	1.61	1.63
98	1.42	1.44	1.46	1.48	1.50	1.52	1.54	1.56	1.58	1.60	1.62	1.64
100	1.43	1.45	1.47	1.50	1.52	1.54	1.56	1.58	1.60	1.62	1.64	1.66
102	1.45	1.47	1.49	1.51	1.53	1.55	1.57	1.59	1.61	1.63	1.65	1.67
104	1.46	1.48	1.50	1.52	1.54	1.56	1.58	1.60	1.62	1.64	1.66	1.68
106	1.47	1.49	1.51	1.53	1.55	1.57	1.60	1.62	1.64	1.66	1.68	1.70
108	1.48	1.50	1.52	1.54	1.57	1.59	1.61	1.63	1.65	1.67	1.69	1.71
110	1.49	1.51	1.54	1.56	1.58	1.60	1.62	1.64	1.66	1.68	1.70	1.72
112	1.50	1.53	1.55	1.57	1.59	1.61	1.63	1.65	1.68	1.70	1.72	1.74
114	1.52	1.54	1.56	1.58	1.60	1.62	1.65	1.67	1.69	1.71	1.73	1.75
116	1.53	1.55	1.57	1.59	1.61	1.64	1.66	1.68	1.70	1.72	1.74	1.76
118	1.54	1.56	1.58	1.60	1.63	1.65	1.67	1.69	1.71	1.73	1.76	1.78
120	1.55	1.57	1.59	1.62	1.64	1.66	1.68	1.70	1.72	1.75	1.77	1.79
122	1.56	1.58	1.60	1.63	1.65	1.67	1.69	1.72	1.74	1.76	1.78	1.80
124	1.57	1.59	1.62	1.64	1.66	1.68	1.71	1.73	1.75	1.77	1.79	1.81
126	1.58	1.60	1.63	1.65	1.67	1.69	1.72	1.74	1.76	1.78	1.80	1.83
128	1.59	1.62	1.64	1.66	1.68	1.71	1.73	1.75	1.77	1.80	1.82	1.84
130	1.60	1.63	1.65	1.67	1.69	1.72	1.74	1.76	1.78	1.81	1.83	1.85
132	1.61	1.64	1.66	1.68	1.71	1.73	1.75	1.77	1.80	1.82	1.84	1.86

124	126	128	130	132	134	136	138	140	142	144	146	148
.808	.818	.827	.837	.846	.855	.864	.874	.883	.892	.901	.910	.919
.845	.855	.865	.875	.884	.894	.904	.913	.923	.933	.942	.952	.961
.880	.891	.898	.911	.921	.931	.941	.951	.961	.971	.981	.991	1.001
.913	.924	.935	.945	.956	.966	.977	.987	.997	1.008	1.018	1.028	1.038
.95	.96	.97	.98	.99	1.00	1.01	1.02	1.03	1.04	1.05	1.06	1.07
.98	.99	1.00	1.01	1.02	1.03	1.04	1.05	1.06	1.08	1.09	1.10	1.11
1.00	1.02	1.03	1.04	1.05	1.06	1.07	1.09	1.10	1.11	1.12	1.13	1.14
1.03	1.04	1.06	1.07	1.08	1.09	1.10	1.12	1.13	1.14	1.15	1.16	1.17
1.06	1.07	1.08	1.10	1.11	1.12	1.13	1.14	1.16	1.17	1.18	1.19	1.20
1.09	1.10	1.11	1.12	1.14	1.15	1.16	1.17	1.19	1.20	1.21	1.22	1.23
1.11	1.12	1.14	1.15	1.16	1.17	1.19	1.20	1.21	1.23	1.24	1.25	1.26
1.13	1.15	1.16	1.17	1.19	1.20	1.21	1.23	1.24	1.25	1.26	1.28	1.29
1.16	1.17	1.19	1.20	1.21	1.23	1.24	1.25	1.27	1.28	1.29	1.30	1.32
1.18	1.20	1.21	1.22	1.24	1.25	1.26	1.28	1.29	1.30	1.32	1.33	1.34
1.20	1.22	1.23	1.25	1.26	1.27	1.29	1.30	1.32	1.33	1.34	1.36	1.37
1.23	1.24	1.25	1.27	1.28	1.30	1.31	1.33	1.34	1.35	1.37	1.38	1.39
1.25	1.26	1.28	1.29	1.31	1.32	1.33	1.35	1.36	1.38	1.39	1.40	1.42
1.27	1.28	1.30	1.31	1.33	1.34	1.36	1.37	1.39	1.40	1.41	1.43	1.44
1.29	1.30	1.32	1.33	1.35	1.36	1.38	1.39	1.41	1.42	1.44	1.45	1.47
1.31	1.32	1.34	1.35	1.37	1.39	1.40	1.41	1.43	1.44	1.46	1.47	1.49
1.33	1.34	1.36	1.38	1.39	1.41	1.42	1.44	1.45	1.47	1.48	1.50	1.51
1.35	1.36	1.38	1.40	1.41	1.43	1.44	1.46	1.47	1.49	1.50	1.52	1.53
1.37	1.38	1.40	1.41	1.43	1.45	1.46	1.48	1.49	1.51	1.52	1.54	1.55
1.39	1.40	1.42	1.43	1.45	1.47	1.48	1.50	1.51	1.53	1.54	1.56	1.58
1.40	1.42	1.44	1.45	1.47	1.49	1.50	1.52	1.53	1.55	1.56	1.58	1.60
1.42	1.44	1.46	1.47	1.49	1.50	1.52	1.54	1.55	1.57	1.58	1.60	1.62
1.44	1.46	1.47	1.49	1.51	1.52	1.54	1.56	1.57	1.59	1.60	1.62	1.64
1.46	1.47	1.49	1.51	1.52	1.54	1.56	1.57	1.59	1.61	1.62	1.64	1.66
1.47	1.49	1.51	1.53	1.54	1.56	1.58	1.59	1.61	1.63	1.64	1.66	1.68
1.49	1.51	1.53	1.54	1.56	1.58	1.60	1.61	1.63	1.64	1.66	1.68	1.69
1.51	1.53	1.54	1.56	1.58	1.59	1.61	1.63	1.65	1.66	1.68	1.70	1.71
1.52	1.54	1.56	1.58	1.59	1.61	1.63	1.65	1.66	1.68	1.70	1.72	1.73
1.54	1.56	1.58	1.59	1.61	1.63	1.65	1.66	1.68	1.70	1.72	1.73	1.75
1.56	1.57	1.59	1.61	1.63	1.65	1.66	1.68	1.70	1.72	1.73	1.75	1.77
1.57	1.59	1.61	1.63	1.64	1.66	1.68	1.70	1.72	1.73	1.75	1.77	1.79
1.59	1.61	1.62	1.64	1.66	1.68	1.70	1.71	1.73	1.75	1.77	1.79	1.80
1.60	1.62	1.64	1.66	1.68	1.69	1.71	1.73	1.75	1.77	1.79	1.80	1.82
1.62	1.64	1.65	1.67	1.69	1.71	1.73	1.75	1.77	1.78	1.80	1.82	1.84
1.63	1.65	1.67	1.69	1.71	1.73	1.74	1.76	1.78	1.80	1.82	1.84	1.86
1.65	1.67	1.68	1.70	1.72	1.74	1.76	1.78	1.80	1.82	1.84	1.85	1.87
1.66	1.68	1.70	1.72	1.74	1.76	1.78	1.79	1.81	1.83	1.85	1.87	1.89
1.68	1.70	1.71	1.73	1.75	1.77	1.79	1.81	1.83	1.85	1.87	1.89	1.90
1.69	1.71	1.73	1.75	1.77	1.79	1.81	1.83	1.84	1.86	1.88	1.90	1.92
1.70	1.72	1.74	1.76	1.78	1.80	1.82	1.84	1.86	1.88	1.90	1.92	1.94
1.72	1.74	1.76	1.78	1.80	1.82	1.84	1.86	1.88	1.89	1.91	1.93	1.95
1.73	1.75	1.77	1.79	1.81	1.83	1.85	1.87	1.89	1.91	1.93	1.95	1.97
1.74	1.76	1.79	1.81	1.83	1.85	1.87	1.89	1.90	1.92	1.94	1.96	1.98
1.76	1.78	1.80	1.82	1.84	1.86	1.88	1.90	1.92	1.94	1.96	1.98	2.00
1.77	1.79	1.81	1.83	1.85	1.87	1.89	1.91	1.93	1.95	1.97	1.99	2.01
1.78	1.81	1.83	1.85	1.87	1.89	1.91	1.93	1.95	1.97	1.99	2.01	2.03
1.80	1.82	1.84	1.86	1.88	1.90	1.92	1.94	1.96	1.98	2.00	2.02	2.04
1.81	1.83	1.85	1.87	1.89	1.92	1.94	1.96	1.98	2.00	2.02	2.04	2.06
1.82	1.84	1.87	1.89	1.91	1.93	1.95	1.97	1.99	2.01	2.03	2.05	2.07
1.84	1.86	1.88	1.90	1.92	1.94	1.96	1.98	2.00	2.02	2.05	2.07	2.09
1.85	1.87	1.89	1.91	1.93	1.96	1.98	2.00	2.02	2.04	2.06	2.08	2.10
1.86	1.88	1.90	1.93	1.95	1.97	1.99	2.01	2.03	2.05	2.07	2.09	2.12
1.87	1.89	1.92	1.94	1.96	1.98	2.00	2.02	2.05	2.07	2.09	2.11	2.13
1.89	1.91	1.93	1.95	1.97	1.99	2.02	2.04	2.06	2.08	2.10	2.12	2.14

Table 7-2. BMR Calculations—Surface Area (Continued)

HEIGHT IN CENTIMETERS

WEIGHT IN KILOGRAMS

kg	150	152	154	156	158	160	162	164	166	168	170	172	174
18	.928	.937	.946	.955	.964	.972	.981	.990	.999	1.007	1.016	1.023	1.033
20	.970	.980	.989	.998	1.008	1.017	1.026	1.035	1.044	1.053	1.063	1.072	1.081
22	1.011	1.020	1.030	1.040	1.049	1.059	1.069	1.078	1.088	1.097	1.107	1.116	1.125
24	1.049	1.059	1.069	1.079	1.089	1.099	1.109	1.119	1.129	1.138	1.148	1.158	1.168
26	1.09	1.10	1.11	1.12	1.13	1.14	1.15	1.16	1.17	1.18	1.19	1.20	1.21
28	1.12	1.13	1.14	1.15	1.16	1.17	1.18	1.19	1.20	1.22	1.23	1.24	1.25
30	1.15	1.16	1.18	1.19	1.20	1.21	1.22	1.23	1.24	1.25	1.26	1.27	1.28
32	1.18	1.20	1.21	1.22	1.23	1.24	1.25	1.26	1.28	1.29	1.30	1.31	1.32
34	1.22	1.23	1.24	1.25	1.26	1.27	1.29	1.30	1.31	1.32	1.33	1.34	1.35
36	1.25	1.26	1.27	1.28	1.29	1.31	1.32	1.33	1.34	1.35	1.36	1.38	1.39
38	1.27	1.29	1.30	1.31	1.32	1.34	1.35	1.36	1.37	1.38	1.40	1.41	1.42
40	1.30	1.32	1.33	1.34	1.35	1.37	1.38	1.39	1.40	1.41	1.43	1.44	1.45
42	1.33	1.34	1.36	1.37	1.38	1.39	1.41	1.42	1.43	1.44	1.46	1.47	1.48
44	1.36	1.37	1.38	1.40	1.41	1.42	1.43	1.45	1.46	1.47	1.49	1.50	1.51
46	1.38	1.40	1.41	1.42	1.44	1.45	1.46	1.47	1.49	1.50	1.51	1.53	1.54
48	1.41	1.42	1.43	1.45	1.46	1.48	1.49	1.50	1.52	1.53	1.54	1.55	1.57
50	1.43	1.45	1.46	1.47	1.49	1.50	1.51	1.53	1.54	1.56	1.57	1.58	1.60
52	1.46	1.47	1.48	1.50	1.51	1.53	1.54	1.55	1.57	1.58	1.60	1.61	1.62
54	1.48	1.49	1.51	1.52	1.54	1.55	1.56	1.58	1.59	1.61	1.62	1.63	1.65
56	1.50	1.52	1.53	1.55	1.56	1.58	1.59	1.60	1.62	1.63	1.65	1.66	1.67
58	1.53	1.54	1.56	1.57	1.58	1.60	1.61	1.63	1.64	1.66	1.67	1.68	1.70
60	1.55	1.56	1.58	1.59	1.61	1.62	1.64	1.65	1.67	1.68	1.69	1.71	1.72
62	1.57	1.58	1.60	1.61	1.63	1.64	1.66	1.67	1.69	1.70	1.72	1.73	1.75
64	1.59	1.61	1.62	1.64	1.65	1.67	1.68	1.70	1.71	1.73	1.74	1.76	1.77
66	1.61	1.63	1.64	1.66	1.67	1.69	1.70	1.72	1.73	1.75	1.76	1.78	1.79
68	1.63	1.65	1.66	1.68	1.70	1.71	1.73	1.74	1.76	1.77	1.79	1.80	1.82
70	1.65	1.67	1.68	1.70	1.72	1.73	1.75	1.76	1.78	1.79	1.81	1.83	1.84
72	1.67	1.69	1.70	1.72	1.74	1.75	1.77	1.78	1.80	1.82	1.83	1.85	1.86
74	1.69	1.71	1.72	1.74	1.76	1.77	1.79	1.81	1.82	1.84	1.85	1.87	1.88
76	1.71	1.73	1.74	1.76	1.78	1.79	1.81	1.83	1.84	1.86	1.87	1.89	1.91
78	1.73	1.76	1.76	1.78	1.80	1.81	1.83	1.85	1.86	1.88	1.89	1.91	1.93
80	1.75	1.77	1.78	1.80	1.82	1.83	1.85	1.87	1.88	1.90	1.92	1.93	1.95
82	1.77	1.78	1.80	1.82	1.84	1.85	1.87	1.89	1.90	1.92	1.94	1.95	1.97
84	1.79	1.80	1.82	1.84	1.85	1.87	1.89	1.91	1.92	1.94	1.96	1.97	1.99
86	1.80	1.82	1.84	1.86	1.87	1.89	1.91	1.92	1.94	1.96	1.98	1.99	2.01
88	1.82	1.84	1.86	1.87	1.89	1.91	1.93	1.94	1.96	1.98	1.99	2.01	2.03
90	1.84	1.86	1.87	1.89	1.91	1.93	1.94	1.96	1.98	2.00	2.01	2.03	2.05
92	1.86	1.87	1.89	1.91	1.93	1.95	1.96	1.98	2.00	2.02	2.03	2.05	2.07
94	1.87	1.89	1.91	1.93	1.95	1.96	1.98	2.00	2.02	2.03	2.05	2.07	2.09
96	1.89	1.91	1.93	1.94	1.96	1.98	2.00	2.02	2.03	2.05	2.07	2.09	2.10
98	1.91	1.93	1.94	1.96	1.98	2.00	2.02	2.03	2.05	2.07	2.09	2.11	2.12
100	1.92	1.94	1.96	1.98	2.00	2.02	2.03	2.05	2.07	2.09	2.11	2.12	2.14
102	1.94	1.96	1.98	2.00	2.01	2.03	2.05	2.07	2.09	2.11	2.12	2.14	2.16
104	1.96	1.97	1.99	2.01	2.03	2.05	2.07	2.09	2.10	2.12	2.14	2.16	2.18
106	1.97	1.99	2.01	2.03	2.05	2.07	2.08	2.10	2.12	2.14	2.16	2.18	2.20
108	1.99	2.01	2.03	2.04	2.06	2.08	2.10	2.12	2.14	2.16	2.18	2.19	2.21
110	2.00	2.02	2.04	2.06	2.08	2.10	2.12	2.14	2.16	2.17	2.19	2.21	2.23
112	2.02	2.04	2.06	2.08	2.10	2.11	2.13	2.15	2.17	2.19	2.21	2.23	2.25
114	2.03	2.05	2.07	2.09	2.11	2.13	2.15	2.17	2.19	2.21	2.23	2.25	2.26
116	2.05	2.07	2.09	2.11	2.13	2.15	2.17	2.19	2.20	2.22	2.24	2.26	2.28
118	2.06	2.08	2.10	2.12	2.14	2.16	2.18	2.20	2.22	2.24	2.26	2.28	2.30
120	2.08	2.10	2.12	2.14	2.16	2.18	2.20	2.22	2.24	2.26	2.28	2.30	2.31
122	2.09	2.11	2.13	2.15	2.17	2.19	2.21	2.23	2.25	2.27	2.29	2.31	2.33
124	2.11	2.13	2.15	2.17	2.19	2.21	2.23	2.25	2.27	2.29	2.31	2.33	2.35
126	2.12	2.14	2.16	2.18	2.20	2.22	2.24	2.26	2.28	2.30	2.32	2.34	2.36
128	2.14	2.16	2.18	2.20	2.22	2.24	2.26	2.28	2.30	2.32	2.34	2.36	2.38
130	2.15	2.17	2.19	2.21	2.23	2.25	2.27	2.29	2.31	2.33	2.35	2.37	2.39
132	2.16	2.18	2.21	2.23	2.25	2.27	2.29	2.31	2.33	2.35	2.37	2.39	2.41

176	178	180	182	184	186	188	190	192	194	196	198	200
1.042	1.061	1.059	1.068	1.076	1.085	1.093	1.101	1.110	1.118	1.127	1.135	1.143
1.090	1.099	1.108	1.116	1.125	1.134	1.143	1.152	1.161	1.169	1.178	1.187	1.195
1.135	1.144	1.153	1.162	1.172	1.180	1.190	1.199	1.209	1.218	1.127	1.236	1.245
1.177	1.187	1.197	1.206	1.216	1.226	1.235	1.245	1.254	1.264	1.273	1.282	1.292
1.22	1.23	1.24	1.25	1.26	1.27	1.28	1.29	1.30	1.31	1.32	1.33	1.34
1.26	1.27	1.28	1.29	1.30	1.31	1.32	1.33	1.34	1.35	1.36	1.37	1.38
1.29	1.31	1.32	1.33	1.34	1.35	1.36	1.37	1.38	1.39	1.40	1.41	1.42
1.33	1.34	1.35	1.36	1.37	1.38	1.40	1.41	1.42	1.43	1.44	1.45	1.46
1.37	1.38	1.39	1.40	1.41	1.42	1.43	1.44	1.45	1.47	1.48	1.49	1.50
1.40	1.41	1.42	1.43	1.44	1.46	1.47	1.48	1.49	1.50	1.51	1.52	1.53
1.43	1.44	1.46	1.47	1.48	1.49	1.50	1.51	1.52	1.54	1.55	1.56	1.57
1.46	1.48	1.49	1.50	1.51	1.52	1.53	1.55	1.56	1.57	1.58	1.59	1.61
1.49	1.51	1.52	1.53	1.54	1.55	1.57	1.58	1.59	1.60	1.61	1.63	1.64
1.52	1.54	1.55	1.56	1.57	1.59	1.60	1.61	1.62	1.63	1.65	1.66	1.67
1.55	1.57	1.58	1.59	1.60	1.62	1.63	1.64	1.65	1.67	1.68	1.69	1.70
1.58	1.59	1.61	1.62	1.63	1.65	1.66	1.67	1.68	1.70	1.71	1.72	1.73
1.61	1.62	1.63	1.65	1.66	1.67	1.69	1.70	1.71	1.73	1.74	1.75	1.76
1.64	1.65	1.66	1.68	1.69	1.70	1.72	1.73	1.74	1.76	1.77	1.78	1.79
1.66	1.68	1.69	1.70	1.72	1.73	1.74	1.76	1.77	1.78	1.80	1.81	1.82
1.69	1.70	1.72	1.73	1.74	1.76	1.77	1.78	1.80	1.81	1.82	1.84	1.85
1.71	1.73	1.74	1.76	1.77	1.78	1.80	1.81	1.82	1.84	1.85	1.87	1.88
1.74	1.75	1.77	1.78	1.80	1.81	1.82	1.84	1.85	1.87	1.88	1.89	1.91
1.76	1.78	1.79	1.81	1.82	1.83	1.85	1.86	1.88	1.89	1.91	1.92	1.93
1.79	1.81	1.82	1.83	1.84	1.86	1.87	1.89	1.90	1.92	1.93	1.95	1.96
1.81	1.82	1.84	1.85	1.87	1.88	1.90	1.91	1.92	1.94	1.96	1.97	1.99
1.83	1.85	1.86	1.88	1.89	1.91	1.92	1.94	1.95	1.97	1.98	2.00	2.01
1.86	1.87	1.89	1.90	1.92	1.93	1.95	1.96	1.98	1.99	2.01	2.02	2.04
1.88	1.89	1.91	1.92	1.94	1.95	1.97	1.99	2.00	2.02	2.03	2.05	2.06
1.90	1.92	1.93	1.95	1.96	1.98	1.99	2.01	2.02	2.04	2.05	2.07	2.08
1.92	1.94	1.95	1.97	1.98	2.00	2.02	2.03	2.05	2.06	2.08	2.09	2.11
1.94	1.96	1.98	1.99	2.01	2.02	2.04	2.05	2.07	2.09	2.10	2.12	2.13
1.96	1.98	2.00	2.01	2.03	2.04	2.06	2.08	2.09	2.11	2.12	2.14	2.15
1.98	2.00	2.02	2.03	2.05	2.07	2.08	2.10	2.11	2.13	2.15	2.16	2.18
2.01	2.02	2.04	2.05	2.07	2.09	2.10	2.12	2.14	2.15	2.17	2.18	2.20
2.03	2.04	2.06	2.08	2.09	2.11	2.12	2.14	2.16	2.17	2.19	2.21	2.22
2.05	2.06	2.08	2.10	2.11	2.13	2.15	2.16	2.18	2.19	2.21	2.23	2.24
2.06	2.08	2.10	2.12	2.13	2.15	2.17	2.18	2.20	2.22	2.23	2.25	2.27
2.08	2.10	2.12	2.14	2.15	2.17	2.19	2.20	2.22	2.24	2.25	2.27	2.29
2.10	2.12	2.14	2.16	2.17	2.18	2.21	2.22	2.24	2.26	2.27	2.29	2.31
2.12	2.14	2.16	2.17	2.19	2.21	2.23	2.24	2.26	2.28	2.29	2.31	2.33
2.14	2.16	2.18	2.19	2.21	2.23	2.25	2.26	2.28	2.30	2.31	2.33	2.35
2.16	2.18	2.20	2.21	2.23	2.25	2.27	2.28	2.30	2.31	2.34	2.35	2.37
2.18	2.20	2.21	2.23	2.25	2.27	2.28	2.30	2.32	2.34	2.35	2.37	2.39
2.20	2.21	2.23	2.25	2.27	2.29	2.30	2.32	2.34	2.36	2.37	2.39	2.41
2.21	2.23	2.25	2.27	2.29	2.30	2.32	2.34	2.36	2.38	2.39	2.41	2.43
2.23	2.25	2.27	2.29	2.30	2.32	2.34	2.36	2.38	2.39	2.41	2.43	2.45
2.25	2.27	2.29	2.30	2.32	2.34	2.36	2.38	2.40	2.41	2.43	2.45	2.47
2.27	2.28	2.30	2.32	2.34	2.36	2.38	2.40	2.41	2.43	2.45	2.47	2.49
2.28	2.30	2.32	2.34	2.36	2.38	2.40	2.41	2.43	2.45	2.47	2.49	2.51
2.30	2.32	2.34	2.36	2.38	2.39	2.41	2.43	2.45	2.47	2.49	2.51	2.52
2.32	2.34	2.35	2.37	2.39	2.41	2.43	2.45	2.47	2.49	2.50	2.52	2.54
2.33	2.35	2.37	2.39	2.41	2.43	2.45	2.47	2.49	2.50	2.52	2.54	2.56
2.35	2.37	2.39	2.41	2.43	2.45	2.47	2.48	2.50	2.52	2.54	2.56	2.58
2.37	2.39	2.41	2.42	2.44	2.46	2.48	2.50	2.52	2.54	2.56	2.58	2.60
2.38	2.40	2.42	2.44	2.46	2.48	2.50	2.52	2.54	2.56	2.58	2.59	2.61
2.40	2.42	2.44	2.46	2.48	2.50	2.52	2.54	2.56	2.57	2.59	2.61	2.63
2.41	2.43	2.45	2.47	2.49	2.51	2.53	2.55	2.57	2.59	2.61	2.63	2.65
2.43	2.45	2.47	2.49	2.51	2.53	2.55	2.57	2.59	2.61	2.63	2.65	2.67

Table 7-3. BMR Calculations—Normals and Rate in Percentage (Adults)

Giving Metabolic Rate in Percent. Above or Below Normal from Calories Obtained

(Aub and DuBois Normal Standards, Cal. per Sq. M. per Hour)

Males Age				70–80		60–70
Females Age	70–80	60–70	50–60		40–50	30–40
Normal	33.0	34.0	35.0	35.5	36.0	36.5
20.0	−39	−41				
21.0	−36	−38	−40			
22.0	−33	−35	−37	−38	−39	−40
23.0	−30	−32	−34	−35	−36	−37
24.0	−27	−29	−31	−32	−33	−34
25.0	−24	−27	−29	−30	−31	−32
26.0	−21	−24	−26	−27	−28	−29
27.0	−18	−21	−23	−24	−25	−26
28.0	−15	−18	−20	−21	−22	−23
29.0	−12	−15	−17	−18	−20	−21
30.0	−9	−12	−14	−15	−17	−18
31.0	−6	−9	−11	−13	−14	−15
32.0	−3	−6	−9	−10	−11	−12
33.0	0	−3	−6	−7	−8	−10
34.0	+3	0	−3	−4	−6	−7
35.0	+6	+3	0	−1	−3	−4
36.0	+9	+6	+3	+1	0	−1
37.0	+12	+9	+6	+4	+3	+1
38.0	+15	+12	+9	+7	+6	+4
39.0	+18	+15	+12	+10	+8	+7
40.0	+21	+18	+14	+13	+11	+10
41.0	+24	+21	+17	+16	+14	+12
42.0	+27	+24	+20	+18	+17	+15
43.0	+30	+26	+23	+21	+19	+18
44.0	+33	+29	+26	+24	+22	+21
45.0	+36	+32	+29	+27	+25	+23
46.0	+39	+35	+31	+30	+28	+26
47.0	+42	+38	+34	+32	+31	+29
48.0	+45	+41	+37	+35	+33	+32
49.0	+48	+44	+40	+38	+36	+34
50.0	+52	+47	+43	+41	+39	+37
51.0	+55	+50	+46	+44	+42	+40
52.0	+58	+53	+48	+47	+44	+42
53.0	+61	+56	+51	+49	+47	+45
54.0	+64	+59	+54	+52	+50	+48
55.0	+67	+62	+57	+55	+53	+51
56.0	+70	+65	+60	+58	+55	+53
57.0	+73	+68	+63	+61	+58	+56
58.0	+76	+71	+66	+63	+61	+59
59.0	+79	+74	+69	+66	+64	+62
60.0	+82	+76	+72	+69	+67	+64
61.0	+85	+79	+74	+72	+69	+67
62.0	+88	+82	+77	+75	+72	+70
63.0	+91	+85	+80	+77	+75	+73
64.0	+94	+88	+83	+80	+78	+75
65.0	+97	+91	+86	+83	+81	+78
66.0	+100	+94	+89	+86	+83	+81
67.0	+103	+97	+91	+89	+86	+84
68.0	+106	+100	+94	+92	+89	+86
69.0	+109	+103	+97	+94	+91	+89
70.0	+112	+105	+100	+97	+94	+92
71.0	+115	+108	+103	+100	+97	+95
72.0	+116	+111	+106	+103	+100	+97
73.0	+121	+114	+109	+106	+103	+100
74.0	+124	+118	+111	+108	+106	+103
75.0	+127	+121	+114	+111	+108	+105
76.0	+130	+124	+117	+114	+111	+103
77.0	+133	+126	+120	+117	+114	+111
78.0	+136	+129	+123	+120	+117	+114
79.0	+139	+132	+126	+123	+119	+116
80.0	+142	+135	+129	+125	+122	+119
81.0	+145	+138	+131	+128	+125	+122
82.0	+148	+141	+134	+131	+128	+125
83.0	+152	+144	+137	+134	+131	+127
84.0	+155	+147	+140	+137	+133	+130
85.0	+158	+150	+143	+139	+136	+133
86.0	+161	+153	+146	+142	+139	+136
87.0	+164	+156	+149	+145	+142	+138
88.0	+167	+159	+151	+148	+144	+141
89.0	+170	+162	+154	+151	+147	+144

CALORIES OBTAINED

AGE and SEX	50-60		40-50	20-40		18-20	16-18	14-16
20-30		18-20			16-18		14-16	
37.0	**37.5**	**38.0**	**38.5**	**39.5**	**40.0**	**41.0**	**43.0**	**46.0**
−38	−39	−40						
−35	−36	−37	−38	−39	−40			
−33	−34	−35	−36	−37	−38	−40		
−30	−31	−32	−33	−34	−36	−38	−40	
−27	−28	−29	−30	−31	−32	−34	−37	−40
−24	−25	−26	−27	−29	−30	−32	−35	−39
−22	−23	−24	−25	−27	−28	−29	−32	−37
−19	−20	−21	−22	−24	−25	−27	−30	−35
−16	−17	−18	−19	−22	−23	−24	−28	−33
−14	−15	−16	−17	−19	−20	−22	−26	−30
−11	−12	−13	−14	−17	−18	−19	−23	−28
−8	−9	−11	−12	−14	−15	−17	−21	−26
−5	−7	−8	−9	−12	−13	−15	−19	−24
−3	−4	−5	−7	−9	−10	−12	−16	−22
0	−1	−3	−4	−6	−8	−10	−14	−20
+3	+1	0	−1	−4	−5	−7	−12	−17
+5	+4	+3	+1	−1	−3	−5	−10	−15
+8	+7	+5	+4	+1	0	−2	−7	−13
+11	+9	+8	+6	+4	+3	0	−5	−11
+14	+12	+11	+9	+6	+5	+2	−2	−9
+16	+15	+13	+12	+9	+8	+5	0	−7
+19	+17	+16	+14	+11	+10	+7	+2	−4
+22	+20	+18	+17	+14	+12	+10	+5	−2
+24	+23	+21	+19	+16	+15	+12	+7	0
+27	+25	+24	+22	+19	+17	+15	+9	+2
+30	+28	+26	+25	+22	+20	+17	+12	+4
+32	+31	+29	+27	+24	+23	+20	+14	+7
+35	+33	+32	+30	+27	+25	+22	+16	+9
+38	+36	+34	+33	+29	+28	+24	+19	+11
+41	+39	+37	+35	+32	+30	+27	+21	+13
+43	+42	+39	+38	+34	+33	+29	+23	+15
+46	+44	+42	+40	+37	+35	+32	+26	+17
+49	+47	+45	+43	+39	+38	+34	+28	+20
+51	+49	+47	+45	+42	+40	+37	+30	+22
+54	+52	+50	+48	+44	+43	+39	+33	+24
+57	+55	+53	+51	+47	+45	+41	+35	+26
+59	+57	+55	+53	+49	+48	+44	+37	+28
+62	+60	+58	+56	+52	+50	+47	+40	+30
+65	+63	+60	+58	+54	+53	+49	+42	+32
+68	+65	+63	+61	+57	+55	+51	+44	+34
+71	+68	+65	+64	+59	+57	+54	+47	+36
+73	+71	+68	+66	+62	+60	+56	+49	+39
+76	+73	+71	+69	+64	+63	+59	+51	+41
+78	+76	+74	+72	+67	+65	+61	+53	+43
+81	+79	+76	+74	+69	+67	+63	+56	+45
+84	+81	+79	+77	+72	+70	+66	+58	+48
+86	+84	+82	+79	+75	+72	+68	+60	+50
+89	+87	+84	+82	+77	+75	+71	+63	+52
+92	+89	+87	+84	+80	+77	+73	+65	+54
+95	+92	+89	+87	+82	+80	+76	+67	+57
+97	+94	+92	+90	+85	+82	+78	+70	+59
+100	+97	+95	+92	+87	+85	+81	+72	+61
+103	+100	+97	+95	+90	+87	+83	+74	+63
+105	+103	+100	+97	+92	+90	+86	+77	+65
+108	+105	+103	+100	+95	+92	+88	+79	+67
+111	+108	+105	+103	+97	+95	+90	+81	+70
+114	+111	+108	+105	+100	+97	+93	+84	+72
+116	+113	+111	+108	+103	+100	+95	+86	+74
+119	+116	+113	+110	+105	+103	+98	+88	+76
+122	+119	+116	+113	+108	+105	+100	+91	+78
+124	+121	+118	+116	+110	+107	+102	+93	+80
+127	+124	+121	+118	+113	+110	+105	+95	+83
+130	+127	+124	+121	+115	+112	+107	+98	+85
+132	+129	+126	+123	+118	+115	+110	+100	+87
+135	+132	+129	+126	+120	+117	+112	+102	+89
+138	+135	+132	+129	+123	+120	+115	+105	+91
+141	+137	+134	+131	+125	+122	+117	+107	+94

Table 7-4. BMR Calculations—Normals and Rate in Percentage (Boys and Girls)

Giving Metabolic Rate in Percent. Above or Below Normal from Calories Obtained

Males Age→	13		12		11		10	
Females Age→		13		12		11		10
Normal→	47.1	42.	47.8	43.4	48.6	44.6	49.5	45.8
24								
25								
26		−39		−40		−41		
27		−36		−38		−39		−41
28	−41	−33	−41	−35		−37		−39
29	−38	−31	−39	−33	−40	−35	−41	−37
30	−36	−29	−37	−31	−38	−33	−39	−35
31	−34	−26	−35	−28	−36	−30	−37	−32
32	−32	−24	−33	−26	−34	−28	−35	−30
33	−30	−21	−31	−24	−32	−26	−33	−28
34	−28	−19	−29	−22	−30	−24	−31	−26
35	−26	−17	−27	−19	−28	−22	−29	−24
36	−24	−14	−25	−17	−26	−19	−27	−21
37	−22	−12	−23	−15	−24	−17	−25	−19
38	−19	−9	−20	−12	−22	−15	−23	−17
39	−17	−7	−18	−10	−20	−13	−21	−15
40	−15	−5	−16	−8	−18	−10	−19	−13
41	−13	−2	−14	−5	−16	−8	−17	−10
42	−11	0	−12	−3	−14	−6	−15	−8
43	−9	+2	−10	−1	−11	−4	−13	−6
44	−7	+5	−8	+2	−9	−1	−11	−4
45	−4	+7	−6	+4	−7	+1	−9	−2
46	−2	+10	−4	+6	−5	+3	−7	0
47	0	+12	−2	+8	−3	+5	−5	+3
48	+2	+14	0	+11	−1	+8	−3	+5
49	+4	+17	+3	+13	+1	+10	−1	+7
50	+6	+19	+5	+15	+3	+12	+1	+9
51	+8	+21	+7	+18	+5	+14	+3	+11
52	+10	+24	+9	+20	+7	+17	+5	+14
53	+13	+26	+11	+22	+9	+19	+7	+16
54	+15	+29	+13	+25	+11	+21	+9	+18
55	+17	+31	+15	+27	+13	+23	+11	+20
56	+19	+33	+17	+29	+15	+25	+13	+22
57	+21	+36	+19	+32	+17	+28	+15	+24
58	+23	+38	+21	+34	+19	+30	+17	+27
59	+25	+41	+23	+36	+21	+32	+19	+29
60	+27	+43	+26	+38	+23	+35	+21	+31
61	+30	+45	+28	+41	+25	+37	+23	+33
62	+32	+48	+30	+43	+28	+39	+25	+35
63	+34	+50	+32	+45	+30	+41	+27	+38
64	+36	+52	+34	+48	+32	+43	+29	+40
65	+38	+55	+36	+50	+34	+46	+31	+42
66	+40	+57	+38	+52	+36	+48	+33	+44
67	+42	+59	+40	+55	+38	+50	+35	+46
68	+44	+62	+42	+57	+40	+53	+37	+49
69	+46	+64	+44	+59	+42	+55	+39	+51
70	+49	+67	+47	+61	+44	+57	+41	+53
71	+51	+69	+49	+64	+46	+59	+43	+55
72	+53	+71	+51	+66	+48	+62	+45	+57
73	+55	+74	+53	+68	+50	+64	+47	+59
74	+57	+76	+55	+71	+52	+66	+49	+62
75	+59	+79	+57	+73	+54	+68	+52	+64
76	+61	+81	+59	+75	+56	+71	+54	+66
77	+63	+83	+61	+78	+58	+73	+56	+68
78	+66	+86	+63	+80	+61	+75	+58	+70
79	+68	+88	+65	+82	+63	+77	+60	+73
80	+70	+90	+67	+85	+65	+79	+62	+75
81	+72	+93	+69	+87	+67	+82	+64	+77
82	+74	+95	+72	+89	+69	+84	+66	+79
83	+76	+98	+74	+91	+71	+86	+68	+81
84	+78	+100	+76	+94	+73	+88	+70	+83
85	+80	+102	+78	+96	+75	+91	+72	+86
86	+83	+105	+80	+98	+77	+93	+74	+88
87	+85	+107	+82	+100	+79	+95	+76	+90
88	+87	+110	+84	+103	+81	+97	+78	+92
89	+89	+112	+86	+105	+83	+100	+80	+94
90	+91	+114	+88	+108	+85	+102	+82	+97

(Left axis label: CALORIES OBTAINED)

374

AGE and SEX									
9		8		7		6		5	
	9		8		7		6		5
50.4	46.9	51.2	48.1	52.	49.3	52.7	50.7	53.	51.6
	−40								
	−38		−40		−41				
−41	−36	−41	−38		−39		−41		
−39	−34	−39	−36	−40	−37	−41	−39		−40
−37	−32	−37	−33	−38	−35	−39	−37	−40	−38
−35	−30	−35	−31	−37	−33	−37	−35	−38	−36
−33	−28	−34	−29	−35	−31	−35	−33	−36	−34
−31	−25	−32	−27	−33	−29	−34	−31	−34	−32
−29	−23	−30	−25	−31	−27	−32	−29	−32	−30
−27	−21	−28	−23	−29	−25	−30	−27	−30	−28
−25	−19	−26	−21	−27	−23	−28	−25	−28	−26
−23	−17	−24	−19	−25	−21	−26	−23	−26	−24
−21	−15	−22	−17	−23	−19	−24	−21	−25	−22
−19	−13	−20	−15	−21	−17	−22	−19	−23	−21
−17	−10	−18	−13	−19	−15	−20	−17	−21	−19
−15	−8	−16	−11	−17	−13	−18	−15	−19	−17
−13	−6	−14	−9	−15	−11	−16	−13	−17	−15
−11	−4	−12	−6	−13	−9	−15	−11	−15	−13
−9	−2	−10	−4	−12	−7	−13	−9	−13	−11
−7	0	−8	−2	−10	−5	−11	−7	−11	−9
−5	+2	−6	0	−8	−3	−9	−5	−9	−7
−3	+4	−4	+2	−6	−1	−7	−3	−8	−5
−1	+7	−2	+4	−4	+1	−5	−1	−6	−3
+1	+9	0	+6	−2	+3	−3	+1	−4	−1
+3	+11	+2	+8	0	+5	−1	+3	−2	+1
+5	+13	+4	+10	+2	+8	+1	+5	0	+3
+7	+15	+6	+12	+4	+10	+3	+7	+2	+5
+9	+17	+7	+14	+6	+12	+4	+8	+4	+7
+11	+19	+9	+16	+8	+14	+6	+10	+6	+9
+13	+22	+11	+19	+10	+16	+8	+12	+8	+10
+15	+24	+13	+21	+12	+18	+10	+14	+9	+12
+17	+26	+15	+23	+14	+20	+12	+16	+11	+14
+19	+28	+17	+25	+15	+22	+14	+18	+13	+16
+21	+30	+19	+27	+17	+24	+16	+20	+15	+18
+23	+32	+21	+29	+19	+26	+18	+22	+17	+20
+25	+34	+23	+31	+21	+28	+20	+24	+19	+22
+27	+36	+25	+33	+23	+30	+21	+26	+21	+24
+29	+39	+27	+35	+25	+32	+23	+28	+23	+26
+31	+41	+29	+37	+27	+34	+25	+30	+25	+28
+33	+43	+31	+39	+29	+36	+27	+32	+26	+30
+35	+45	+33	+41	+31	+38	+29	+34	+28	+32
+37	+47	+35	+43	+33	+40	+31	+36	+30	+34
+39	+49	+37	+46	+35	+42	+33	+38	+32	+36
+41	+51	+39	+48	+37	+44	+35	+40	+34	+38
+43	+54	+41	+50	+38	+46	+37	+42	+36	+40
+45	+56	+43	+52	+40	+48	+39	+44	+38	+41
+47	+58	+45	+54	+42	+50	+40	+46	+40	+43
+49	+60	+47	+56	+44	+52	+42	+48	+42	+45
+51	+62	+49	+58	+46	+54	+44	+50	+43	+47
+53	+64	+50	+60	+48	+56	+46	+52	+45	+49
+55	+66	+52	+62	+50	+58	+48	+54	+47	+51
+57	+69	+54	+64	+52	+60	+50	+56	+49	+53
+59	+71	+56	+66	+54	+62	+52	+58	+51	+55
+61	+73	+58	+68	+56	+64	+54	+60	+53	+57
+63	+75	+60	+70	+58	+66	+56	+62	+55	+59
+65	+77	+62	+73	+60	+68	+58	+64	+57	+61
+67	+79	+64	+75	+62	+70	+59	+66	+58	+63
+69	+81	+66	+77	+63	+72	+61	+68	+60	+65
+71	+83	+68	+79	+65	+74	+63	+70	+62	+67
+73	+86	+70	+81	+67	+76	+65	+72	+64	+69
+75	+88	+72	+83	+69	+78	+67	+74	+66	+71
+77	+90	+74	+85	+71	+81	+69	+76	+68	+72
+79	+92	+76	+87	+73	+83	+71	+78	+70	+74

Source: "Consolidated Tables for McKesson Recording Metabolers," McKesson Appliance Company, Toledo, Ohio.

375

and exhalation is considered the vital capacity and is measured in cubic inches of air.

Another test is one for *tidal air*. Tidal air is the amount of oxygen taken into the lungs and expired with each normal respiration. The height of an average respiration during the regular BMR breathing test is measured and recorded in liters of oxygen.

The results of the BMR test may be used to measure *minute volume*. Minute volume is the total volume of air breathed per minute. It is equal to the tidal air multiplied by the number of respirations per minute as seen in the regular breathing pattern in the BMR test.

DISEASES AFFECTING THE BMR

The BMR is affected by several different diseases. Some of the diseases characterized by a high metabolic rate are hyperthyroidism, toxic adenoma, hyperpituitarism, lymphatic and myelogenous leukemia, severe anemia, Graves' disease, severe acidosis, some malignant tumors, arterial hypertension, and moderate diabetes mellitus. A high metabolic rate is also seen with fever and after administration of stimulating drugs.

Diseases and conditions characterized by a low metabolic rate are hypothyroidism, hypopituitarism, myxedema, cretinism, endocrine obesity, epilepsy, arterial hypotension, anorexia nervosa, and cachexia. A low metabolic rate is also seen after the use of depressing drugs.

. BIBLIOGRAPHY

Anthony, Catherine P.: "Textbook of Anatomy and Physiology," 5th ed., The C. V. Mosby Company, St. Louis, 1959.

Boothby, Walter M., and Irene Sandiford: Normal Values of Basal or Standard Metabolism, *Am. J. Physiol.,* 90:291, 1929.

Du Bois, Eugene F.: "Basal Metabolism in Health and Disease," 3d ed., Lea & Febiger, Philadelphia, 1936.

Goldman, Mervin J.: "Principles of Clinical Electrocardiography," 6th ed., Lange Medical Publications, Los Altos, California, 1967.

Peters, J. P., and D. D. Van Slyke: "Quantitative Clinical Chemistry," vol. I, "Interpretations," The Williams & Wilkins Company, Baltimore, 1932.

———— and ————: "Quantitative Clinical Chemistry," vol. II, "Methods," chap. V, The Williams & Wilkins Company, Baltimore, 1932.

Roe, Joseph H.: "Principles of Chemistry," 9th ed., The C. V. Mosby Company, St. Louis, 1963.

Watson, C. J.: "Outlines of Internal Medicine," pt. III, 8th ed., Wm. C. Brown Company, Dubuque, Iowa, 1955.

————: "Outlines of Internal Medicine," pt. II, 10th ed, Wm. C. Brown Company, Dubuque, Iowa, 1962.

Index

A₁ antigen, 274
ABO blood group system, 269, 272–279
  immune antibody, 276–277
  inheritance, 272–273
  natural antibodies, 274, 276–277
  subgroups, 276
  typing, 273, 274, 276
  typing reactions, table, 275
Accidents, first aid for (*see* First aid)
Accuracy:
  in chemical analyses, 73
  means of ensuring, 73, 78–79
  (*See also* Reliability of results)
Acetest, 226–227
Acetoacetic acid (*see* Ketone bodies, urinary)
Acetone (*see* Ketone bodies, urinary)
Acetone bodies (*see* Ketone bodies, urinary)
Acetylmethylcarbinol, 329
Acid-alcohol reagent, 325
Acid-base balance (*see* Plasma chloride)
Acid cleaning solution, 6, 57
Acid-fast bacteria, 325
Acid-fast staining method, 324–325
Acid hematin, 72
Acidosis, 225
Aerobe, 312
Agar, 313
Agar-agar, 312
Agar slants, 328
Agglutination in blood banking, 271
Albumin, urinary (*see* Protein, urinary)
Albumin-active antibody, 284, 285
Albuminuria, 216
Albustix, 223
Albutest, 222
Alcohol-acetone decolorizer, 323

Alkaline copper reagent, 90
Allele, 266, 280
Alpha streptococci, 332
American Chemical Society, reagent grade, 14
Ammonia-free water, 17–18, 103
Ammonium and potassium oxalate, anticoagulant, 69
  composition, 113
  use in hematology, 112–116
Ammonium biurate crystals, 254
Ammonium sulfate standard solution, 99, 100
Amorphous material, urinary, 251–255
  identification, 259, 260
  reporting results, 252, 259, 260
Amorphous phosphates, 196, 254
Amorphous urates, 196, 252–253
Anaerobe, 312, 327
Analytical balance, 38
  automatic type, 38, 44–45
  care of weights, 40
  general care, 39
  manual type, 38, 42–44
  parts, 39–41
  procedure for use, 41–42
  sensitivity, 39
  types available, 38
  use of vernier scale, 41, 43
Analytical reagent grade, 14
Anemia, 122
  definition of, 169
  occurrence, 122
  osmotic fragility of erythrocyte in, 174
  types, 122
  use of red blood cell indicies in, 176–177

Anisocytosis, 148
Antibiotics in microbiology, 304, 315
Antibody, 265–272
  albumin-active, 284, 285
  blocking, 285
  chemical composition, 269
  classification, 288
  complete, 284, 288
  formation, 267, 268
  immune (*see* Immune antibody)
  incomplete, 284, 288
  irregular (*see* Irregular antibodies)
  natural (*see* Natural antibody)
  physical types, 269
  response, 268–269
  Rh-Hr system (*see* Rh-Hr blood group
    system)
  saline-solution active, 284, 285
  screening, 297
  titer, 268, 269, 276–278, 294
  typing, 268, 274, 287
  univalent, 284, 288
Anticoagulant:
  general reaction, 161
  for hematology, 112, 142–143
  types available, 69–70
Antigen, 265–272
  chemical composition, 267
  Rh-Hr system (*see* Rh-Hr blood group
    system)
  specificity, 267
  strength, 267
  typing, 274
Antigen-antibody reaction, 267
  detection of, 270–272
Antiglobulin crossmatch, 297, 298
Antihemophilic factor (AHF), 161
Antihemophilic globulin (AHG) [*see*
  Antihemophilic factor (AHF)]
Anti-human globulin (AHG) reagent,
  289
Anti-human globulin (AHG) test, reac-
  tion, 284, 286, 288–291, 298
Antiserum, 270
  preparation of, 270
  requirements, 270
  Rh-Hr, 285
Anuria, 193
Aqua regia, 6
Arnold sterilizer, 308
Arsenomolybdate color reagent, 91
Autoclave, 308–309, 313
Autoimmune anemia, 290

Back typing, 274
Bacteria:
  colonial characteristics, 314–315
  cultural requirements, 311–314
  morphology, 310–311
  size, 310
  staining, 310
  urinary, 196, 245, 257
Bacterial infection, urinary, 245
Bacteriology (*see* Microbiology)
Balance:
  Cent-o-Gram type, 47
  torsion type, 45–46
  triple-beam type, 46–47
    Harvard, 46
  (*See also* Analytical balance)
Balanced oxalate (*see* Ammonium and
    potassium oxalate, anticoagulant)
Barium hydroxide reagent, 90, 97
Barometric pressure, 358
  correlation with gas factor, 364
  standard conditions of, 364
Basal metabolic rate (BMR):
  calculating, 364–371
  definition of, 353
  factors influencing, 354–355, 359
  laboratory procedures, 359–364
  machine for measuring: basic parts,
    355–358
    operation of, 361–364
    (*See also* McKesson Recording
      Metaboler)
  methods of measuring, 355
  normal values, chart for, 372–375
  percentage values, chart for, 372–375
  (*See also* Basal metabolic rate test)
Basal metabolic rate test:
  calculations for, 364–375
    use of gas factor, 364
    use of normal values, 365, 372–375
    use of percentage values, 365,
      372–375
    use of surface area, 365, 368–371
    use of temperature correction, 365,
      367
  drawing oxygen consumption line for,
    356–357, 363
  operating machine for, 361–364
    (*See also* McKesson Recording
      Metaboler)
  patient connection to machine for,
    362–363

Basal metabolic rate test:
  patient preparation for, 359–361
    blood pressure, 360–361
    pulse rate, 360
    rest period, 359
    temperature, 359–360
    weight and height, 359
  technical factors to note in, 367
  use for measurement of minute volume, 376
  use for measurement of tidal air, 376
  use for measurement of vital capacity, 376
  [See also Basal metabolic rate (BMR)]
Basophil:
  description of, 120, 151–152
  development (see Granulocytes)
  differential counting and classification (see Blood film)
  normal value, 151
Basophilic stippling, 148
Batch of determinations, 73
Beer-brown color, 230
Beer-Lambert law, 49
Beer's law (see Beer-Lambert law)
Bellows for BMR machine, 355–356
Benedict's qualitative reagent, 212
Benedict's qualitative test, 210–213, 215, 226
  principle, 211–212
  procedure, 212–213
  reagent, 212
Benzidine, 237
Benzidine filter paper test, 238–239
Benzoic acid, saturated solution, 90
Beta-hydroxybutyric acid (see Ketone bodies, urinary)
Beta streptococci, 332
Bilazo, 232
Bile pigments, breakdown product of erythrocyte, 118
Bilirubin, 229–230
  in blood, 293
  urinary, 194, 198, 230–232
    laboratory procedures, 231–232
Biliverdin, 230, 231
  urinary, 194
Binary fission, 314
Biopsy, kidney, 246
Bipolar leads, 342–344
Blank solutions, 54, 77, 78

Bleeding time tests, 162–164
  Duke method, 162–164
  Ivy method, 162–164
  normal values, 163–164
  precautions to note in, 164
Blocking of antibody, 285
Blood:
  capillary (see Capillary blood)
  circulatory function of, 107
  collection of, 68, 110–115
    capillary, 110–112
    venous, 110, 112–115
  composition of, 107, 263
    layers after settling, when preserved, 116
  factors, 264, 266
  protein, precipitation of, 72–73
    (See also Protein precipitation)
  specimens (see Specimens, blood)
  type, 264, 270
  unit, 263
  urinary and fecal (see Hemoglobin, urinary and fecal)
  venous (see Venous blood)
  volume, 263
Blood banking:
  errors, 299
  laboratory procedures (see Procedures, laboratory, blood banking)
  negative reaction, 271
  organization, 299
  positive reaction, 271
Blood cast, 249
Blood cells:
  enumeration of, 121–137
  formation of, 118
  morphology of, 142–155
  production by bone marrow, 118
  (See also Erythrocytes in blood; Leukocytes in blood; Thrombocytes in blood)
Blood film, 142–154
  classification and differential count of leukocytes, 149–150
  description of leukocytes, 150–153
  evaluation of, 147–150
  examination of, 146–150
  feather edge of, 143–145
  general appearance of cells, 147
  morphology of blood cells, 142, 153–154
  preparation of, 142–144
    use of spreader slide, 143

Blood film:
  source of blood for, 142
  staining, 144–146
Blood group:
  ABO system (see ABO blood group
    . system)
  inheritance, 265–266
  introduction, 264
  Rh-Hr system (see Rh-Hr blood group
    system)
  systems, 264
  tests, 272, 274, 284–287
Blood pressure:
  definition of, 360
  diastolic, 360
  procedure for obtaining, 360–361
  systolic, 360
  use of sphygmomanometer in, 361
  use of stethoscope in, 361
Blood pressure cuff, 361
  procedure for use, 361
Blood smear (see Blood film)
Blood transfusion (see Transfusion,
  blood)
Body fluid (see Extravascular fluids)
Boiling water, sterilization by, 308
Bordeaux red color, 228
Bordet-Gengou agar (BG), 333
Bordetella pertussis, 333
"Brick dust," 197, 253
Brilliant cresyl blue dye, 140–141
Broad casts, 250–251
Broad-spectrum antiglobulin reagent, 289
Broth, 312
Buffy coat, 116
Bumintest, 219, 221–222
  principle, 221
  procedure, 222
Buret, 32, 37, 64
  care of, 64
  cleaning, 66–67
  definition of, 64
  general use of, 63–67
  (See also Titration)
Burning, sterilization by, 307

Cable cord, patient, 350
Calcium carbonate crystals, 254
Calcium oxalate crystals, 254
Calcium phosphate crystals, 254
Calculations, 18–26
  dilution factors, 19

Calculations:
  proportion problems, 18
  significant figures, 19
  solution concentration: by chemical
    units, 23–26
    by physical units, 20–23
    by proper name, 20
    (See also Molarity; Normality)
Calibrating:
  burets, 37
  diluting pipets, 123–124, 171
  glassware, volumetric, 32
  photometer for hemoglobinometry,
    171–173
  photometer cuvettes, 49–53, 55–57
  pipets, general types, 36
  standards for glassware, 32–33, 35
Calibration curve (see Standard curve)
Calorie, 353
Capillary blood:
  collection procedure, 110–112
    equipment used, 111, 112
    precautions to note in, 112
  pipetting for hematologic tests, 112
Carbolfuchsin stain, 325
Cardiac waves, 340–341
Casts, urinary, 217, 243, 246–251
  blood, 249
  broad, 250–251
  cellular, 248–249
  classification, 247
  clinical significance, 246–247
  coarsely granular, 250
  epithelial, 249
  fatty, 247, 250
  formation, 246
  granular, 249–250
  hyaline, 247–248
  identification, 247, 251, 259, 260
  narrow, 250–251
  red blood cell, 249
  reporting results, 259, 260
  true blood, 249
  waxy, 249–251
  white blood cell, 249
Catheter, 190
Catheterized urine, 242
CBC (complete blood count), 142, 168
CDE nomenclature, 279, 280
Cell typing, 274
Cellular casts, 248–249
Cent-O-Gram balance, 47

Centrifuge, 7–8
  balancing of, 8
  microhematocrit, 7, 157
  tubes for, 8
Cerebrospinal fluid:
  examination of, 181–182
    chloride, 83, 86
    clinical implication of, 181
    erythrocyte count, 181–182
    glucose, 91, 94
    leukocyte count, 182
    leukocyte differential, 182
  specimens, 181
    handling, 181
    obtaining, 181
  (See also Extravascular fluids)
Chemical analysis:
  accuracy of, 73–80
  for chloride, 80–86
  for glucose, 86–95
  for urea nitrogen, 95–105
Chemical sterilization, 309
Chemicals:
  grades of, 14, 15
  storage of, 15
Chemistry laboratory procedures (see
    Procedures, laboratory, chemistry)
Cherry-red color, 234
Chest leads, 344–345
Chloride, plasma (see Plasma chloride)
"Chloride shift," 80
Chocolate agar, 332–333
Cholesterol crystals, 255
Christianson's urea slant, 330–331
Chromosome, 265
Clark-Lubs broth, 328–329
Clinistix, 210, 214–215
  principle, 214
  procedure, 215
Clinitest, 210, 213–215
  principle, 213
  procedure, 214
Clot retraction tests, 165
Clotting (see Coagulation)
Clotting time tests (see Lee-White
    venous clotting time test)
Coagulation:
  contraction of blood vessels in, 160
  factors in, 160–161
  general studies of, 160, 162
  role for platelets in, 160
  tests for, 164–168
Coarsely granular casts, 250

"Coffin-lid" crystals, 254
Coleman Junior Spectrophotometer,
    52–56
  calibration for hemoglobinometry,
    171–173
  cuvettes for, 56
    (See also Cuvettes)
  operation of, 52–54
  parts of, 52
Coliforms, 331, 334
Collecting specimens (see Specimens)
Colonial characteristics of bacteria,
    314–315
Color, urine, 193–196
  (See also Urine, color)
Colorimeter (see Photometer)
Colorimetry (see Photometry)
Colors of light, 48
Combistix, 200
Compatibility testing (see Crossmatch-
    ing)
Complement, 271–272, 289
Complete antibody, 284, 288
Complete blood count (CBC), 142, 168
Compound microscope, 9
Condenser, microscope, 9
Conjugated bilirubin, 229, 230, 233
Constant boiling hydrochloric acid, 67
Containers and receivers (see Glass-
    ware)
Control specimens, 78–79
  acceptable values for, 78
  allowable limits for, 78
  for blood glucose procedure, 91
  calculation of acceptable limits for,
    79
  general use of, 78
  for hemoglobinometry, 170–171
  for osmotic fragility of erythrocyte
    test, 175
  preparation of, 78
  for prothrombin time test, 167–168
  quality control chart for, 79
  for urea nitrogen procedure, 100, 101
  for urine and fecal hemoglobin, 239
Coombs crossmatch, 298
Coombs reagent, 289
Coombs test [see Anti-human globulin
    (AHG) test]
Coproporphyrin, 233
Corynebacterium diphtheriae, 331
Counting chamber (see Hemacytometer)

Crenation, 117, 243
   (*See also* Hemolysis)
Crossmatch:
   major, 297
   minor, 297
Crossmatching, 290, 295–298
Crossover, 281
Crystal violet stain, 323
Crystals, urinary, 251–255
   abnormal, 254–255
   identification, 259, 260
   normal, 252–254
   reporting results, 252, 259, 260
Cuff test, 162
Cultural requirements of microorganisms, 311–314
Culture and transfer of microorganisms, 317–319
Culture medium, 311
Cuvettes:
   calibrated for photometer, 49–53
   calibrating, 55–57
Cyanmethemoglobin method, 170–174
   Drabkin's reagent, 170–171
   procedure, 173
   reaction occurring, 170
   standardization of photometer for, 171–173
   use of control solution in, 170
Cylindroids, 247, 251
Cystine crystals, 255

D^{11} varient, 286, 287
Dark-field microscope, 13
Decastello, ABO blood group system, 272
Decomposition of urine specimens, 189
Deionized water, 17
Denis, 263
Deoxyribonucleic acid (DNA), 265
Dextrose:
   blood (*see* Glucose, blood)
   urinary (*see* Sugar, urinary)
Diabetes mellitus, 208, 224, 225
   increased glucose in blood, 95
Diabetic coma, 95
Diacetic acid (*see* Ketone bodies, urinary)
Diazo reagent, 232
Differential media, 315
Differential staining methods, microbiologic, 322–325

Diluents, hematologic, 117, 122–123
Diluting pipet (*see* Thoma pipet)
Dilution factors (*see* Calculations)
Diphenylcarbazone indicator, 82–83
Direct AHG test, 289–290
Direct typing, 274
Disinfection, 309
Distilled water, 17
Diuresis, 193
Döhle bodies, 151
Dominent, 266
Double distilled water (*see* Ammonia-free water)
Double oxalate, anticoagulant (*see* Ammonium and potassium oxalate, anticoagulant)
Drabkin's reagent, 170
   preparation of, 170
Dry heat, sterilization by, 307
Duke method (*see* Bleeding time tests)
"Dumbbell" crystals, 254
Duplicate determinations, use, 79
Dysentery, 334

ECG [*see* Electrocardiogram (ECG); Electrocardiography]
EDTA (*see* Sequestrene)
Ehrlich-reactive compounds, 234
Ehrlich's qualitative aldehyde reaction, 234–236
Ehrlich's reagent, 234
Einthoven's equation, 342
EKG [*see* Electrocardiogram (ECG); Electrocardiography]
Electrical interference, 347–348
Electrocardiogram (ECG), 338
   cardiac waves in, 340–341
   interpretation of, 341–342, 351
   Master two-step test, 352–353
   pathway of electric impulse in, 338
   routine procedure for obtaining: coding the leads, 345
      labeling, 351
      leads used, 342–345
      operation of machine, 350–351
      patient preparation, 342, 349–350
      placement of electrodes, 342–343, 349
      use of electrode paste or jelly, 343, 349
   standardization of, 345–346, 350

Electrocardiogram (ECG):
  technical difficulties in, 346–349
    (*See also* Electrical interference; Jittery baseline; Somatic tremor; Wandering baseline)
    (*See also* Electrocardiograph)
Electrocardiograph:
  checking polarity of, 350
  general operation of machine, 350–351
  paper used for, 338–339, 345
  pathway of electric impulse in, 338
  standardization of, 345–346, 350
  types of machines, 350
    [*See also* Electrocardiogram (ECG)]
Electrocardiography:
  cardiac waves in, 340–341
  definition of, 337
  heart, function of (*see* Heart)
  laboratory procedures, 349–351
  machines used for test, 338, 350
    [*See also* Electrocardiogram (ECG); Electrocardiograph]
Electrode paste or jelly, 349
Electrodes:
  chest, 349
  limb, 349
  paste, or jelly for, 349
  placement of, 349
Electrolyte balance (*see* Plasma chloride)
EMB agar, 333–334
End product, 97
English measurement system, 29
Enrichment media, 315
Enterococci, 331
Envelope crystals, 254
Enzyme crossmatch, 298
Enzymes:
  general laws governing, 98
  inhibitors of, 98
  in urea nitrogen procedure, 95–98
Eosinophilia, 137
Eosinophils:
  counting, 137–139
    blood sample for, 138
    calculations, 138
    counting chamber used, 138
    description of cells, 138
    diluent used, 137–138
    precautions to note, 138
    procedure for, 138
  description of, 120, 151

Eosinophils:
  development of (*see* Granulocytes)
  differential counting and classification (*see* Blood film)
  normal value, 151
Epithelial cell cast, 249
Epithelial cells, urinary, 245–246, 249, 251, 256
Equivalent weight (*see* Normality)
Equivalents (*see* Normality)
Erythroblastosis foetalis (*see* Hemolytic disease of the newborn)
Erythrocyte sedimentation rate (ESR):
  clinical use, 158–159
  definition of, 157–158
  methods, 159
    (*See also* Westergren method for erythrocyte sedimentation rate)
  normal values, 159
  specimens for, 159
Erythrocytes:
  in blood: appearance on stained blood film, 119
  association with reticuloendothelial system, 119
  counting (manual method), 121–134
    calculating the cell count, 130
    counting the cells, 132
    counting chamber, 126–130
      (*See also* Hemacytometer)
    diluents used, 122–123
      (*See also* Hayem's solution)
    diluting procedure, 125–126
    mounting the sample, 128–130
    pipets used, 123–125
      (*See also* Thoma pipet)
    precautions to note in, 126, 133–134
  description of, 118
  destruction of, 118
  development of, 154
  evaluation from stained blood film, 147
    alterations seen, 148–149
    morphologic changes, 154
    terms used, 148–149
  formation of, 118
  indices for, 176–177
    calculation of, 176–177
    use of, 176
  normal value, 133
  osmotic fragility of, 174
  use in body of, 118

Erythrocytes:
  in blood: waste products from, 118
  urinary (see Red blood cells, urinary)
Erythrocytosis, 169
Esbach protein test for body fluids, 180
Escherichia coli, 333
Exchange transfusion, 294
Exton's sulfosalicylic acid test, 219,
    221–222
  principle, 221
  procedure, 222
Extravascular fluids:
  definition of, 185
  examination of, 178–181
    cell counts, 179
    mucin test, 180–181
    protein test, 181
    specific gravity, 180
    stained smear analysis, 180
  exudates, 179
  transudates, 179
  (See also Cerebrospinal fluid)
Exudates, 179
Eyepiece, microscope (see Ocular,
    microscope)

Factor, blood, 264, 266
Factor V (see Proaccelerin)
Factor VII (see Proconvertin)
Factor VIII [see Antihemophilic factor
    (AHF)]
Factor IX [see Plasma thromboplastin
    component (PTC)]
Factor X (see Stuart-Prower factor)
Factor XI [see Plasma thromboplastin
    antecedent (PTA)]
Facultative anaerobe, 312
Fasting blood specimens for glucose pro-
    cedure, 87
Fasting state for basal metabolism test,
    354
Fat, urinary, 197
Fat bodies, oval, 250, 256, 257
Fat droplets, urinary, 250, 256
Fat metabolism, 223
Fatty casts, 250, 257
Featheredge, 143, 145
Fecal hemoglobin (see Hemoglobin, uri-
    nary, and fecal)
Fermentation in microbiology, 327
Ferroprotoporphyrin, 9, 233

Fibrin:
  clot, 161–162
  formation, 161
Filtrate (see Protein-free filtrate)
Filtration, 72
  sterilization by, 309
Finely granular casts, 249
Fingerprick:
  equipment for, 111–112
  pipetting from, 112
  procedure for, 110–112
  (See also Capillary blood)
First aid, 2
  burns, 2
  eye injury, 2
  general rules of, 2–3
  minor cuts, 2
Fisher and Race CDE nomenclature,
    279, 280
Fisher and Race Rh-Hr inheritance,
    280–281
Fixing bacteria, 321–322
Flora, intestinal, 315
Foam, urinary, 198, 230
Foam test, 230–231
Folin-Wu filtrate, 72
  Hayden modification, 72, 73
Folin-Wu tubes, 91, 92
Formalin, 190, 242
Fouchet's reagent, 231
Fractional sterilization, 308
Fragility of erythrocyte test (see Osmotic
    fragility of erythrocyte)
Free bilirubin, 229, 230
Front typing, 274
Fuchs-Rosenthal ruling, 128
  use in eosinophil count, 138

Galactosuria, 208, 210
Galvanometer:
  in Coleman Junior spectrophotometer,
    53
  in electrocardiograph machine, 338
  in photometers, 51
  viewing scale, 54
Gamma globulin, 268
Gamma streptococci, 332
Gas factor, 364–365
  chart for calculating, 366
Gastric carcinoma, 237
Gelatin, 312

Gene, 265
Genotype, 266, 273, 286, 292
Gerhardt's test, 225, 227–228
Ghost red blood cells, 243
Glass:
  alkali resistant, 31
  borosilicate, 31
  cutting, 3
  kinds of, 31
Glassware:
  breakage and replacement, 7
  beakers, 33, 34
  burets, 37
  calibration of, 32, 33
    procedure used for, 32
    standards applied for, 32–33
  cleaning of, 4
    acid cleaning solution, 6
    diluting pipets, 6
    general pipets, 6
    methods used, 5
  cylinders, graduated, 35, 36
  diluting pipets, 123–125
  erlenmeyer flasks, 33, 34
  general care of, 3
  general pipets, 36, 57–61
  reagent bottles, 35
  test tubes, 34
  volumetric flasks, 35
Glomerular filtrate, 216, 217
Glomerulitis, 249
Glomerulonephritis, 249
Glucose:
  blood, 86–95
    clinical significance, 94, 95
    function in body, 86
    glycolysis of, 88
      (See also Sodium fluoride, anti-
        coagulant)
    methods for quantitative determina-
      tion of, 88–89
      (See also Nelson-Somogyi glucose
        method)
    reducing properties of, 86–87
    specimens for analysis of, 87
      (See also under Fasting)
  urinary (see Sugar, urinary)
Glucose oxidase, 88, 89, 210, 214–216
Glucose standard solution, 90, 91
  use of benzoic acid, 90
Glucuronic acid, 229
Glycogen, 224

Glycolysis in blood, 88
  prevention of, 88
  use of sodium fluoride to inhibit, 88
Glycosuria, 208
Gmelin's test, 231
Gonorrhea, 333
Graduated pipets, 59–60
Gram equivalent, 24–25, 64
Gram iodine solution, 324
Gram-negative, 323
Gram-negative rods, 329
Gram-positive, 323
Gram staining method, 322–324
Granular casts, 249–250
Granulocytes:
  description of, 120, 154
  formation of, 118, 154
  (See also Basophil; Eosinophils; Neu-
    trophil)
Graph paper (see Semilogarithmic graph
  paper)
Group, blood (see Blood group)
Group-specific blood, 278, 279, 293
Gum guaiac, 237
Gum guaiac filter paper test, 238

H substance, 276
Harrison's test, 231
Harvey, William, 263
Hayem's solution, 122–123
Heart:
  basic anatomy for electrocardiography,
    339–340
  impulses sent out by, 339–342
Heat and acetic acid test, 220–221
  principle, 220
  procedure, 220
Heller's test, 219
Hemacytometer:
  description of, 127
  Nebauer ruled areas, 127–128
  types in use, 127–128
    Fuchs-Rosenthal ruling, 128, 138
    Levy-Hausser, 127–129
    Spencer Brightline, 128, 135
  use of microscope with, 130
Hemastix, 239–240
Hematin, acid, 72
Hematocrit:
  clinical use, 155
  correlation with hemoglobin value,
    157

Hematocrit:
definition of, 155
microhematocrit test (see Microhematocrit test)
normal values, 155
use in calculation of erythrocyte indices, 176–177
Wintrobe method (see Wintrobe
hematocrit test)
Hematologic tests:
anticoagulants used for, 116, 142
"routine" tests, 107
specimen requirements for, 116–117,
142
Hematology:
laboratory procedures (see Procedures,
laboratory, hematologic)
origin of word, 107
Hematoma, 115
Hematopoiesis, 118
Hematuria, 236, 242, 243
Hemoglobin:
in blood: abnormal types of, 168
clinical importance of, 168–169
correlation of value with hematocrit, 157
equipment for analysis of, 171
function of, 168
makeup of molecule of, 168
methods for analysis of, 169
cyanmethemoglobin (see Cyanmethemoglobin method)
gasometric, 169
oxyhemoglobin (see Oxyhemoglobin method)
Sahli (see Sahli hemoglobin
method)
standard chart used for reading result, 173
standardization of photometer for
analysis of, 171–173
use of K factor, 172–173
use of value in calculation of erythrocyte indices, 176–177
urinary, 195
and fecal, 236–240
controls, 239
laboratory tests, 238–240
reliability of tests, 237
sensitivity of tests, 237
Hemoglobinuria, 236, 242
Hemolysis, 71, 230, 242
appearance, 71, 116

Hemolysis:
in blood banking, 271
causes of, 71, 116–117
crenation of red blood cell and, 117
in osmotic fragility of erythrocyte test,
174
relationship to osmotic pressure, 117
Hemolytic anemia, 122, 290
Hemolytic disease of the newborn, 269,
277, 279, 286, 290–295
Hemolytic transfusion reaction (see
Transfusion, reaction, hemolytic)
Hemophilus, 332
Hemostasis:
definition of, 160
tests for study of, 162–168
(See also Bleeding time tests; Clot
retraction tests; Coagulation; Cuff
test; Lee-White venous clotting
time test; Prothrombin time test)
Heparin, 70
Heterozygous, 266, 280, 287
High-protein crossmatch, 297–298
Hippuric acid crystals, 255
Homogentisic acid, urinary, 195
Homozygous, 266, 280, 287
Howell-Jolly bodies, 139, 148
Hucker modification of gram
stain, 323–324
Hyaline casts, 247–248
β-Hydroxybutyric acid (see Ketone
bodies, urinary)
Hypochromasia, 148
Hypotonic solution, 117
of sodium chloride for erythrocyte os-
motic fragility test, 175

Ictotest, 232
IgA (γ-A) antibody, 269, 270
IgD (γ-D) antibody, 269
IgE (γ-E) antibody, 269
IgG (γ-G) antibody, 269, 270, 277, 284,
285, 288, 291–293
IgM (γ-M) antibody, 269, 270, 277, 284,
288, 293
Immersion oil, 12, 147
Immune antibody, 269, 276–277, 283
Immunity, 267
Immunization, 268, 270
Incomplete antibody, 284, 288
Indices, erythrocyte, 176–177
calculation, 176–177

Indices, erythrocyte: mean corpuscular
    hemoglobin (MCH), 176–177
    mean corpuscular hemoglobin con-
        centration (MCHC), 177
    mean corpuscular volume, 176
    use in classifying anemias, 176–177
Indirect AHG test, 290, 298
Indirect typing, 274
Indole medium, 328
Indole test, 328
Indoxyl, 234
Infection, urinary, 245
Inflammation, 245
Inoculating loop or needle, 307
    use of, 316–317
Insulin, 209, 225
Insulin shock, 95
Intact red blood cells in urine, 243
Intermediate Ehrlich-reactive com-
        pounds, 234
International Bureau of Weights and
        Measures, 29
International standard for electrocardio-
        gram, 345–346
    time standardization, 345
    voltage standardization, 345–346
Intestinal flora, 229, 233, 315
In vitro, 270
In vivo, 270
Iris diaphragm, 9
Irregular antibodies, 270, 283, 295, 296
Isoelectric point, 218, 220
Isolation of bacterial colonies, 318
Isolation technique:
    for electrocardiography, 352
    for obtaining blood samples, 110
    protective, 110
    strict, 110
Isotonic solution, 117, 243
    (See also Saline solution, isotonic)
Ivy method (see Bleeding time tests)

Jaundice, 71, 194, 229, 230, 293
Jittery baseline, 348
Jolly bodies (see Howell-Jolly bodies)

K factor, 172–173
Ketogenic diet, 224
Ketone bodies, urinary, 223–229
    laboratory procedures, 226–228

Ketone bodies, urinary:
    physiology and significance, 223–226
Ketonuria, 224
Ketosis, 224, 225
Ketostix, 227
Kidney biopsy, 246
Kidney damage, 95, 96, 104, 105, 246,
        249, 252
Kidney failure, 267, 277
Kidney function tests, 96, 104–105
Kidney stone formation, 252
Kinyoun acid-fast method, 325
Kligler's iron agar, 330
Kovac's reagent, 328
Kupffer cells, 229

Laboratory procedures (see Procedures,
        laboratory)
Lactose-positive microorganisms, 334
"Lake," 324
Landsteiner, Karl, ABO system, 272
Landsteiner and Weiner, Rh system, 282
LE cell test, 178
    procedure for, 178
    use of, 178
Leads for ECG (see Bipolar leads; Chest
        leads; Limb leads; Unipolar leads)
Lectin, 276
Lee-White venous clotting time test,
        165–166
    normal value, 165
    precautions to note in, 165–166
    procedure, 165
    specimens for, 165
Leprosy, 324
Leucine crystals, 255
Leukemia, classification of, 122
Leukocytes:
    in blood: appearance on stained blood
        film, 119, 120
        counting (manual method) 121–134
        calculating cell count, 130
        counting cells, 130
        counting chamber, 126–130
            (See also Hemacytometer)
        diluents used, 123
            (See also Two percent acetic
                acid)
        diluting procedure, 125–126
        mounting the sample, 128–130
        pipets used, 123–125
            (See also Thoma pipet)

Leukocytes:
   in blood: counting (manual methods):
      precautions to note in, 126, 133–134
      description of, 119–120
      differential and classification of (*see* Blood film)
      estimate of count from stained blood film, 147
      morphologic changes, 154
   formation of, 118, 154–155
   function of, 119
   normal values, 121
   types, 119, 120, 150–153
      (*See also* Basophil; Eosinophils; Lymphocyte; Monocyte; Neutrophil)
   in urine (*see* White blood cells, urinary)
Leukocytosis, 122
Leukopenia, 122
Levine and Stetson, Rh system, 282
Levine's methylene blue agar (EMB), 333–334
Levy-Hausser hemacytometer, 127–129
Limb leads, 342–344
Linear graph paper, 75
Linkage, 266, 280
Lipemia in plasma and serum, 71
Liquifiable solid media, 312
Lithiasis, 252
Litmus milk, 331–332
Litmus paper, 200
"Live" steam, sterilization by, 307, 308
Liver, 229
Liver damage, 233
Liver function tests, 230, 233
Locus, 265
Loeffler's slant, 331
"Low titer" blood, 278
Lupus erythematosus cell test (*see* LE cell test)
Lymphocyte:
   description of, 120, 152–153
   development of, 154
   differential counting and classification (*see* Blood film)
   normal value, 152

MacConkey's agar (Mac), 334
McKesson Recording Metaboler, 355
   basic parts of, 355, 358

McKesson Recording Metaboler:
   chart paper, 356
   checking for leaks in, 362
   operation of, 361–364
   patient connection to, 356–358, 362
   used for tidal air value, 376
   used for vital capacity test, 367, 376
Macrocytosis, 148
Major crossmatch, 297
Major transfusion reaction, 277, 296
Master test (*see* Master two-step test)
Master two-step test, 352–353
   clinical importance of, 352, 353
   general procedure for, 353
Mean corpuscular hemoglobin (MCH) (*see* Indices, erythrocyte)
Mean corpuscular hemoglobin concentration (MCHC) (*see* Indices, erythrocyte)
Mean corpuscular volume (MCV) (*see* Indices, erythrocyte)
Measuring pipets, 59–60
Meat-free diet, 237
Media, microbiologic: buffers, 313
   described, 325–335
   differential, 315
   enrichment, 315
   in Petri dishes, 332–335
   pH, 313
   physical types, 312–313
   preparation, 319–321
   selective, 315
   storage, 314
   in test tubes, 326–332
Melanin, urinary, 195
Meningitis, 333
Mercuric nitrate, reagent, 82
Metabolism, 353
   [*See also* Basal metabolic rate (BMR)]
Methyl red medium, 328–329
Methylene blue staining method, 322
Metric system, 29
   standards for, 29–30
   units in, 29–30
Microaerobe, 312
Microbiologic, laboratory procedures (*see* Procedures, laboratory)
Microbiology:
   bacterial morphology, 310–311
   colonial characteristics, 314–315
   cultural requirements, 311–314

Microbiology:
　isolation of individual colonies, 318
　media (*see* Media, microbiologic)
　plate cultures and transfers, 317-319
　protection of personnel, 305–309
　special equipment, 316
　special techniques, 316
　specimens (*see* Specimens, micro-
　　biologic)
　staining, 310
　staining techniques, 321–325
　sterilization (*see* Sterilization)
　tube culture and transfers, 317
Microcytosis, 148
Microhematocrit test, 156–158
　centrifuge for, 157
　precautions, 157
　procedure, 157
　reading result of, 157
　specimens, 157
　tubes, 156
Microorganism:
　distribution, 302
　pathogenic, 303
　pure culture, 304, 313
Microscope, 8–13
　basic parts, 9
　binocular, 9
　care of, 10–11
　compound, 9
　dark-field, 13
　general procedure for use of, 11–13
　monocular, 9
　objectives for, 10
　phase, 13
　use of: in counting blood cells, 130,
　　132
　　in examining blood films, 146
　　in examining urine sediment,
　　　258–260
　　in microbiology, 302
Microscopic examination of the urinary
　　sediment, 258–260
Milky urine, 245
Milliequivalents, 25, 67
Minor crossmatch, 297
Minor transfusion reaction, 277–278, 296
Minute volume, 376
Miscellaneous structures, urinary sedi-
　　ment, 255–260
Mohr pipets, 59–60
Moist heat, sterilization by, 307

Molarity:
　calculation, 23–24
　definition of, 23
　mole, 23
　molecular weight, 23
Mold in urine sediment, 251
Mole (*see* Molarity)
Monocyte:
　description, 120, 153
　development, 155
　differential and classification (*see*
　　Blood film)
　normal value, 153
Mordant, 324
Morphology:
　bacterial, 310–311
　of blood cells (*see* Blood cells)
Motility test medium, 331
Mucin, urinary, 196, 219, 220
Mucous, 247
Mucous threads, urinary, 196, 251
Myoglobin, urinary, 195, 236, 239
Myohemoglobin, urinary, 195

Narrow casts, 250–251
National Bureau of Standards, 32–36,
　123
Natural antibody, 269, 273, 274, 276–277
Negative reaction in blood banking, 271
Neisseria, 333
Nelson-Somogyi glucose method, 89–94
　calculation of results, 92, 93
　control solution used for, 91
　dilution of filtrates, 94
　normal values, 94
　principle, reaction taking place, 89
　procedure, 91–92
　reagents used, 89–91
　reporting results, 94
　sources of error in, 93, 94
　technical factors in, 93, 94
　(*See also* Glucose, blood)
Nephritis, urea nitrogen level in, 104
Nephron, 246
　definition of, 185
Nephrosis, 250
Nesslerization method for blood urea
　　nitrogen, 98–105
　calculation of results, 102, 103
　dilution of filtrates, 104
　normal values, 104
　principle, 99

Nesslerization method for blood urea
  nitrogen:
  procedure, 100–102
  reagents used for, 99, 100
  reporting results, 104
  sources of error in, 103, 104
  technical factors in, 103, 104
  use of recovery solution in, 100, 103
  (*See also* Urea nitrogen, blood)
Nessler's reagent, 97, 100
Neubauer ruling, 127, 128
Neutrophil:
  description, 120, 150–151
  development (*see* Granulocytes)
  differential counting and classification
    (*see* Blood film)
  normal values, 150
Neutrophilia, 150, 151
New methylene blue dye, 140–141
Nichrome, 316
Nitrazine paper, 200
Nocturia, 193
Nonglucose reducing substances
    (NGRS), 87, 209–211
Nongranulocyte, description, 120
  (*See also* Lymphocyte; Monocyte)
Nonlactose fermenting microorganisms,
    334
Nonprotein nitrogen, 95, 96
Normality:
  calculation, 24–26
  definition of, 24
  equivalent weight in, 24–25, 64
Normoblast:
  correcting leukocyte count for, 148,
    149
  description, 148, 153
Normochromasia, 148
Numerical system nomenclature, 279

Objective, microscope, 10
  high-power, 10
  low-power, 10
  oil-immersion, 10
Obstructive jaundice, 230
Occult blood, 236–240
  (*See also* Hemoglobin, urinary, and
    fecal)
Ocular, microscope, 9
Odor, urine, 197–198
Oliguria, 193
Origin, graph paper, 75

Orthostatic proteinuria, 217
Orthotolidine, 237, 239
Osmolality, 203
Osmosis (*see* Osmotic pressure)
Osmotic fragility of erythrocyte:
  definition of, 174
  method of testing, 175
Osmotic pressure:
  definition of, 117
  of hypertonic solutions, 117
  of hypotonic solutions, 117
  of isotonic solutions, 117
  principles applied in hematologic tests,
    117
Ostwald-Folin pipets (*see* Ostwald
    pipets)
Ostwald pipets, 60
Oval fat bodies, 250, 256, 257
Ovalocytes, 148
Oxygen consumption line, 356, 357, 363
Oxygen slope line (*see* Oxygen consump-
    tion line)
Oxyhemoglobin method, 168–174
  procedure, 174
  reagents for, 170–171
  standardization of photometer for,
    171–173
  use of control solution in, 170
  (*See also* Hemoglobin)

Paratyphoid, 334
Parfocal, 10
Pasteur pipet, 155, 156
Pathogenic microorganisms, 303
Patient approach, 108–110
  for basal metabolism test, 359
  for electrocardiography, 349
  for obtaining blood samples, 108–110
    adult patient, 109
    nursery patient, 109
    pediatric patient, 109
  using isolation technique, 110, 352
Peptone water with tryptophan, 328
Percent transmission:
  on galvanometer viewing scale, 54
  plotting readings on graph paper, 77
  reading to nearest one-quarter, 54
  use in photometry, 52
Pericardial fluid (*see* Extravascular
    fluids)
Peripheral blood (*see* Capillary blood)

Peritoneal fluid (*see* Extravascular fluids)
Peroxidase activity, 237–240
Petri dish, 317
pH, urinary, 198–200, 246
  clinical significance, 199
  definition of, 198
  methods of measuring, 200
  normal values, 199
Phase microscope, 13
Pheneen, 305, 306
Phenol, 305, 306
Phenol poisoning, 195
Phenolphthalein, 64–66
Phenotype, 266, 273
Phenylethyl alcohol agar (PEA), 333
Phosphate buffer:
  for staining blood films, 144–145
  in urea nitrogen procedure, 99
Photoelectric cell, photometer, 51
Photometer, 50
  Coleman Junior Spectrophotometer
    (*see* Coleman Junior Spectro-
    photometer)
  cuvettes for, 49–51
    calibration of, 55
  diffraction grating, 51
  filters, 50–51, 55
  general care, 54
  general essential parts of, 50
  photoelectric colorimeter, 50
  spectrophotometer, 52–54
  use in hemoglobinometry, 170
  use of light in, 11
  (*See also* Photometry)
Photometry:
  Beer-Lambert law, 49
  fundamentals of color in, 48, 49
  standard calibration curves, 74–77,
    171–173
  standard solutions used in, 50, 74–77
  use of blank solution in, 54, 77, 78
  wavelengths of light in, 48
  (*See also* Photometer)
Physical properties of urine (*see* Urine,
  physical properties)
Physiologic solution (*see* Isotonic solution)
Pipet, 36, 57–61
  calibrating, 32–36, 123–124
  cleaning, 6, 57
  shaker for diluting, 128

Pipet:
  types: blowout, 58
    diluting, 123–125
    graduated, 59, 60
    measuring, 59, 60
    Mohr, 59, 60
    Ostwald, 60–61
    Ostwald-Folin, 60–61
    Sahli, 171
    serologic, 61
    stopcock, 61
    to-contain, 33, 58–60
    to-deliver, 33, 58
    transfer, 58
    volumetric, 58
Pipetting:
  general procedure for, 61–63
  precautions in, 2–3
  procedure for cell counts, 125–126
Placenta, 269
Plasma cell, 150
Plasma chloride, 80–86
  acid-base balance, 80
  chloride shift, 80
  distribution in body of, 81
  electrolyte balance, 81
  function in body, 80
  methods for quantitative analysis, 82
    (*See also* Schales and Schales chlo-
    ride method)
  specimens for analysis, 81–82
Plasma specimens:
  appearance, normal and abnormal,
    70–71
  collection, 68
  preservation, 70
  protein precipitation of, 72–73
    (*See also* Plasma chloride)
Plasma thromboplastin antecedent
  (PTA), 161
Plasma thromboplastin component
  (PTC), 161
Platelet in blood (*see* Thrombocyte in
  blood)
Pleural fluid (*see* Extravascular fluid)
Poikilocytes, 148
Poikilocytosis (*see* Poikilocytes)
Polychromasia, 148
Polycythemia, 155, 169
Polymorphonuclear neutrophil leukocyte
  (PMN) (*see* Neutrophil)
Polyuria, 193
Poorly defined baseline, 348, 349

Porphobilinogen, 233–234
    laboratory procedures, urinary,
        234–235
Porphyrias, 233–234
Porphyrins, urinary, 195, 233
Positive reaction in blood banking, 271
Postabsorptive state for BMR test,
    353–354
Potassium gluconate, reagent, 100
Potassium oxalate, anticoagulant, 69
    in chloride procedure, 81
    in urea nitrogen procedure, 96
Potassium persulfate, reagent, 100
Pour plate, 318
Preservation:
    of blood specimens, 70, 115–116
    of urine specimens, 189–190
Proaccelerin, 161
Procedures, laboratory:
    basal metabolic rate, 359–364
    blood banking: ABO typing,
        273–276
        antiglobulin reaction (Coombs
            test), 288–291
        compatibility testing, 295–298
        crossmatching, 295–298
        Rh typing, 284–287
    chemistry: blood glucose (Nelson-
        Somogyi method), 91–93
        blood urea nitrogen (direct nes-
            slerization method), 100–103
        plasma chloride (Schales and
            Schales method), 83–85
        preparation of protein-free fil-
            trate, 72–73
    electrocardiography, 349–351
    hematologic: blood film preparation
        and evaluation (see Blood film)
        clot retraction, 164
        cuff test, 162
        Duke bleeding time, 163
        eosinophil count, 138
        erythrocyte count, manual
            method, 125, 128, 129, 132
        erythrocyte sedimentation rate,
            159
        examination of cerebrospinal fluid
            (see Extravascular fluids)
        examination of extravascular fluid
            (see Extravascular fluids)
        fingerprick, 111, 112
        hemoglobin, cyanmethemoglobin,
            173–174

Procedures, laboratory:
    hematologic: indices, calculation,
        176–177
        Ivy bleeding time, 163, 164
        LE cell test, 178
        Lee-White venous clotting time,
            165
        leukocyte count, manual method,
            125, 128–131
        leukocyte differential and classi-
            fication, 146, 149, 150
        microhematocrit, 157
        osmotic fragility of erythrocyte,
            175
        platelet count, manual method,
            136
        prothrombin time, 167, 168
        reticulocyte count, 141
        venipuncture, 113–115
        Wintrobe hematocrit, 156–157
    microbiologic: acid-fast stain,
        324–325
        gram stain, 322–324
        inoculating needle and loop, use
            of, 316–317
        methylene blue stain, 322
        plate cultures and transfers,
            317–319
        preparation of artificial culture
            media, 319–321
        staining techniques, 321–325
        tube cultures and transfers, 317
    urinalysis: Acetest, 226–227
        Albustix, 223
        Albutest, 222
        Benedict's qualitative test,
            211–213
        benzidine test, 238–239
        for bilirubin, 231–232
        Bumintest, 221–222
        Clinistix, 214–215
        Clinitest, 213–214
        Combistix, 200
        Ehrlich's qualitative aldehyde re-
            action, 234–235
        Exton's sulfosalicylic acid test,
            221–222
        Gerhardt's test, 227–228
        gum guaiac test, 238
        Harrison's test, 231
        heat and acetic acid test,
            220–221

Procedures, laboratory:
  urinalysis: Hemastix, 239–240
    for hemoglobin, urinary and
      fecal, 238–240
    Ictotest, 232
    for ketone bodies, 226–228
    Ketostix, 227
    litmus paper, 200
    microscopic examination of the
      urinary sediment, 258–260
    nitrazine paper, 200
    for pH, 200
    for protein, 220–223
    Rothera's test, 226
    Schlesinger's test, 235
    for specific gravity, 207–208
    for sugar, 211–216
    Tes-Tape, 215–216
    urinometer, 207–208
    for urobilin, 235
    for urobilinogen, 234–236
Proconvertin, 161
Protection of personnel in microbiology,
  305–309
Protective immunity, 267
Protein, urinary, 216–223, 240, 243, 246
  classification of tests, 218–220
  laboratory procedures, 220
  pH indicator tests, 218–220
  precipitation or coagulation tests,
    218–219
Protein error of pH indicators, 218, 219,
  223
Protein-free filtrate, 71–73
  agents used to prepare, 72
  in blood glucose procedure, 89, 91
  in blood urea nitrogen procedure, 101
  in chloride procedure, 83, 84
  Folin-Wu filtrate, 72
    Hayden modification, 72–73
  preparation of, 71–73
Protein nitrogen, 95
Protein precipitation, 71–73
  agents used, 72
  Folin-Wu filtrate, 72
  Hayden modification, 72
  procedure, 72–73
  reaction occurring, 73
  (See also Protein-free filtrate)
Proteinuria, 216
  orthostatic, 217
Proteus, 334

Prothrombin time test, 166–168
  clinical value, 166
  normal values, 166
  procedure, 167–168
    agreement of replicates, 167
    precautions, 168
  reagents for, 166–167
  specimens, 166
  use of control specimen in, 167–168
Pseudomonas aeruginosa, 333
Pulse rate, patient: definition of, 360
  procedure for obtaining, 360
Pure culture of microorganisms, 304,
  313
Pus, urinary, 197
Pus cells in urine (see White blood cells,
  urinary)
Pyuria, 245

Qualitative tests, urine: definition of, 191
  for ketone bodies, 226
  for sugar, 211, 213
Quality control:
  for blood glucose procedure, 91
  chart, 79
  general use, 78
  specimens for, 78–79
  use in hemoglobinometry, 170–171
  use in prothrombin time test, 167–168
Quantitative measurement:
  for blood glucose, 86–95
  for blood urea nitrogen, 95–105
  definition of, 191
  photometry, 49, 50
  for plasma chloride, 80–86
  titration, 63–64, 67
  for urine urobilinogen, 236
Quantitative transfer, 15

Rabbit blood agar (RB), 332
RE system [see Reticuloendothelial (RE)
  system]
Reagent:
  checking, 17
  containers, 16
    labeling of, 16
  definition of, 13
  preparation of, 13–16
    use of quantitative transfer, 15–16
  "ready made," 14
Recessive, 266

Recovery solutions:
  general use of, 79–80
  use in urea nitrogen procedure, 100
  calculation of recovery, 103
Red blood cell (*see* Erythrocytes, in
  blood)
Red blood cell cast, 249
Red blood cell indices (*see* Indices,
  erythrocyte)
Red blood cells, urinary, 195, 197, 236,
  239, 242–245
  forms possible, 243
  identification, 243, 260
  reporting results, 245–260
  significance, 242–243
Rees-Ecker solution, 135
Refractive index, 203
Refractometer, 203
Refrigeration:
  of blood specimens, 70
  of urine specimens, 189
Regurgitative jaundice, 230
Renal damage, 246, 249, 252
Renal epithelial cells, urinary, 256
Renal failure, 267, 277
Renal stasis, 250, 251
Renal threshold, 209
Reliability of results, means of ensuring,
  73–80
  blank solutions, 77–78
  control solutions, 78–79
  duplicate determinations, 79
  recovery solutions, 79–80, 100
  standard calibration curve, 74–77
  standard solutions, 78–79
Resazurin, 327
Respiratory quotient, 354, 364
Retentive jaundice, 230
Reticulocyte, 139–141
  counting, 139–141
    blood sample for, 140
    calculations, 141
    methods for, 140
    precautions, 141
    procedure, 141
    stains used, 140–141
      (*See also* Brilliant cresyl blue
        dye; New methylene blue dye)
  description, 139
  normal values, 139
  production, 139
  relationship to anemia therapy,
    139–140

Reticuloendothelial (RE) system:
  general function, 119
  involving erythrocyte destruction, 119
  monocyte formation, 155
Rh system nomenclature, 279, 280
Rh-Hr blood group system, 279–288
  antibody: characteristics, 283–284
    classification, 283–284
  antigen, characteristics, 283
  antiserum, 285
  factors, 279–281
  historical information, 282
  inheritance, 279–281
  nomenclature, 279
  transfusion, 285
  typing procedures, 284–287
Rh-negative, 282–283, 295
Rh-positive, 282–283, 295
Rhesus monkey red blood cells, 282
Roberts' test, 219
Rosenfield et al. numerical nomenclature,
  279
Rothera's test, 225, 226
Rouleau formation, 149
Rounded red blood cells, 243

Sabourands agar, 335
Safety, laboratory, 1–4
  fire, 2
  general rules for, 2–4
  reference library available for, 4
  safety goggles, 3–4
Safety goggles, 3–4
Safranin counterstain, 323
Sahli hemoglobin method, 169
Sahli hemoglobin pipet, 171
Saline solution, isotonic, 117
  use in hematology, 117
Saline solution or serum crossmatch, 297
Saline solution-active antibody, 284, 285
Salmonella, 315, 331, 334
Salmonella-Shigella agar (SS), 334
Saturated benzoic acid, reagent, 90
Schales and Schales chloride method,
  82–86
  calculation of results, 84–85
  normal values, 86
  principle, 82
  procedure, 83–84
  reagents, 82–83
  reporting results, 86
  sources of error in, 85

Schales and Schales chloride method:
  specimens for, 81–83
  technical factors in, 85
Schlesinger's test, 235
Screening tests:
  for occult blood, 237
  for urine: definition of, 190–191
    for sugar, 211, 215
Sediment, urinary, 240–260
  amorphous material, 251–255, 259–260
  casts, 246–251, 259, 260
  composition of, 241
  crystals, 251–255, 259, 260
  decomposition of, 242
  microscopic examination of, 241,
    258–260
  miscellaneous structures, 255–260
  organized, 241, 242, 245, 246
  red blood cells, 242–245, 260
  specimen requirements, 241–242
  unorganized, 241, 251
  white blood cells, 244–246, 260
Sedimentation rate [see Erythrocyte sedimentation rate (ESR)]
Selective media, 315
Selenite broth, 331
Semilogarithmic graph paper, 75
Semisolid media, 313
Sensitization, 268, 270
Sequestrene, 69
  use in hematology, 113, 116
Serologic pipet, 61
Serum specimens:
  appearance, normal and abnormal, 70
  collection, 68–70
  preservation, 70
  protein precipitation of, 72–73
Serum typing, 274, 276
Shadow red blood cells, 243
Sheep blood agar (SB or BA), 332
Shigella, 315, 331, 334
Shock, insulin, 95
Shrunken red blood cells, 243
Sickle cells, 148
Siderocytes, 148
Significant figures (see Calculations)
Simmons citrate agar, 328
Simple staining procedures, 322
Single oxalate, anticoagulant (see Potas-
  sium oxalate, anticoagulant)
Slant tube, 321
  figure, 320
Smith's test, 231

Soda lime for BMR machine, 357
Sodium chloride standard solution, 83
Sodium citrate, anticoagulant, 69–70
Sodium fluoride, anticoagulant, 69
  in blood glucose procedure, 88
  as enzyme inhibitor, 96, 98
Sodium tungstate, reagent, 72, 82, 97–99
Somatic tremor, 346–347
Specific gravity, urinary, 200–208
  clinical application, 202–203
  definition of, 200–202
  methods of measuring (see Uri-
    nometer)
  normal values, 202–203
  other measures of, 203
Specimens:
  blood: appearance, 70–71, 116
    for blood glucose determination, 87
    collection of, 68, 110–115
      general precautions, 68–69
    fasting, 87
    for hematologic tests, 115–117, 142,
      143
    labeling, 108
    for plasma chloride determination,
      81–82
    preparation of protein-free filtrate
      from, 72–73
      (See also Protein-free filtrate)
    preservation of, 70, 115–116
    for urea nitrogen determination, 96
    use of anticoagulants in, 69, 116
  extravascular fluid, 178–179
    (See also Extravascular fiuids)
  microbiologic: colection, 303–305
    storage, 305
    types, 303–305
  plasma (see Plasma specimens)
  serum (see Serum specimens)
  urine: catheterized, 190, 242
    collection, 188–189, 190
    containers, 189
    decomposition, 189
    after eating, 189
    first morning, 188, 241
    freely voided, 190
    fresh, 242
    preservation, 189–190, 242
    random, 188
    sediment, 241
    24-hour, 188
Spencer Brightline Hemacytometer, 128,
  135

Spherocytes, 148
Sphygmomanometer (see Blood pressure cuff)
Spinal fluid (see Cerebrospinal fluid)
Spirometer dial, 363
Spores, 308, 312
Spreader slide, 143
Squamous epithelial cells, urinary, 256
Staining microorganisms, 310
Staining procedures:
  hematologic: for blood films, 144–146
    for reticulocytes, 140
  microbiologic, 321–325
Standard curve, 74
  in blood glucose procedure, 92, 93
  construction, 75–77
  criteria for use, 75
  in hemoglobinometry, 171–173
  labeling, 75
  linear graph paper for, 75
  semilogarithmic graph paper for, 75
  in urea nitrogen procedure, 102
  use of, 75–77
  use of K factor in, 172–173
Standard solutions, 74–77
  of ammonium sulfate, 99, 100
  of glucose, 90, 91
  for hemoglobinometry, 171–172
  for photometry, 50, 74–77
  of sodium chloride, 83
  for titration, 67
Steam under pressure, sterilization by, 307–309
Sterilization, 305–309
  of inoculating loops and needles, 316
Stopcock pipet, 61
Streak plate, 318
Streptococci, 332
Struli, ABO system, 272
Stuart-Prower factor, 161
Substrate, 97
Sugar:
  blood (see Glucose, blood)
  urinary, 208–216, 257
    classification of tests, 209
    laboratory procedures, 211–216
    nonspecific tests, 209–211, 213
    qualitative tests, 211, 213
    quantitative tests, 211
    screening tests, 211, 215
    specific tests, 209, 210–211, 214
Sugars, microbiologic media, 327–329
Sulfonamides, 252, 255

Supravital staining, reticulocyte count, 140
Surface area:
  for calculation of BMR, 354, 359, 368–371
  chart for calculating, 368–371
  Du Bois formula, 365
Swollen red blood cells, 243
Synovial fluid:
  mucin test, 180–181
  procedure for general examination, 178–179
Syringe for collecting venous blood, 113
  (See also Venipuncture; Venous blood)

Tarry black specimen, 236
Temperature:
  for bacterial culture, 313
  correction applied for BMR calculation, 365–366
  of oxygen for BMR test, 363–364
    reading from spirometer dial, 363
  of patient, 354
    procedure for obtaining, 359–360
  scales: centigrade, 30, 31
    conversion formulae for, 31
    Fahrenheit, 30, 31
Tergitol number 7, 325
Tes-Tape, 210, 215–216
  principle, 215
  procedure, 216
Thioglycolate (Thio broth), 327
Thoma pipet, 124–125
  brand names, 124
  description of, 124
  dilution procedure, 125
  units of volume in, 124–125
"Thorn apple" crystals, 254
Thrombin:
  in blood coagulation, 161
  formation, 161
Thrombocytes in blood:
  counting (manual method), 135–137
    blood sample, 136–137
    calculations, 136
    counting chamber, 135–136
      (See also Spencer Brightline Hemacytometer)
    diluents, 135
      (See also Rees-Ecker solution)
    pipets, 135

Thrombocytes in blood:
counting (manual method): precautions to note, 137
procedure, 136
description, 120, 136
evaluation from stained blood film, 149
morphologic changes seen, 154
function, 120, 134, 160–162
normal values, 134
precursor, 120, 134
Thrombocytopenia, 134
Thrombocytosis, 134–135, 150–151
Thromboplastin, 161
reagent for prothrombin time test, 166–167
Thromboplastinogen [see Antihemophilic factor (AHF)]
Thymol, 190
Tidal air, 376
Titer, 268, 269, 276–278, 294
Titration, 63
calculations, 67
equipment, 64
(See also Buret)
general procedure, 63–67
indicator solutions for, 64–66
(See also Phenolphthalein)
methods (see Plasma chloride)
requirements, 63
standard alkalies for, 67
standard acids for, 67
use of normality in, 64, 67
uses for, 68
Toluene, 189–190, 242
Toluol, 190
Torsion balance, 45
procedure for use, 45, 46
Tourniquet, procedure for use, 113, 114
Transfer needle (see Inoculating loop or needle)
Transfer pipet, 58
Transfusion:
blood, historical background, 263–264
exchange, 294
reaction, 278
hemolytic, 262, 267, 274, 282, 283
major, 277, 296
minor, 277–278, 296
Rh-Hr type, 285
selection of blood, 295
Transparency, urine, 196–197, 240
Transudates, 179

Triple-beam balance, 46–47
Cent-O-Gram type, 47
general procedure for use, 47
Triple phosphate crystals, 254
Triple sugar iron agar (TSI), 329–330
True blood cast, 249
Trypticase soy broth (Tryp broth), 326
TS meter, 203n.
TSI slants, 329–330
Tuberculosis, 324
Two percent acetic acid, reagent, 123
Tyndallization, 308
Type, blood, 264, 270
Type-specific blood, 278, 279, 293
Typhoid, 334
Typing (see Blood group, tests)
Tyrosine crystals, 255

Ulcers, 237
Unipolar leads, 344
Unit of blood, 263
Univalent antibody, 284, 288
Universal donors, 277–278, 296, 297
Universal recipients, 277–278, 296
Urea, 96, 104
recovery solution, 99, 100
Urea nitrogen, blood, 95–105
clinical significance, 104–105
function in body, 95
methods for quantitative determination, 97
principle, 97
reactions taking place, 97
use of enzyme urease, 97
(See also Nesslerization method for blood urea nitrogen)
nonprotein nitrogen, 95, 96
protein nitrogen, 95
specimens, 96
urea, 96
Urease, 96–100
Uremia, 104
Uric acid crystals, 253
Urinalysis:
classification of tests, 190–191
consists of, 186–187
definition of, 186–187
procedures (see Procedures, laboratory)
purpose of, 187
qualitative tests, definition of, 191

Urinalysis:
    quantitative tests, definition of, 191
    screening tests, definition of, 190–191
Urinary system, definition of, 185
Urine:
    albumin (see Protein, urinary)
    bilirubin (see Bilirubin, urinary)
    casts (see Casts, urinary)
    cloudiness (see transparency below)
    color, 193–196
        abnormal, 194–196
        normal, 193–194
    composition of, 187–188
    definition of, 185
    dextrose (see Sugar, urinary)
    foam, 198
        (See also Foam, urinary)
    glucose (see Sugar, urinary)
    hemoglobin (see Hemoglobin, urinary
        and fecal)
    ketone bodies (see Ketone bodies, uri-
        nary)
    obtaining the specimen, 190
    odor, 197–198
    pH (see pH, urinary)
    physical properties: definition of, 191
        summarized, table, 192
    protein (see Protein, urinary)
    red blood cells (see Red blood cells,
        urinary)
    sediment (see Sediment, urinary)
    specific gravity (see Specific gravity,
        urinary)
    specimens (see Specimens, urine)
    sugar (see Sugar, urinary)
    transparency, 196–197, 240
    urobilinogen (see Urobilinogen, uri-
        nary)
    volume, 193
    white blood cells (see White blood
        cells, urinary)
Urinometer, 204–208
    abnormal substance correction,
        206–207
    calibration, 204–205
    definition of, 202
    procedure, 207–208
    temperature corrections, 205–206
Urobilin, 229, 233, 234
    urinary, 194, 195
        laboratory procedures, 235–236
Urobilinogen, 229, 230
    urinary, 195, 232–236

Urobilinogen:
    urinary: laboratory procedures,
        234–236
    physiology and significance, 232–234

V factor, 332, 333
Vacuum tube for collecting venous
    blood, 113
    (See also Venipuncture; Venous
        blood)
Venipuncture:
    choice of vein for, 113
    position of patient for, 113
    syringe method, 113
    use of tourniquet, 113
        procedure, 113, 114
    vacuum tube method, 113
Venous blood:
    collection procedure, 113–115
        syringe method, 113
        use of tourniquet, 113, 114
        vacuum tube method, 113
    use of anticoagulant with, 112
Venous clotting time tests (see Lee-
    White venous clotting time test)
Vernier scale, 41, 43
Visual colorimeter, 55
Visual colorimetry, 55
    disadvantages of, 55
    methods, 169
Vital capacity test, 367, 376
Voges-Proskauer medium, 328–329
Volume, urine, 193
Volumetric glassware:
    flasks, 35
    pipets, 36, 58–59

Wandering baseline, 348
Warm aldehyde reaction, 234
Water, 17–18
    ammonia-free, 17–18, 103
    deionized, 17
    distilled, 17
    double-distilled, 17–18, 103
Wavelengths of light, 48
Waxy cast, 249–251
Westergren method for erythrocyte sedi-
    mentation rate, 159–160
    equipment, 159
    precautions to note, 159–160
    procedure, 159

Westergren method for erythrocyte sedimentation rate:
reading results, 159
[*See also* Erythrocyte sedimentation rate (ESR)]
Whetstone, 253
White blood cell (*see* Leukocytes, in blood)
White blood cell cast, 249
White blood cells, urinary, 197 244–246, 257
clinical significance, 245
identification, 245, 260
reporting results, 246, 260
Whooping cough, 333
Wiener Rh-Hr inheritance, 280–281
Wiener Rh nomenclature, 279, 280
Wintrobe hematocrit test, 155–158
calculations for, 156
equipment, 155–156

Wintrobe hematocrit test:
precautions to note, 157
procedure, 156
specimens, 157
Wintrobe tube, 155
Wright's stain:
preparation, 144–145
use, 144–146

X factor, 332, 333

Yeast, urinary, 244–245, 257

Zeihl-Neelsen acid-fast method, 325
Zeta potential, 284, 285, 288
Zinc sulfate, reagent, 90, 97